ROUTLEDGE LIBRARY [illegible]
HEALTH, DISEASE & S[illegible]

Volume 19

DISEASE, MEDICINE, AND EMPIRE

DISEASE, MEDICINE, AND EMPIRE

Perspectives on Western Medicine and the Experience of European Expansion

Edited by
ROY MACLEOD and
MILTON LEWIS

Routledge
Taylor & Francis Group
LONDON AND NEW YORK

First published in 1988 by Routledge

This edition first published in 2022
by Routledge
4 Park Square, Milton Park, Abingdon, Oxon OX14 4RN

and by Routledge
605 Third Avenue, New York, NY 10158

Routledge is an imprint of the Taylor & Francis Group, an informa business

British Library Cataloguing in Publication Data
A catalogue record for this book is available from the British Library

ISBN: 978-0-367-52469-2 (Set)
ISBN: 978-1-032-23539-4 (Volume 19) (hbk)
ISBN: 978-1-032-23554-7 (Volume 19) (pbk)
ISBN: 978-1-003-27824-5 (Volume 19) (ebk)

DOI: 10.4324/9781003278245

DISEASE, MEDICINE, AND EMPIRE

PERSPECTIVES ON WESTERN MEDICINE AND THE EXPERIENCE OF EUROPEAN EXPANSION

Edited by
ROY MACLEOD AND MILTON LEWIS

Routledge
London and New York

First published in 1988 by
Routledge
11 New Fetter Lane, London EC4P 4EE
29 West 35th Street, New York, NY 10001

Printed and bound in Great Britain by Mackays of Chatham PLC, Kent
Phototypeset in 10pt Times Roman by
Mews Photosetting, Beckenham, Kent

British Library Cataloguing in Publication Data

Disease, medicine and empire.
1. Colonies, Medicine, 1800–1950
I. MacLeod, Roy, *1941-* II. Lewis,
Milton *1940-* .
610

Library of Congress Cataloging-in-Publication Data
Disease, medicine, and empire: perspectives on Western medicine and the experience of European expansion / edited by Roy MacLeod and Milton Lewis.
p. c.m.
Includes bibliographies and index.
1. Medicine — Europe — Colonies — History. 2. Medicine — Great Britain — Colonies — History. 3. Medicine — History — 19th century. 4. Medical policy — Europe — Colonies — History. 5. Medical policy — Great Britain — Colonies — History. 6. Medical policy — History — 19th century. I. MacLeod, Roy M. II. Lewis, Milton James.
[DNLM: 1. Health Policy — history — Europe. 2. History of Medicine. 19th cent. 3. Social Control, Informal. WZ 60 D611]
R484.D57 1988
610'.9'034 — dc19
DNLM/DLC
for Library of Congress 88-11330

ISBN 0-415-00685-6 CIP

Contents

Notes on contributors

Neil Andersson is Director of the Centre for Tropical Disease Research and Professor of Tropical Medicine at the Universidad Autónoma de Guerrero in Acapulco, Mexico, and a Clinical Lecturer at the London School of Hygiene and Tropical Medicine.

Geoffrey Bilson was born in Wales and educated at the University College of Wales, Aberystwyth, and Stanford University. He was until his death in 1987 Professor of History at the University of Saskatchewan, Saskatoon, Canada. His research interests were in Canadian medical history. He was the author of *A Darkened House: Cholera in Nineteenth Century Canada* (Toronto: University of Toronto Press, 1980) and a number of articles on public health in Canada. By his colleagues and by us he will be sorely missed.

Donald Denoon was born in Scotland in 1940, brought up in South Africa and educated at Natal University and Queens' College, Cambridge. He has taught at Makerere University in Uganda, Ibadan University in Nigeria, and the University of Papua New Guinea, and is now a Senior Research Fellow in Pacific History at the Australian National University.

Diana Dyason was educated at the Melbourne Church of England Girls Grammar School and the University of Melbourne, where she held appointments in Physiology and the History and Philosophy of Science. She retired in 1985 and is currently an honorary research associate in the HPS Department, working on the public health of the Colony of Victoria.

Wolfgang U. Eckart is Professor for History of Medicine at the Medizinische Hochschule Hannover, Federal Republic of Germany. Born in 1952 in Schwelm, Germany, he studied medicine and history at the University of Münster. His PhD thesis was on Daniel Sennert (1572–1636): 'Grundlagen des medizinischwissenchaftlichen Erkennens bei Daniel Sennert' (Schwelm, 1978). His research and teaching activities embrace the history of science in early modern Europe; medical iconography of the seventeenth century; the history of medical ethics; and medicine and German colonial imperialism. He completed his *habilitation* in the History of Medicine in May 1986.

Raeburn Lange graduated MA in History from the University of Auckland, and PhD from the University of Otago. His doctoral research was in the social and medical history of the Cook Islands. He taught history at the University of Otago, Dunedin, New Zealand, and since 1984 has been a Lecturer in History at the Pacific Theological College, Suva, Fiji, where he teaches Christian history and Pacific history.

Milton Lewis is a graduate of the University of New South Wales and the Australian National University. He has held teaching and research posts in

Australia, the United Kingdom and New Guinea. He is currently Senior Lecturer in Preventive and Social Medicine in the School of Public Health and Tropical Medicine at the University of Sydney.

Maryinez Lyons is a graduate of the University of California, Los Angeles, where she earned an MA in African Studies and, in 1987, a PhD in History. Her thesis, 'The colonial disease: sleeping sickness in the social history of Northern Zaire, 1903–1930', is an examination of the roles of disease, medicine and public health policy in the early colonial history of Zaire. She is currently a Research Fellow of the Institute of Commonwealth Studies and an Honorary Fellow of the London School of Hygiene and Tropical Medicine.

Roy MacLeod is a graduate of Harvard and Cambridge, and has held academic positions at Sussex, London, Amsterdam and Paris. He is the author of several books and papers in the social history of science and medicine. He is at present Professor of History at the University of Sydney, where he teaches imperial history, military history, and the history of science and medicine.

Anne Marcovich is a graduate of the Ecole des Hautes Etudes en Sciences Sociales (Paris) in social psychology and in historical sociology. She has worked at the Centre de Recherche en Gestion at the Ecole Polytechnique of Paris where she specialized in sociology of sciences. She spent a year in the Department of History and Social Studies of Sciences (University of Sussex) where she specialized in the social history of medicine. She has collaborated at various times with the Musée des Sciences des Techniques et des Industries du Parc de la Villette (Paris). She is now working on the introduction and development of acupuncture in France.

Shula Marks is Director of the Institute of Commonwealth Studies and Professor of Commonwealth History at the University of London. She has written extensively on the history of South Africa, and is the author of *Reluctant Rebellion. The 1906–8 Disturbances in Natal* (Oxford: Clarendon Press, 1970) and *The Ambiguities of Dependence in South Africa: Class, Nationalism and the State in Twentieth Century Natal* (Baltimore and Johannesburg: Johns Hopkins University Press and Ravan Press, 1985). She is the co-editor (with A.E. Atmore) of *Economy and Society in Preindustrial South Africa* (London: Longman, 1980); (with R. Rathbone) of *Industrialisation and Social Change in South Africa: African Class Formation, Culture and Consciousness, 1870–1930* (London: Longman, 1982); and (with S. Trapido) *The Politics of Race, Class and Nationalism in Twentieth Century South Africa* (London: Longman, forthcoming). Her main current research interest is on the history of late nineteenth- and twentieth-century South Africa, and in particular the impact of industrialization on women and health.

Alan Mayne graduated from the Australian National University with a BA degree in history, and moved to the Research School of Social Sciences to write his doctorate. He was a tutor in history at the University of Queensland for two years, and then worked in the University of Cambridge for a year. He is now a Lecturer in History at the University of Melbourne. He is the author of articles on late-nineteenth-century urban social history, and of *Fever, Squalor and Vice: Sanitation and Social Policy in Victorian Sydney* (St Lucia: University of Queensland Press, 1982).

Radhika Ramasubban, MA, PhD (Bombay) has been engaged in teaching and research in the area of science and technology policy for many years. Her research contributions cover the organization of science, the emergence of scientific specialities, grassroots scientific initiatives and various aspects of the public health situation in India. She has been on the faculty of the School of Planning, Ahmedabad and the Department of Sociology at the University of Bombay, Visiting Fellow at the Science Policy Research Unit, University of Sussex and a Senior Fellow of the Indian Council of Social Science Research, Delhi. She is currently with the Centre for Social and Technological Change, Bombay.

Rodney Sullivan is Senior Lecturer in History at James Cook University. His biography of Dean C. Worcester is currently being prepared for publication by the University of Michigan's Centre for South and Southeast Asian Studies. It is expected to appear in 1988 under the title *'Exemplar of Americanism': The Philippine Career of Dean C. Worcester*.

Diane Sydenham completed her PhD at the Johns Hopkins University. She has lectured at Monash University, has been a Research Fellow at the Australian Institute of Multicultural Affairs, and is currently preparing a history of the pharmaceutical company, Glaxo Australia Pty Ltd.

Helen R. Woolcock graduated in occupational therapy from the University of Queensland and practised in Australia, Britain, India, and Canada. Here her interest in history was stimulated. She completed an MA at the University of Western Ontario and a PhD in medical history at the University of London. Since then she has lectured part-time in Canada and Australia, while continuing research into the medical aspects of nineteenth-century migration. Her book on this subject was published by Tavistock in 1986.

Michael Worboys is a graduate of Manchester and Sussex (PhD), where he read biology and the social studies of science. He is currently a Lecturer in History at Sheffield City Polytechnic. His main research has been on science in relation to British colonial imperialism, and on the development of the biomedical sciences between 1880 and 1914.

Preface

It has been many years since George Rosen, the distinguished medical historian, drew attention to what he described as the prevailing perspective in the history of western, principally European, medicine — a preoccupation with medical theory, literature, and practice, which gave little attention to the significance of social and economic factors in the development and direction of medicine and its professional obligations. No student of the subject today would recognize this description, as the history of modern medicine has been steadily recast in the direction of understanding more about the role, authority, and influence of the profession and its changing relationship with science and technology. In this newer perspective, few dimensions of professional development have been left unexplored. But among those regions which still lack a coherent agenda, let alone an agreed theoretical basis, must surely be the history of medicine in its relation to empire. This neglect no single volume of essays can alone redress. But as that relationship comes to bear closely upon our understanding of medical practice and policy in the post-colonial world, the task of reconstructing its influence becomes all the more important.

Every true historian, Benedetto Croce reminded us, is to some degree a contemporary historian; and to a generation now contemplating epidemic autoimmune diseases and retroviruses, the ties that bind the 'periphery' of the Third World to the metropolitan centres of former European empires are not hard to locate. Similarly, European medicine can no longer be considered an 'accident' of empire, nor can its particular forms be construed as accidental to the purposes of colonization — including the survival of the white races, and the social control of native populations. European medicine, and its handmaiden, public health, served as 'tools of Empire', of both symbolic and practical consequence, and as images representative of European commitments, variously to conquer, occupy or settle. To prompt discussion of the historical realities underlying contemporary rhetoric, to show how medicine served as an instrument of empire, as well as an imperializing cultural force in itself, is the object of this book. In the widest sense, it is about the experience of European medicine overseas, in colonies established by conquest, occupation and settlement.

In the context of European, and particularly British, colonial experience, our authors have been invited to consider issues which arise from their specialized knowledge of medical history and their understanding of the relationship of European precept and colonial practice. They have in different ways explored the tensions between the 'medical occupier' and the occupied; the ideology underlying tropical and colonial medicine, the preferences and politics of imperial medical research, and the dramatic effects of new sciences and new technologies on the experience of 'Europe overseas'. Upon such a vast canvas, reaching from tropical to temperate regions, from eighteenth-century colonial America to twentieth-century South Africa, it is difficult and invidious to impose generalizations. There is, therefore, no single thesis unifying this volume. Instead, our purpose is to reveal the scope of work now under way on the political, racial, economic, and military objectives that involved medicine during the 'Expansion of Europe', particularly during the nineteenth century; on the characteristics of European medicine in certain 'settler colonies' of the British Empire; and on the influence of epidemic disease and theories of race in their effect upon the posture and status of European medicine.

Our point of departure lies in an Australian — itself, within recent memory, a colonial — perspective. We have sought to balance conventional accounts of colonial medicine, as seen from the metropolis, with commentaries from scholars on the 'periphery'. We have in common the practice of social and medical history, rather than medicine; a qualification which serves to disqualify in some circles, but one which we believe essential to the investigative enterprise that medical history has become. Inevitably, several regions of the world — even many corners of the British Empire — are absent from our map. Their important lessons deserve separate treatment, as do those of other regions — notably Latin America, the West Indies, West Africa and Egypt, and the whole of Asia — whose experience of imperialism reaches beyond our limited framework of colonial rule. We cannot claim to have exhaustively treated even those regions and times we have touched.

In two other respects we recognize inherent limitations. First, in setting the agenda, we reflect the dominant legacies of European occupation. However, it is well known that the reality of 'medicine' in many parts of the world is not yet, or not yet wholly, European (or American); and that indigenous systems of medical belief and treatment form an important and growing body of alternative experience. Second, the history of colonial medicine is still seen from a 'victors' perspective, defined in terms of the survival of Europeans in foreign lands. That the certainties of this victory are themselves problematic in those large parts of the world where malaria is still endemic, and where three-quarters of mankind still suffer from anaemia, malnutrition and debilitating diseases, involves representations that form the subtext of this book. Third, we write from the knowledge that imperialism has historically taken many shapes, some important examples of which are non-European in origin; and recognizing that the manifestation of any invasive cultural influence — whether in language, science, art, music, or commerce, by war or in peace — must carry within it corresponding implications and contradictions. The imperial history of European medicine is significant, however, in that it speaks both to the imagery of a self-appointed civilizing vector, and to a degree of authority that transcends politics. Arguably, even in a world of instant global influence this historical mission should not be left neglected in the shadow of lesser gods.

This book forms part of a series of studies in the social history of medicine and empire, and in the history of colonial medicine in Australasia since 1788. To the Trustees of the Clive and Vera Ramaciotti Foundations of Sydney, who sponsored this work, we express our warm appreciation. It is a pleasure also to record our thanks to the staff of the Public Health Library, and the Fisher Library at the University of Sydney; and to acknowledge with gratitude the generous help of Dr Anthea Hyslop, of the University of Adelaide; Dr Diane Sydenham, of the University of Melbourne; Mr William Mackenzie, of the Department of Foreign Affairs, Canberra; Mr William Schupbach, of the Wellcome Institute of the History of Medicine; Mr Hilary Bettinson of the Wellcome Institute for Tropical Medicine; Miss Mary Gibson of the London School of Hygiene and Tropical Medicine; Ms Catherine Crawford of the History Faculty, Oxford University; and Professor Dr H. Schadewalt, of the University of Dusseldorf. While individual authors will record their separate acknowledgements, we extend our collective thanks to Ms Melanie Oppenheimer and Ms Ruth Bennett, of Sydney University; and to Ms Gill Davies of Routledge, who had the vision that made this voyage possible.

Sydney
Empire Day,1987

Introduction

Roy MacLeod

Western medicine, as we know it, is a cultural force. At the same time, it has become a culture in itself. For these reasons, the interplay between medicine and culture, today figures prominently on the research agenda of modern medical history. Medicine, in its conceptual, professional and political dimensions, is both shaping and shaped by the cultural circumstances that surround it, and that give it at any time its particular character. Nowhere is the reciprocal process more evident than in the history of western medicine transmitted overseas. In this process of transmission, medicine acquired a new dimension, acting both as a cultural agency in itself, and as an agency of western expansion.

Over the last ten years, it has been fashionable to criticize western medicine as having promoted a scarce commodity, which developing countries and foreign assistance have inequitably distributed. These critics have been joined by scholars who have challenged the image of medicine as morally neutral, essentially 'benign', an activity which merely deploys effective techniques for curing diseases and reducing suffering and pain.[1] But scientific knowledge, as applied through medicine, is not merely factual knowledge; it also comprises a set of social messages wrapped up in technical language. For decades, medical history traditionally dwelt upon the history of disease, emphasizing less the political or cultural environment of disease, and more the conquest of disease itself.[2] This emphasis coincided with a view of medicine as a progressive influence, developing from art and craft to science; and so carefully served the legitimating interests of the medical profession.[3] Where it addressed problems of disease and illness, the operation of this discourse had the effect of 'depoliticizing' them, rendering the false impression that all problems of health are responsive to technical solutions, where instead political and economic action may be required.[4] However, as historians have moved away from an exclusive attention to medical theory, to systematic engagement with practice, so the political and economic dimensions of medical activity have become more evident.[5] Today the study of medicine as heroic intervention against disease is giving way, thanks to the work of Charles Rosenberg, John Harley Warner, and others, to a perspective which interprets medicine and the treatment of disease as structurally embedded in contemporary political and social thought.[6] Medicine, as practised, is more evidently today an institution of culture, and typically of western culture. As a cultural institution, it has the power to redefine (or 'medicalize') concepts into the terms of its own discourse. Thus, 'medical imperialism', in the colloquialism of our day, now encompasses not only the conquest of new diseases, but also the extension of what has been called the 'bio-medical' model to the non-medical world.[7] It also implies the extension of western cultural values to the non-western world.

It is widely observed that the nature and consequences of imperialism constitute one of the central questions of our time.[8] Despite its long history in political economy, imperialism remains an imprecise concept; possibly, as W.K. Hancock reminds us, it is too imprecise for definition, yet too important to neglect.[9] If by imperialism we mean the extension of international systems of domination — by economic, cultural, or political means — it is clear that medicine has a place in this definition.[10] In the history of medicine, the concept of imperialism has come to serve as much as a tool of apologetics as a domain of scientific enquiry. If medicine, viewed as technology, helps illuminate *methods* by which European expansion took place, then medicine, as a system of practice, suggests how, within knowable limits, its *objectives* could be achieved. The history of European medicine overseas, particularly within the 'classic' period of nineteenth-century colonialism, from 1815 to the Second World War, thus offers a perspective on the twinned relations of political and professional power.

If the history of *imperialism in medicine* can be taken to comprise the expansion of medical attitudes, beliefs and practices to non-medical domains, then the history of *medicine in empire* refers to the complementary history of medical regimes as participants in the expansion and consolidation of political rule. In the latter aspect, the last twenty years have seen an outpouring of case studies, often more custodial than critical. But there is, as yet, little coherent perspective on the relations between medicine and empire.

There are at least three senses in which this relationship may be construed. First, we may consider medicine in its direct relation with the political, commercial and military expansion of the imperial powers.[11] In this sense, medicine embodies both a 'tool' of empire[12] and a form of practice within the European colonies. Within the picture of European expansion, we can to some extent distinguish between developments in tropical and in temperate climates. In both cases, medicine enabled Europeans to conquer distant corners of the globe and, in certain areas, to remain. In both, European medicine developed administrative forms congruent with imperial government. These are implicit in the 'navalism' and explorations of the eighteenth century, and become more explicit with the establishment of the colonial empires in the nineteenth century.[13] In the history of tropical colonies we find systems of medical ideas and practice often stimulated by the necessities of military conquest and administration; and enduring patterns of disease control confined to the tropics and to maladies which exhibit special features in those areas.[14]

However, the presence of transmissible and debilitating disease also forced imperial powers to establish increasingly more systematic sanitary and medical services. Notably in India, Africa, South-East Asia and the Pacific, 'colonial medicine' became the professional activity of 'colonial medical services', which formed in turn an arm of colonial authority.[15] Each European power addressed the provision of medical services differently. In the British case, the Indian Medical Service, tracing its origins from 1714, served the interests of the British community in the subcontinent, and grew in direct association with military and political necessity. In Africa, the Colonial Medical Service, beginning in 1927 and by the 1940s embracing all British Africa, grew from the private enterprise of missions and West African trading 'companies'.[16] In the case of France and Germany, medical officers were the officers of imperial governments, trained and appointed as civil servants.[17] In either case, distinctions between the medical officers' professional and public duties became difficult to draw. Colonial medical services which enforced the 'sanitary order' were no less part of the political order they helped maintain.[18] Imperialism, both as impulse and as attitude, required the operation of a set of skills and rules. These European medicine undoubtedly complemented. As Frantz Fanon put it, in the colonial context, 'going to see the doctor, the administrator, the constable or the mayor [became] identical moves'.[19]

Finally, we may consider medicine in its imperial practice within what Donald Denoon calls the 'settler colonies'. The colonial medical services in British, French, Belgian and German Africa, the Caribbean, South East Asia and the Pacific began by serving imperial military, political, and trading interests, and only by slow degrees moved towards the needs of indigenous inhabitants.[20] While medical services became permanent, individual offers were, in principle if not always in fact, provisional; and the practice of colonial medicine had constant reference to the imperial metropolis for its authority, training, and recognition. In the more temperate climates, and in the 'white dominions' of the British Empire, however, the practice of imperial medicine soon acquired its own colonial dynamic. Practitioners of colonial medicine in this respect drew closer to the original Latin meaning of colonists, as settlers tilling foreign fields. Familiar institutions were adopted, and given new shape, as 'transplanted' Europeans took up permanent settlement in lands where professional niceties and therapeutic distinctions, acceptable at 'home', did not always apply.[21]

If imperial medicine provided the metropolitan 'push', so to these practitioners the problems of colonial medicine represented a peripheral 'pull'. But from Atlantic America to the Australasian antipodes, in the French and Spanish colonies as in the British sphere, governments and their medical representatives sought to replicate the structures of Old World medicine in the New.[22] Meeting similar patterns of disease, set against the foreign circumstances of frontier life, colonial medicine eventually came to compare itself, and later compete with, its professional parents. A common culture of medicine — sustained by the image of science as the universal agent of progress, and scientific medicine as its servant — became the hallmark of European empires throughout the world.

In each of these relationships, medicine has served a different aspect of empire, and a different aspect of European expansion. In the circumstances it seems strange that these 'imperial relations' of medicine have attracted so little comparative interest, in contrast to the increasing attention being paid to the historical development of 'imperial science' and the relationships between technology and empire.[23] Many have drawn attention to the ways in which the European 'metropolis' influenced colonial intellectual and material development, and to the extent to which the 'periphery' shared or reshaped metropolitan assumptions. In medical history, these relationships are still far from clear. If scholars today are generally familiar with the movements and patterns of disease that formed part of the 'Columbian exchange',[24] few have placed medicine within the economic and political 'terms of trade' that arose during three centuries of European contact with the worlds of America, Africa, Asia, Oceania and Australasia.[25] In ways yet to be fully established, European medicine, playing upon a distant stage, formed a lasting part of the colonial legacy, the discourse of conquest, and the quixotic politics of deference and resistance.

II

In viewing what may become themes in the historiography of imperial medicine, it is convenient to consider the writing of recent years in four sequential but overlapping phases, each continuing in some form to the present day. In tropical medicine, there has been a long, heroic history, commemorating the epochal movements through which the newly constituted specialty progressed from legend, mystery, and medical geography[26] in the eighteenth century, to the organized colonial efforts of the 1880s.[27] The 1950s and early 1960s saw continued interest in the history of epidemic diseases as agents of potential change,[28] and a substantial revival of 'participants' history', including a profusion of biographical accounts and autobiographical memoirs by leading players in colonial medical administration, for whom the previous half-century had been their finest hour.[29] The language of these accounts spoke of revolutionary 'milestones' in the triumphal march against disease. That march is still far from finished, as references to the campaign against malaria readily acknowledge.[30]

In the early 1960s, post-war decolonization reached the agenda of imperial historians, and the role of disease and medicine in imperial history, so long taken for granted, became a subject of interest in its own right. Ann Beck, Philip Curtin, and others working on Africa, began to explore the imagery and consequences of the 'white man's grave' for the institutions that focused and administered European medicine during the most rapid period of European expansion in the late nineteenth century.[31] In many cases, such histories of European confrontation with disease took the form of 'case histories' — notably of malaria, dysentery, parasitic diseases and sleeping sickness — and began to view disease within a wider, political frame of reference.[32] These accounts, generally by no means critical of western medicine, formed part of the resource base enjoyed by the new discipline of development studies, and the advocates of modernization theory.[33] H.C. Squires was early, but not alone, in referring to the history of the Sudan Medical Service as an 'experiment in social medicine'.[34] From the 1960s onwards, however, historical journals as well as medical and medical historical journals joined in recognizing the political contingencies of medicine as pivotal aspects of empire.[35]

With the early 1970s, the contradictions of 'modernization' and the persisting economic consequences of colonial dependency reached the conscience of the world. A new and vigorous analytical tradition, *marxisant sinon marxiste*, forced attention to connections between medical practice and colonial rule. Some saw little distance between medicine and the factors inherent in western domination generally, whether in Europe, America or the Third World. The *International Journal of Health Services*, beginning in 1970, became a continuing critic of the traditional accountancy of western medicine in overseas enterprise.[36] Other authors brought within range the 'newer imperialism' of the League of Nations, WHO and the Rockefeller Foundation.[37] By the late 1970s, the political economy of medicine as a whole, mediating between the advance of industrialized nations and the Third World, became the target. Western medicine was considered to be in a state of 'cultural crisis'.[38] That this 'crisis' was associated with contemporary critiques of capitalism and military interventionism in Asia and Africa was perhaps inevitable; just as its near-exclusive focus on the activities of Western countries, to the neglect of socialist imperialism, was regrettable. In the event,'imperial medicine', past and present, fell into disfavour. The future of rational and humane medical policy was to be determined not by models of the past — not simply by supplying scientific 'know-how' and resources in ever-increasing quantities — but by deciding who would control and distribute the resources supplied.

This revisionist historiography unavoidably focused upon the tropical regions. From the 1940s to the 1960s, 'the conquest of epidemic disease' could still be regarded by public health reformers as principally a 'chapter in the history of ideas'.[39] By the early 1980s, the study of tropical diseases had passed, in the phrase of Clive Wood, from 'Romance to Reality'.[40] Strategies for the future were needed, to answer the many questions left by the previous decade of rapid decolonization.[41] Alongside this political agenda came a new historical consciousness. Beginning in the late 1970s and early 1980s, a fourth phase opened, characterized by a new cultural vigour, but also by an eclecticism which has so far escaped easy definition. Fresh interest in tropical medicine was sustained by accounts of the pro-consular figures of colonial medicine.[42] Within the British Commonwealth, this was then extended to the Crown Colonies, the 'white settlements' and India, where colonial medical history has been rediscovered and given a place in the vanguard of recent colonial historiography.[43] Meanwhile, political and imperial historians and historians of science, principally in Britain, Australia, and the United States, today see tropical medicine emerging as a discipline, conceived in the schools and laboratories of London and Liverpool,[44] baptized at American military camp fires in Cuba and the Philippines,[45] and reaching maturity in French and British Africa,[46] and in the 'secondary imperialism' of Australia in Papua New Guinea.[47] Historians of western medicine in the non-western world have begun to query the distinction implied by the imperial division between 'temperate' and 'tropical' medicine, and to look instead to the 'struggles for control' they embraced.[48] A generation ago, scholars were conditioned to regard epidemic and debilitating tropical diseases as of climatic or genetic character, rather than as the product of circumstances in which people live, and where race, poverty and 'deficiency diseases' seemed synonymous. Today, many recognize the spread of epidemic physical disease as a product of remediable neglect, whether in tropical or in temperate regions. Tropical diseases, once defined geographically, are now seen as diseases of poverty rather than of place.[49] The distinction between temperate and tropical medicine becomes increasingly political and economic: in the temperate colonies, needs for adequate housing, fresh water, sanitation and nutrition were met; and in place of the devastations of malaria, came the so-called 'diseases of affluence', with their different political economies.

In many ways, it must be said, this recent scholarship on medicine and empire has yet to sway or even seriously to engage the prejudices of past generations. European medicine fostered a powerful discourse of authority and progress, committed to the extension of 'expert' control over otherwise intractable social systems.[50] In former colonies, these assumptions, together with the research and reward patterns of metropolitan medicine, have fostered enduring dependencies, in ideas, individuals and institutions. That these dependencies today produce sophisticated medical techniques for the wealthy few, and Primary Health Care schemes for the impoverished many, speaks to a continuation of practices that the patristic figures of European medicine could never have envisaged.[51]

III

If the respective conditions of tropical and temperate colonies, which unified the imperial world from 'palm to pine', help to shape our perspectives today, the history of medicine and empire must reflect both these dimensions and their differences. The tension between them provides a subtext running through this book. The language of 'settler medicine' is the language of practical public health and professional advancement. But the discipline and practice of tropical medicine encompasses a very different set of concepts and historiography. That history is the language of military and political conquest; the history of conflict in biblical dimensions, between the heroic endeavours of human beings and the vast microscopic armies and resources of the animal kingdom. Memoirs of tropical doctors are the journals of medical Caesars confronting microbial Gauls, in lands never more than half won. This message moves with passion through R.W.

Cilento's *Triumph in the Tropics* and Aldo Castellani's *Microbes, Men and Monarchs*.[52] Theirs was the history of the 'insect wars' — for which Cloudsley-Thompson's *Insects and History* and J.R. Busvine's *Insects, Hygiene and History* provide tactical treatises, both worthy successors to Hans Zinsser's famous *Rats, Lice and History*.[53] In these wars of attrition, primitive organisms formidably oppose frail human attempts at understanding and control. Their conduct involved, throughout, the linking of military and medical metaphor — from Benjamin Kidd's *The Control of the Tropics*[54] to the Rockefeller hookworm 'campaign' of 1925, and the 'campaign' against malaria in our own day.[55]

This imagery of armed struggle seems foreign to the language of laboratories, test tubes, and white coats; yet its usage comes compellingly to historians who view the advent of Europeans in the tropics as marking the inception of a crusade against disease, a hundred years' war without pause or armistice. The six principal British expeditions to West Africa between 1805 and 1841 suffered an average mortality of nearly 50 per cent. Between 1881 and 1887, the annual death rate of European civilians employed by the governments of the Gold Coast and Nigeria averaged between 5 and 8.5 per cent.[56] As Sir Robert Boyce put it candidly in 1909, it was a question of 'mosquito or man?'.[57] As late as the 1920s, in John L. Todd's words, the 'future of imperialism lay with the microscope'. Whether there would be a 'Europe in the tropics' was reduced to the resolve of men against the tsetse fly. To some historians, the struggle against the tsetse fly *became* the struggle for Africa.[58]

It is not surprising that the struggle of men against disease should be mirrored in the struggle of men for recognition in the field. In a history with generals and victors, the language of combat and conquest parallels the language of colonial development. From Joseph Chamberlain to Alfred Milner,[59] the discipline of tropical medicine was given marching orders — to secure the safety and improve the productivity of the British Empire. The French, Belgians, and Germans soon joined the fray.[60] From the 1880s, the practice of medicine in the empire became a history of techniques and policies — of education, epidemiology, and quarantine — the discovery of pathogens and vectors and the segregation of races. Simultaneously, tropical medicine became a history of *mentalités*, shaped by the Pasteurian revolution, which lent a conceptual strategy to complement Europe's political mission. European medicine after Pasteur espoused a set of doctrines — a model, based upon the discovery of specific etiologies and disease-causing mechanisms.[61] From the West Indies to West Africa, Egypt to Asia, medical doctrine and public health administrators pursued policies which sustained European control, and which had increasingly to focus on diseases which affected the economic activity of entire populations.

From the late 1870s, this tropical medicine — its ideology European, its instrument the microscope, its epistemology the germ theory of disease — served the interests of dominant economic groups and obscured the relationship of disease to social structure. In Africa and India, despite the work of missionaries and individual doctors, the health of indigenes inevitably remained subordinate to the economic and political interests of governments. Unlike most of the diseases endemic in East Africa, malaria and sleeping sickness impinged directly on metropolitan interests, and so became the main focus for colonial medical activity. In French Africa, the very concept of *médecine coloniale* embraced the policy and the priorities of European health in uncongenial climates.[62] By the early years of the twentieth century, with the *Annales d'Hygiène et Médecine Coloniale* (established 1897) and the *Journal of Tropical Medicine and Hygiene* (established 1895), and with a Royal Society of Tropical Medicine and Hygiene (established 1906), the discipline had won an established place.[63]

Levels of death and disease among indigenous inhabitants of the tropical colonies were very high even before Europeans arrived. While little is definitively known, it seems that with wider contact between regions, stimulated by new technologies and transport, colonial contact may have accelerated the spread of infectious diseases.[64] Nevertheless, colonial medicine, in the strict sense, remained reserved to expatriate populations for nearly three generations. The principal efforts made by the Colonial Office to foster medical research in colonial territories did not occur until the Second World War.[65] As such, it generally had little to say to, and sadly little to learn from, the traditional medical cultures with which it came into contact.[66]

In 1904 an Advisory Committee for the Imperial Defence Research Fund was established to advise the Colonial Office, and the Imperial Diseases Bureau was founded, as the first of several imperial bureaux assisting colonial research. In 1909 the Secretary of State for the Colonies appointed an Advisory Medical and Sanitary Committee for Tropical Africa. Following the exhaustion of Europe between 1914 and 1918, a belief that Europe's overseas estates should be formally developed arose again, and met little resistance. With Lord Lugard's 'dual mandate'[67] came the convenient view that Britain's imperial responsibilities lay jointly on behalf of her colonial subjects and on behalf of the civilized world.[68] The 'prime object' of development, said Leo Amery, Colonial Secretary, in 1919, 'must be the welfare of the inhabitants of these regions. . . . But I am sure . . . that we cannot develop them and help them without an overspill of wealth . . . that would be an immense help to this country.'[69] In 1922 the functions of this Committee were extended to all other dependencies, and a Colonial Advisory Medical and Sanitary Committee was established. In 1926 the first Chief Medical Adviser to the Colonial Office was created, to advise the Colonial Office and the British Government.[70] With their own *mission civilisatrice*, the French and Belgians established comparable bodies in their provinces *d'outre-mer*. In most cases, however, their record was to prove disappointing. Economic initiative was left to the colonies, or to private enterprise; and rarely did 'colonial development' become, in Bernard Porter's phrase, more than 'a pious wish'.

Elsewhere in the British Empire, 'colonial medicine' characteristically claimed to represent the extension of a framework of scientific medicine to the colonized world. In the 'old Empire', and the 'settler colonies' of Canada, Australia, New Zealand, and South Africa, the surgeons and physicians who served the army or navy were also employed to serve the needs of white citizens. As civil society developed, private practitioners replaced government doctors, and the white populations eventually enjoyed a health status comparable to that of European populations. For demographic and geographical reasons, general practitioners were more important than specialist surgeons or physicians in the colonies. But with the growth of medical schools and hospitals in such large cities as Toronto, Melbourne, and Sydney, a division into elite groups of specialists and rank-and-file practitioners, not unlike that in England, began to occur. The extension of the medical profession in the colonies thereafter became a struggle for 'internal' reforms to regulate professional behaviour and entry to the profession, and 'external' campaigns, involving the profession's relationship with the state and the community.

In 'settler medicine', certain issues bound the metropolis to the periphery. Such were medical claims that governmental and professional interests coincided in the history of registration and education, in the transmission of an urban conception of public health, and in extending to all the apparatus of the 'sanitary state'. But at the periphery there were also different priorities. Environments were harsh and unfamiliar, with small European populations living at great distances over large areas. In consequence, colonial specialities developed, to offset the 'tyranny of distance', and intercolonial and imperial ties were strengthened. In government medical policy, the strengths of these ties grew more, rather than less, prominent. At the end of the nineteenth century, European medicine witnessed a changing vision of the sanitary idea, with environmental policies giving way to policies centred on individual diseases and personal hygiene, selectively applied to the rhetoric of racial advantage.[71] At the imperial periphery, the trend was mirrored and then magnified, in ways which had far-reaching consequences for colonial medicine. In Queensland, the Australian Institute of Tropical Medicine set out to discover means by which to promote the health of whites in the tropics, in order that long-term white settlement areas could be assured. But the Australian government exhibited a deep absence of concern for the health of Aborigines until the 1960s. In Papua New Guinea, at least until the 1930s, medical efforts were almost wholly directed towards protecting the health of expatriates and native males employed in European economic interests. In South Africa, public health improvement was used to justify urban segregation of whites from non-whites. Only in New Zealand was medical knowledge directly applied to the task of improving the health of the non-white population.[72] In ways which this book only begins to address, the consequences of these disparities remain with us today.

IV

The essays in this volume illustrate the broad spectrum of issues that were present in the expansion of European medicine overseas, and formative in the institution of colonial policy, in both tropical and temperate regions. Viewing developments over two centuries, and confronting such an enormous variety of imperial experience, it is impossible to seek or present a unified thesis. From the diversity of these cases, however, reviewed within a common framework, arise interpretations which are central to the rewriting of imperial history. While concentrating principally on the British Empire, cases are also drawn from French, Belgian and German experience; these in some ways qualify, in others confirm, the main directions of this task.

In some respects, this volume could be considered three books in one, linked by the common experience of Europeans overseas. In Part I, we find histories of conflict and arguments, not only between men and pathogens, but also between rival schools of thought. We find confrontation and conciliation between imported and indigenous systems of medical belief; and we see controversy and injustice, where medical men are torn between commercial, military and governmental regulations, professional standards and expectations, and their ignorance of local rites and practices. We see the primacy of military motives in India, and of commerce and statecraft in Algeria, South-East Asia and the Pacific. We see, too, the unfolding prospect of medical policy, once merely handmaiden to political purpose, becoming equal, independent and in some cases, pre-eminent in the rituals of imperial order and control.

Colonial medicine in the 'white empire' has yet to find a unifying Commonwealth perspective and the cases we offer unavoidably fall short of a comprehensive picture. However, when we turn, in Part II, to semi-tropical and 'temperate medicine' in the settler colonies, we confront what must be a more general picture of formal similarities and fundamental contrasts. In colonial practice, from the Carolinas to the antipodes, we see the medical profession preserved in a colonial chrysalis, from which it slowly, even reluctantly, emerged. Seeking professional independence, yet coveting metropolitan recognition, British doctors in these colonies confronted an intersection of economic and political requirements, and resolved those requirements to their advantage. With this advantage came the consolidation of professional attitudes, fostering the identity of professional goals with the language of colonial and imperial progress.

With the politics of race and epidemic disease, tensions inherent in colonial medicine become most vivid, and questions that underlie medical roles in colonial society are indelicately revealed. In Part III we examine selected crises — smallpox in Sydney, cholera in Manila, typhus at the Cape, sleeping sickness in the Congo — that challenged the medical and political order. Historians and novelists are long accustomed to viewing epidemics as similar in more than one respect to political revolution. In Evan Stark's phrase, epidemics are 'social events', producing a flood of documentation through which the workings of society are revealed.[73] Where civil *potentia* is threatened, victims of epidemics are not limited to those who succumb to disease. In combating epidemics, medical men (and rarely, women), alongside engineers and to a varying extent missionary clergy, became necessary arms of the occupying and settling power. When they threatened the *status quo*, epidemics also created conditions favourable to the consolidation of imperial or government rule. Almost unavoidably they also threatened established medical practice and contributed to the emergence of new medical regimes, 'modern' and reformist in medical technology and highly custodial in their social application. Empires which based their claims of occupation and settlement in part on the moral superiority of European civilization, and saw an obligation to secure the safety of their subjects, found their credibility as purveyors of European culture and rational government intricately tied to their power to control the spread of disease. Similarly, medical men who spoke in defence of public health were not spared the associations between health and race. In struggling for public health in the competition among nations, the medical profession often employed its power selectively; and did so in the interest of what was defined as the 'public good'. That we see ambiguity in that definition today speaks to our capacity for wisdom after the event.

V

The composition of this volume inevitably exposes many lacunae — some structural, some analytical. In Part I we find the instrument of western medicine, shaping expectations in tropical lands, sometimes appearing as a weapon aimed at disease, but coincidentally falling upon passive, helpless masses. But this description masks many territorial and epistemological interplays between colonizers and the colonized, between European benevolence and colonial dominion. First, the political uses of medical knowledge are not unambiguously one-sided; its effects are not simple. Medical historians have only begun to expose the complex relationships between traditional and western medical belief systems in colonial contexts; if our essays recognize this problem, they also, regrettably, pass by on the other side. Second, the impact of colonial medicine must be measured against the nature and extent of diseases not only within selected cases and colonies (as we do), but comparatively, throughout the world. Since the great works of historical epidemiology earlier this century, the exercise of relating disease to colonial circumstances has yet to be attempted. It is to be hoped that the accumulation of 'vertical' cases, such as those we present, will now lead to 'horizontal' comparisons of political diseases and their colonial consequences within and between rival imperial structures, and between Europe and the rest of the world.

Third, the imperial role of western medicine, just as the success (or otherwise) of empire, cannot be judged by simply equating its existence with its acceptance, or with the abandonment of alternatives. In the case of western therapeutics, this is strikingly clear. The major advances in western preventive medicine were only beginning to occur towards the end of the period our essays address; and then, as now, medicine in the colonies could not in itself be more effective than that practised in Europe. Since McKeown's work in Britain,[74] few historians look to medical practice as having been more effective in saving lives than were the advances of the last century in nutrition, housing and sanitation. Arguably, in those areas colonial medicine could have improved its 'effectiveness'; but it is in these areas that development is, in many cases, still waiting to occur.

Finally, there is a residual sense in which any cultural critique of medicine, as an instrument-shaping culture, implies a critique of western medicine itself. But, as our exploration of colonial history suggests, while medical practice may reinforce dependence and sustain political hegemonies, it does not create them. It is clearly possible to examine the culture of western medicine without questioning the benefits of modern science; and this the following essays demonstrate. At the same time, the consequences of imperial expansion created obligations which western medicine and the advanced industrial world can still do much to fulfil. The history of medicine in its relation to empire is no longer bounded by the past experience of rulers, colonists, and medical men. Today it looks toward the future action of nations to meet the political and economic challenges of hunger, poverty, racism, and disease. These also in part form the history of medicine and empire.

NOTES

1. Meredith Turshen, *The Political Ecology of Disease in Tanzania* (New Brunswick, N.J.: Rutgers University Press, 1984). Cf. L. Doyal and I. Renwell, *The Political Economy of Health* (London: Pluto Press, 1979); I. Kennedy, *The Unmasking of Medicine* (London: Allen & Unwin, 1981).
2. In the English-speaking world, Henry E.Sigerist's *History of Medicine* (New York: Oxford University Press, 1951) marked a transition towards viewing medicine in its social, political, and economic context. At about the same time, Richard Shryock took a similar path, in his *The Development of Modern Medicine: An Interpretation of the Social and Scientific Factors Involved* (London: Gollancz, 1948). George Rosen applied this perspective in *A History of Public Health* (New York: MD Publications, 1958).
3. N. Jewson, 'The disappearance of the sick man from medical cosmology, 1770–1870', *Sociology, 10* (2) (1976), 225–44; H.S. Berliner and J.W. Salmon, 'The holistic alternative to scientific medicine: history and analysis', *International Journal of Health Services, 10* (1) (1980), 133–47; E.R. Brown, *Rockefeller Medicine Men: Medicine and Capitalism in America* (Berkeley: University of California Press, 1979); T.S. Pensabene, *The Rise of the Medical Practitioner in Victoria* (Canberra: Australian National University Press, 1980).
4. Cf. John Ehrenreich (ed.), *The Cultural Crisis of Modern Medicine* (New York: Monthly Review Press, 1978); Vicente Navarro (ed.), *Imperialism, Health and Medicine* (London: Pluto Press, 1982).
5. A major revision began with Edwin Clarke (ed.), *Modern Methods in the History of Medicine* (London: Athlone Press, 1971), and continues with Gert H. Brieger, 'History of medicine', in Paul T. Durbin (ed.), *A Guide to the Culture of Science* (New York: The Free Press, 1980), 121–94, and Russell Maulitz, 'Disciplinary perspectives in the history of medicine: a view for the 1980s', in Jerome J. Bylebyl (ed.), *Teaching the History of Medicine at a Medical Center* (Baltimore: Johns Hopkins University Press, 1982).
6. See Charles E.Rosenberg, *The Cholera Years: The United States in 1832, 1849, and 1866* (Chicago: University of Chicago Press, 1962) and C.E. Rosenberg (ed.), *Healing*

and History: Essays for George Rosen (Folkestone: W. Dawson, 1979); John Harvey Warner, *The Therapeutic Perspective: Medical Practice, Knowledge and Identity in America, 1820–1885* (Cambridge, Mass.: Harvard University Press, 1987).

7. Berliner and Salmon, op. cit., n. 3 above; and A. Briggs and J.H. Shelley (eds), *Science, Medicine and the Community. The Last Hundred Years* (Amsterdam: Excerpta Medica, 1986).

8. For a general consideration of imperialism in its wider bearings, see Michael Barrett Brown, *The Economics of Imperialism* (Harmondsworth: Penguin, 1974).

9. W.K. Hancock, 'The moving metropolis', in A.R. Lewis and T.F. McGann, *The New World Looks at History* (Austin: University of Texas Press, 1963), 135–41.

10. Clearly the belief of Vicente Navarro, 'The nature of imperialism and its implications in health and medicine', in Navarro, op. cit., n. 4 above, 5–9.

11. As considered, for example, by Robert V. Kubicek, *The Administration of Imperialism: Joseph Chamberlain at the Colonial Office* (Durham, N.C: Duke University Press, 1969).

12. The phrase made famous by Daniel Headrick, *The Tools of Empire: Technology and European Imperialism in the Nineteenth Century* (New York: Oxford University Press, 1981); see also Rondo Cameron, 'Imperialism and technology' in Melvin Kranzberg and Carroll W. Pursell, Jnr, (eds), *Technology in Western Civilization* (New York: Oxford University Press, 1967), 692–706.

13. Cf. Benjamin Moseley, *A Treatise upon Tropical Diseases; on Military Operations; and on the Climate of the West Indies* (London: T. Cadell, 3rd edn, 1792); Sir John Pringle, *Observations on the Diseases of the Army in Camp and Garrison* (London, 7th edn, 1775) and *Discourse upon some Late Improvements of the Means for Preserving the Health of Mariners* (London, 1776); Sir Alexander Murray Tulloch and H. Marshall, 'Statistical report on the sickness, mortality and invaliding among the troops in the West Indies; prepared from the records of the Army Medical Department and War Office returns', *Parliamentary Papers* (Great Britain), 1837–38, XL, 417; Sir Neil Cantlie, *A History of the Army Medical Department*, 2 vols (Edinburgh: Churchill Livingstone, 1974).

14. Cf. H. Harold Scott, *A History of Imperial Medicine*, 2 vols (London: Edward Arnold, 1939–42); Paul Brau, *Trois siècles de médecine coloniale française* (Paris: Vigot Frères, 1931); A. Balfour and H.H. Scott, *Health Problems of the Empire: Past, Present and Future* (London: Collins, 1924); F.K. Mostofi, 'Contributions of the Military to tropical medicine', *Bulletin of the New York Academy of Medicine, 44* (1968), 702–20.

15. David Arnold, 'Medical priorities and practice in nineteenth century British India', *South Asia Research, 5* (2) (1985), 167–83; and 'Cholera and colonialism in British India', *Past and Present*, no. 113 (1986), 118–51; R. Ramasubban, *Public Health and Medical Research in India: Their Origins under the Impact of British Colonial Policy* (Stockholm: SAREC, 1982); Edmund Burrows, *A History of Medicine in South Africa up to the End of the Nineteenth Century* (Cape Town, Amsterdam: Balkema, 1958); A. Beck, 'The role of medicine in German East Africa', *Bulletin of the History of Medicine, 45* (1971), 170–8. The history of the Colonial Medical Service in Africa, from its 'prehistory' in the 1870s to the 1960s, has yet to be fully written. For impressions, see Sir Alan Burns, *Colonial Civil Servant* (London: Allen & Unwin, 1949); A.D. Milne, 'The rise of a Colonial Medical Service', *Kenya and East African Medical Journal, 5* (1928–9), 50–8; and the stimulating critique in 'The development of the dependent Empire' in Henry L. Hall, *The Colonial Office: A History* (London: Longman, 1937).

16. S.G. Browne, 'The contribution of medical missionaries to tropical medicine. Service-training-research', *Transactions of the Royal Society of Tropical Medicine and Hygiene, 73* (1979), 357–60; A. Beck, *A History of the British Medical Administration of East Africa, 1900–1950* (Cambridge, Mass.: Harvard University Press, 1970); T.P. Eddy, 'The evolution of British colonial hospitals in West Africa', *Transactions of the*

Royal Society of Tropical Medicine and Hygiene, 77 (1983), 563–4; Guiseppe Bucco and Angelo Natoli, *L'Italia in Africa: L'organizzazione sanitaria nell'Africa Italiana* (Rome: Instituto Poligrafico dello Stato, 1965).

17. Cf. M.A. Vaucel, 'Le Service de santé des troupes de marine et la médecine tropicale française', *Transactions of the Royal Society of Tropical Medicine and Hygiene, 59* (1965), 226–33; D. Domergue, 'French Sanitary Services on the Ivory Coast', *Revue française histoire outre-mer, 65* (1979), 40–63; W. Eckart, 'Der ärztliche Dienst in den Ehemaligen Deutschen Kolonien', *Arzt und Krankenhaus*, no. 10 (1981), 422–6; Albert Diefenbacher, *Psychiatrie und Kolonalismus. Zur 'Irrenfürsorge' in der Kolonie Deutsch-Ostafrika* (Frankfurt: Campus Verlag, 1985).

18. M.W. Swanson, 'The sanitation syndrome: bubonic plague and urban native policy in the Cape Colony, 1900–1909', *Journal of African History, XVIII* (3) (1977), 387–410.

19. Frantz Fanon, 'Medicine and colonialism', in Ehrenreich, op. cit., n. 4 above.

20. Patrick A. Twumasi, 'Colonialism and international health; a study in social change in Ghana', *Social Science and Medicine, 15 B* (1981), 147–51.

21. C.J. Cummins, *A History of Medical Administration in New South Wales, 1788–1973* (Sydney: Health Commission of NSW, 1979); N.R. Barrett, 'Contributions of Australians to medical knowledge', *Medical History, 11* (1967), 321–33.

22. F. Guerra, 'Medical colonisation of the New World', *Medical History, 7* (1963), 147–55; Ronald L. Numbers (ed.), *Medicine in the New World: New Spain, New France and New England* (Knoxville: Tennessee University Press, 1987); Raymond Fery, 'Colonisation et médecine', *Presse Médecine, 63* (1955), 1245; Teodora V. Tiglao and Wilfredo L. Cruz, *Seven Decades of Public Health in the Philippines, 1898–1972* (Tokyo: South East Asian Medical Information Centre, 1975).

23. Roy M. MacLeod, 'On visiting the "moving metropolis": Reflections on the architecture of imperial science', *Historical Records of Australian Science, 5* (1982), 1–16.

24. A.W. Crosby, *The Columbian Exchange: Biological and Cultural Consequences of 1492* (Westport, Conn.: Greenwood Publishers, 1972).

25. A notable exception is Philip Curtin. See his *The Image of Africa: British Ideas and Action, 1780–1850* (Madison: University of Wisconsin Press, 1964). But also see Michael Gelfand, *Tropical Victory. An Account of the Influence of Medicine on the History of Southern Rhodesia* (Cape Town: Juta Press, 1953); Nancy E. Gallagher, *Medicine and Power in Tunisia, 1780–1900* (Cambridge: Cambridge University Press, 1983); and Dennis E. Carlson, *African Fever: A Study of British Science, Technology and Politics in West Africa, 1787–1864* (Canton, Mass.: Science History Publications, 1984).

26. In the phrase of Ackerknecht, medical geography became tropical medicine which, in his view, meant 'colonial medicine, i.e. that branch of medicine dealing with diseases that for the most part were not tropical *per se*, but were prevalent in tropical countries and which therefore were of intense interest to colonial powers'. E.H. Ackerknecht, *History and Geography of the Most Important Diseases* (New York: Hafner, 1965), 4–5.

27. R. Fleming Jones, 'Tropical diseases in British New Guinea', *Transactions of the Royal Society for Tropical Medicine and Hygiene, V* (1910–11), 93–105.

28. Cf. E. Ford, 'The malaria problem in Australia and the Australian Pacific Territories', *Medical Journal of Australia* (10 June 1950) (1), 749–60; St Julien Ravenel Childs, *Malaria and Colonization in the Carolina Low Country, 1526–1696* (Baltimore: Johns Hopkins University Press, 1940); and John Duffy, *Epidemics in Colonial America* (Baton Rouge: Lousiana State University Press, 1953).

29. Cf. R. Foskett (ed.), *The Zambesi Doctors: David Livingstone's Letters to John Kirk, 1858–1872* (Edinburgh: Edinburgh University Press, 1964); Sir Leonard Rogers, *Happy Toil: Fifty-five Years of Tropical Medicine* (London: Muller, 1950); J.S.K. Boyd, 'Fifty years of tropical medicine', *British Medical Journal* (1950) (i), 37; J. Rowland, *The Mosquito Man: The Story of Sir Ronald Ross* (London: Lutterworth Press, 1958);

M. Gelfand, *Lakeside Pioneers: a Socio-Medical Study of Nyasaland, 1875–1920* (Oxford: Blackwell, 1964); P.C.C. Garnham, 'Britain's contribution to tropical medicine, 1868–1968, *Practitioner, 201* (1968), 153–61; V.G. Heiser, 'Reminiscences on early tropical medicine', *Bulletin of the New York Academy of Medicine, 44* (1968), 654–60; P.E.C. Manson-Bahr, 'The march of tropical medicine during the last fifty years', *Transactions of the Royal Society of Tropical Medicine and Hygiene, 52* (1958), 483–99; 'Then and now: memoirs of colonial medicine, Part 4', *British Journal of Clinical Practice, 14* (1960), 300–1, 324; *Patrick Manson: The Founder of Tropical Medicine* (London: Nelson, 1962); Balfour and Scott, op. cit., n. 14 above.

30. E. Ford, op. cit., n. 28 above; Eli Chernin (ed.), 'A bicentennial sampler: milestones in the history of tropical medicine and hygiene', *American Journal of Tropical Medicine and Hygiene, 26*, Supplement (1977), 1053–104.

31. Cf. P.D. Curtin, '"The White Man's Grave": image and reality', *Journal of British Studies, 1* (1961), 94–110.

32. R.E. Dumett, 'The campaign against malaria and the expansion of scientific, medical and sanitary services in British West Africa, 1898–1910', *African Historical Studies, 1* (1968), 153–99; J.N.P. Davies, 'The cause of sleeping sickness', *East African Medical Journal, 39* (1962), 81–99, 145–60; W.H. Ewers, 'Malaria in the early years of German New Guinea', *Journal of the Papua New Guinea Society, VI* (1973), 3–30.

33. Cf. S. May, 'Economic interest in tropical medicine', *American Journal of Tropical Medicine and Hygiene, 3* (1954), 412–21; Gwendolyn Z. Johnson, 'Health conditions in rural and urban areas of developing countries', *Population Studies, 17* (1964), 293–309; C.C. Hunter and J.M. Hunter, 'Disease and development in Africa', *Social Science and Medicine, 3* (1970), 443–93; James Paul, 'Medicine and imperialism in Morocco', *Middle East Research and Information Project Board*, no. 60 (1977), 3–12; I. Maddocks, 'Medicine and colonialism', *Australian and New Zealand Journal of Sociology, XI* (1975), 27–33.

34. H.C. Squires, *The Sudan Medical Service: An Experiment in Social Medicine* (London: Heinemann, 1958).

35. See the 'Secondary Sources' section of the Bibliography at the end of this volume.

36. Cf. H. Leng Chee, 'Health status and the development of health services in a colonial state: the case of British Malaya', *International Journal of Health Services, 12* (3) (1982), 397–417; Kader A. Parahoo, 'Early colonial health developments in Mauritius', *International Journal of Health Services, 16* (3) (1986), 409–23.

37. E.R. Brown, 'Public health and imperialism in early Rockefeller programs at home and abroad', *American Journal of Public Health, 66* (1976), 897–903; H. Cleaver, 'Malaria and the political economy of public health', *International Journal of Health Services, 7* (4) (1977), 557–79; D. Fisher, 'Rockefeller philanthropy and the British Empire: the creation of the London School of Hygiene and Tropical Medicine', *History of Education, 7* (2) (1978), 129–43.

38. Ehrenreich, op. cit., n. 4. above.

39. C.E.A. Winslow, *The Conquest of Epidemic Disease: A Chapter in the History of Ideas* (Princeton: Princeton University Press, 1943, 1967).

40. C. Wood (ed.), *Tropical Medicine: From Romance to Reality* (London: Academic Press, 1978).

41. R.A. Douglas, 'Dr Anton Breinl and the Australian Institute of Tropical Medicine', *Medical Journal of Australia* (17, 14, 21 May 1977) (1), 713–16, 748–51, 784–90; A.J. Duggan, 'Bruce and the African trypanosomes', *American Journal of Tropical Medicine and Hygiene, 26* (1977), 1080–1; P.G. Janssens, 'The colonial legacy: health and medicine in the Belgian Congo', *Tropical Doctor, 11* (3) (1981), 132–40; T.A. Aidoo, 'Rural health under colonialism and neo-colonialism: a survey of the Ghanian experience', *International Journal of Health Services, 12* (4) (1982), 637–57.

42. Roger Joyce, *Sir William MacGregor* (Melbourne: Oxford University Press, 1971);

Leonard Jan Bruce-Chwatt, 'Ronald Ross, William Gorgas and malaria eradication', *American Journal of Tropical Medicine and Hygiene, 26* (1977), 1071–9.

43. Lee Young Kiat, *The Medical History of Early Singapore* (Tokyo: South East Asian Medical Information Centre, 1978); G.R. Gupta, 'Indigenous medicine in 19th and 20th century Bengal', in C.M. Leslie (ed.), *Asian Medical Systems: A Comparative Study* (Berkeley: University of California Press, 1976); G.R. Gupta (ed.), *The Social and Cultural Context of Medicine in India* (New Delhi: Vikas Publishing House, 1981); O.P. Jaggi, 'Indigenous systems of medicine during British supremacy in India', *Studies in History of Medicine, 1* (4) (1977), 320–47; Roger Jeffery, 'Recognizing India's doctors: the institutionalization of medical dependency, 1918–39', *Modern Asian Studies, 13*(2) (1979), 301–26.

On the settler colonies, see: Cf. F.S. MacLean, *Challenge for Health: A History of Health in New Zealand* (Wellington: Owen, 1964); N.R. Barrett, 'Contributions of Australians to medical knowledge', *Medical History, 11* (1967), 321–33; P.W. Laidler and M. Gelfand, *South Africa. Its Medical History, 1652–1898: A Medical and Social Study* (Cape Town: Struik, 1971); T.S. Pensabene, *The Rise of the Medical Practitioner in Victoria* (Canberra: Australian National University Press, 1980); B. Gandevia, 'Medical history in its Australian environment', *Medical Journal of Australia* (18 November 1967) (2) 941–6; M. Lewis and R. MacLeod 'A workingman's paradise? Reflections on urban mortality in colonial Australia, 1860–1900', *Medical History* 31 (1987), 387–402; M. Lewis and R. MacLeod, 'Medical politics and the professionalisation of medicine in New South Wales, 1850–1901', *Journal of Australian Studies* no. 22 (1988), 69–82. Charles G. Roland (ed.), *Health, Disease and Medicine: Essays in Canadian History* (Toronto: The Hannah Institute for the History of Medicine, 1984). We await further studies of the 'fatal contact' between white men and indigenous inhabitants. J.Campbell, 'Smallpox in Aboriginal Australia, 1829–31', *Historical Studies, 20* (81) (1983), 536–56; and 'Smallpox in Aboriginal Australia in the early 1830s', *Historical Studies, 21* (84) (1985), 336–58.

44. Cf. M. Worboys, 'The emergence of tropical medicine: a study in the establishment of a scientific speciality', in G. Lemaine *et al.* (eds), *Perspectives on the Emergence of Scientific Disciplines* (The Hague: Mouton, 1976), 75–98; M. Worboys, 'Science and British Colonial imperialism, 1895–1940' (Unpublished D. Phil thesis, University of Sussex, 1979); Ira Klein, 'Death in India, 1871–1921', *Journal of Asian Studies, 32*(4) (1973), 639–59; John Chandler Hume, 'Colonialism and sanitary medicine: the development of preventive health policy in the Punjab, 1860 to 1900', *Modern Asian Studies, 20* (4) (1986), 703–24.

45. Charles M. Wilson, *Ambassadors in White: The Story of American Tropical Medicine* (New York: Kennikat Press, 1942); N.Stepan, 'The interplay between socio-economic factors and medical science: yellow fever research, Cuba and the United States', *Social Studies of Science, 8* (1978), 397–423.

46. See eg. L. Spitzer, 'The mosquito and segregation in Sierra Leone', *Canadian Journal of African Studies, 11*(1986), 49–61.

47. Donald Denoon, 'Medical services in Papua New Guinea, 1884–1984', in S. Latukefu (ed.), *Papua New Guinea: A Century of Colonial Impact, 1884–1984* (Port Moresby: University of Papua, 1988).

48. Steven Feierman, 'Struggles for control: the social roots of health and healing in modern Africa', *African Studies Review, 28* (2/3) (1985), 73–147.

49. J.M. Janzen, *The Quest for Therapy in Lower Zaire* (Berkeley: University of California Press, 1978); Cf. Leonard Jan Bruce-Chwatt, 'The rise of tropical medicine: milestones of discovery and application' in C.G. Bernbard *et al.*(eds.), *Science, Technology and Society in the Time of Alfred Noble* (Stockholm: Pergamon, 1982), 167–85. There are, however, hopeful signs. See K. David Patterson, *Health in Colonial Ghana: Disease, Medicine and Socio-Economic Change, 1900–1955* (Waltham, Mass.: Crossroad Publishing Company, 1981).

50. Cf.World Health Organisation, *Apartheid and Health* (Geneva: WHO, 1983).

51. Cf. Ann Johnston and Albert Sasson (eds), *New Technologies and Development* (Paris: UNESCO, 1986), ch. 4, 'Health care technologies and health care delivery systems'.

52. R.W. Cilento and C. Lack, *Triumph in the Tropics: An Historical Sketch of Queensland* (Brisbane: Smith & Patterson, 1959); Aldo Castellani, *Microbes, Men and Monarchs: A Doctor's Life in Many Lands* (London: Gollancz, 1960).

53. J.L. Cloudsley-Thompson, *Insects and History* (London: Weidenfeld & Nicholson, 1976); J.R. Busvine, *Insects, Hygiene and History* (London: Athlone Press, 1976); Hans Zinsser, *Rats, Lice and History* (Boston: Little, Brown, 1935).

54. Benjamin Kidd, *The Control of the Tropics* (New York: Macmillan, 1898).

55. G. Harrison, *Mosquitoes, Malaria and Man: A History of Hostilities since 1880* (London: John Murray, 1978).

56. Bruce-Chwatt, op. cit., n. 49 above, 169; E.E. Sabben-Clare *et al.* (eds), *Health in Tropical Africa during the Colonial Period* (Oxford: Clarendon Press, 1980).

57. Sir Robert W. Boyce, *Mosquito or Man?*(London: H.K. Lewis, 1909).

58. J.J. McKelvey, *Man Against Tsetse: Struggle for Africa* (Ithaca, N.Y.: Cornell University Press, 1973).

59. Kubicek, op. cit., n. 11 above; M. Worboys, 'Science and British colonial imperialism, 1895–1940', n. 44 above.

60. G. Roelants, 'The Belgian Society of Tropical Medicine', *Journal of Tropical Medicine and Hygiene, 77* (1974), 103–5; Edmond Sergent, 'La Médecine française en Algérie', *Archives de l'Institut Pasteur d'Algérie, XXXIII* (1955), 281–5; Edmond Sergent and L. Parrot, *Contribution de l'Institut Pasteur d'Algérie à la connaissance humaine du Sahara, 1900–1960* (Algiers: Institut Pasteur, 1961); M.A. Vaucel, 'Les acquisitions de la médecine tropicale dans ces cinquant dernières années', *Annales Société Belge de Médecine Tropicale, 36* (1956), 655–64; J. Tachon, 'La Revue Médecine Tropicale — retrospective', *Médecine tropicale, 40* (1980), 639–41. For comparison between the French and British systems, see the articles by Montague Yudelmen and Michael Crowder in P. Duignan and L.H. Gann, (eds) *Colonialism in Africa, 1870–1960. Vol. 4: The Economics of Capitalism* (Cambridge: Cambridge University Press, 1975). 320–54.

61. Claire Salomon-Bayet *et al.*, *Pasteur et la Révolution Pastorienne* (Paris: Payot,1986).

62. Fery, op. cit., n. 22 above, 1245; Frantz Fanon, *A Dying Colonialism* (New York: Grove Press, 1965).

63. Cf. C.V. Foll, 'Seventy five years old — the "Journal of Tropical Medicine and Hygiene"', *Journal of Tropical Medicine and Hygiene, 76* (1973), 217–22. The *Annales de la Société Belge de Médecine Tropicale* was begun in 1920, and the *American Journal of Imperial Medicine and Hygiene* in 1951.

64. Cf. G.W. Hartwig and K.D. Patterson (eds), *Disease in African History* (Durham, N.C.: Duke University Press, 1978); W.H. McNeill, *Plagues and Peoples* (Oxford: Blackwell, 1977); Oliver Ransford, *Bid the Sickness Cease: Disease in the History of Black Africa* (London: John Murray, 1983).

65. Sir Charles Jeffries (ed.), *A Review of Colonial Research, 1940–1960* (London: HMSO, 1964), 77.

66. B. Porter, *Critics of Empire: British Radical Attitudes to Colonialism in Africa, 1895–1914* (London: Macmillan, 1968).

67. F.D. Lugard, *The Dual Mandate in British Tropical Africa* (London: Blackwood, 1922).

68. Duncan Pederson and Veronica Baruffati, 'Health and traditional medical cultures in Latin America and the Caribbean', *Social Science and Medicine, 21* (1) (1985), 5–12; K. David Patterson, 'Disease and medicine in African history: a bibliographical essay', *History in Africa, 1* (1974), 141–8.

69. Porter, op. cit., n. 66 above, 278.

70. In 1940 the Colonial Development and Welfare Act presaged the extension of imperial scientific and medical research advice, and in 1942 a Colonial Research Committee was established. In 1945 this was joined by the Colonial Medical Research Committee. Cf. Sir George Fiddes, *The Dominions and Colonial Offices* (London and New York: G.P. Putnam's Sons, 1926), 32–8; Sir Charles Jeffries, *The Colonial Empire and its Civil Service* (Cambridge: Cambridge University Press, 1938), ch. 2; (ed.) *A Review of Colonial Research, 1940–1960* (London: HMSO, 1964); *Whitehall and the Colonial Service: An Administrative Memoir, 1939–1956* (London: Athlone Press, 1972), ch. 5; and Sir Cosmo Parkinson, *The Colonial Office from Within, 1909–1945*, (London: Faber & Faber, 1945), ch. 3.

71. G.R. Searle, *The Quest for National Efficiency: A Study in British Politics and Political Thought, 1899–1914* (Oxford: Blackwell, 1971); B. Semmel, *Imperialism and Social Reform: English Social-Imperial Thought, 1895–1914* (London: Allen & Unwin, 1960); S. Tesh, 'Political ideology and public health in the nineteenth century', *International Journal of Health Services, 12* (2) (1982), 321–42.

72. See Donald Denoon, Chapter 6 in this volume: P. Moodie and E.B. Pedersen, *The Health of Australian Aborigines: An Annotated Bibliography with Classifications by Subject Matter and Locality* (Sydney: School of Public Health and Tropical Medicine, 1966); J. Waterford, 'A fundamental imbalance: Aboriginal ill-health', in J. Reid (ed.), *Body, Land and Spirit. Health and Healing in Aboriginal Society* (St Lucia: University of Queensland Press, 1982), 8–30; Maynard W. Swanson, 'The sanitation syndrome: bubonic plague and urban native policy in the Cape Colony, 1900–1909', *Journal of African History, XVIII* (3) (1977), 387–410; Shula Marks and Neil Andersson, chapter 13 in this volume; P.D. Curtin, 'Medical knowledge and urban planning in tropical Africa', *American Historical Review, 90* (3) (1985), 594–613; R.T. Lange, 'The revival of a dying race: a study of Maori health reform, 1900–1918, and its nineteenth century background' (Unpublished MA thesis, University of Auckland, 1972); F.S. MacLean, *Challenge to Health: A History of Health in New Zealand* (Wellington: Owen, 1964).

73. Evan Stark, 'The epidemic as a social event', *International Journal of Health Services, 7* (1977), 681–705.

74. T. McKeown and R.G. Record, 'Reasons for the decline of mortality in England and Wales during the nineteenth century', *Population Studies, 16* (2) (1962), 94–122; T. McKeown, *Medicine in Modern Society. Medical Planning Based on Evaluation of Medical Treatment* (London: Allen & Unwin, 1965), ch. 2; T. McKeown, *The Role of Medicine. Dream, Mirage or Nemesis?* (Oxford: Blackwell, 1979), ch. 3.

Part I

European Medicine and Imperial Experience

1

Manson, Ross and colonial medical policy: tropical medicine in London and Liverpool, 1899–1914

Michael Worboys

INTRODUCTION

In 1899, there were two dominant figures in the newly emerging medical specialism of tropical medicine in Britain. There was Patrick Manson, who, with an established reputation in parasitological research, was the leading metropolitan authority on tropical diseases, who had been the first medical adviser to the Colonial Office since 1897, and who had recently been appointed head of the new London School of Tropical Medicine.[1] There was also Ronald Ross, Director of the equally new Liverpool School of Tropical Medicine, a national celebrity who had shown in the previous year that malaria was transmitted by mosquitoes, and who was soon to become the first Briton to win one of the newly instituted Nobel Prizes.[2] In 1899 Manson and Ross were in no sense rivals; indeed, they had been collaborators on the mosquito-malaria theory, and were identified as the twin leaders in the exciting new area of tropical medicine. However, by 1903 the two men were in open public dispute, and in 1912 their differences resulted in a libel action. Why did relations between these two men, who had worked so closely together, become so acrimonious?

I have elsewhere suggested that the differences between Manson and Ross reflected rival traditions associated with different facets of the medical profession.[3] Manson was representative of a new curative, reductionist, and research-based 'laboratory medicine', whereas Ross acted within an older, preventive, holist, and sanitary tradition. In retrospect, it is doubtful whether such exclusive medical categories existed, and it is difficult to place an individual exclusively in one or the other. It is also perhaps unfair to describe Manson and Ross as passive and unchanging symbols of particular traditions engaged in a general dispute abstracted from their personal and institutional contexts. The intention of this chapter is to offer a fresh perspective on the differences between the two men, which situates their personal and professional rivalry in the specific context of British colonial medical policy between 1899 and 1914.

THE ESSENTIAL TENSION

By 1900, the specialism of tropical medicine had become institutionalized independently of the medical schools of Britain. Although the field eventually became a medical specialism, initially it was closer to being a biological subject because of its dependence on morphology and natural history. Structured around the life-cycle of parasites, tropical medicine required detailed knowledge of the taxonomy of vector species and ecological management, which found application in the tropical environment. Work at home and in the field depended upon resources from colonial and economic interests looking for practical benefits in the fight against tropical disease. In the language of today, tropical medicine was a 'mission oriented', postgraduate specialism.

A decade ago, Johnson and Robbins distinguished between two 'ideal types' of scientific disciplines: those that are 'collegiate controlled' and those that are 'patron controlled'.[4] 'Collegiate control', in their view, tends to produce autonomous disciplines, with distinguishable cognitive structures and technical resources, generating 'universal' or theoretical-oriented knowledge. 'Patron control', on the other hand, tends to be associated with isolated and locally oriented disciplines, with research which is problem- or subject-based, and with knowledge that is particular and empirical. Typically, a specialism may move from 'patron control' in its early years to a more autonomous pattern of 'collegiate control' as it becomes established and secure. In the long term, this is what happened in tropical medicine, but at different rates in different settings.

The professional rivalry between Manson and Ross reflected the different professional pressures operating upon them in London and Liverpool. In London, tropical medicine moved very quickly towards 'collegiate control', while in Liverpool, 'patron control' persisted for many years. Indeed, the policies and priorities of the Colonial Office in London, and of entrepreneurs in Liverpool, produced significantly different kinds of institutions, practitioners and research programmes at Britain's two most important schools of tropical medicine. Manson and Ross both exemplify, and were influenced by, these differences.

MANSON AND ROSS

Patrick Manson and Ronald Ross met in London in April 1894, when Ross approached Manson for advice on the investigation of tropical diseases. At that time Ross was a Surgeon-Major in the Indian Medical Service on leave in Britain. Unusually for a member of the Indian Medical Service, he was interested in sanitary matters and military hygiene, and had been the first member of the service to take the Diploma of Public Health in 1889. At that time, the germ theory opened immense possibilities for the discovery of causative agents of infectious disease, and for the redefinition of disease itself. Where, as Temkin observed, 'Diseases could be bound to definitive causes', a knowledge of the 'cause' elevated 'a clinical entity or a syndrome to the rank of a disease'.[5] From such a perspective, the current state of knowledge of tropical diseases was quite unsatisfactory. There were many vaguely defined fevers whose causes were unknown or were still explained in environmental or climatic terms. Malaria, the most dangerous tropical disease facing Europeans, had been clearly differentiated; a pathogenic parasite had been clearly identified, and quinine prophylaxis was widely practised.[6] However, the aetiology of the disease remained a mystery, and it was on this matter that Ross sought Manson's advice.

Manson in 1894 was fast becoming Britain's leading authority on tropical diseases. In 1883, while serving in the Imperial Maritime Customs Service in China, he had shown that elephantiasis was caused by a filarial worm that was transmitted by mosquitoes.[7] This was the first demonstration of the insect-borne transmission of disease, and was to provide tropical medicine, and Ross in particular, with a fruitful etiological model. After a period in Hong Kong, Manson returned to Britain in 1889 and set up a consulting practice in London, where he found his experience of tropical diseases much in demand. At the turn of the century, up to 20 per cent of British medical graduates practised in tropical and sub-tropical climates.[8] Manson was soon appointed visiting physician in the Maritime Hospital at Greenwich and a lecturer in tropical diseases at various London medical schools.[9] In fact, London provided enough clinical and biological material for Manson to continue his principal interests in scientific investigation. In 1893 he had suggested that the mode of infection with malaria might be analogous to that found with elephantiasis, and it was this hypothesis, together with associated microscopic and experimental techniques, that Manson persuaded Ross to pursue on his return to India.

The story of Ross's protracted investigations and their outcome has become a classic of popular science. Ross's lengthy letters to Manson convey the excitement of the chase, the moments of despair, and the final elation. They also reveal the close confidence shared between the two men.[10] Ross was an isolated investigator, making his discovery of the mosquito borne transmission of malaria in spite of the obstructions of the Raj and in circumstances unconducive to experimental work. Manson offered advice and encouragement throughout, and pulled strings at the India Office in London to prevent postings that might have interrupted Ross's work. Manson also facilitated publication of this work, which appeared solely under Ross's name. As the mosquito-malarial hypothesis had first been propounded by Manson, it was possible for contemporaries to say that 'Manson was the real discoverer and Ross the tame disciple',[11] but whatever was being said by others, relations between the two men continued cordially well into 1899.

By early 1899, however, Ross was uncertain of his future. His letters suggest different intentions: to retire to Italy and continue research; to adopt literature, so as to 'look after those essential parts of clothing — the pockets'; or to work on the prevention of malaria.[12] Manson had obtained a lectureship for him at the newly founded Liverpool School of Tropical Medicine, expecting that Ross would use this as a lever to obtain a better position in the Indian Medical Service.[13]

Tellingly, however, the Indian Medical Service was unconcerned at losing its most famous officer, while Ross himself was tired of India and the tropical climate.[14] Instead, as he later wrote, in Liverpool he hoped to find businessmen who 'would not be slow to learn the great advantages which my methods of malaria prevention would confer . . . on their plantations, factories and trade'.[15]

Unlike Manson, Ross had a lifelong commitment to practical sanitary reform. But he also had a reputation, according to Gibson, for being 'conceited, quick to take offence and greedy for fame and money'.[16] For him, scientific priority was both of personal and financial significance. His Indian Army pension was not large and his small salary at Liverpool was a constant grievance. When he was awarded the Nobel Prize in 1901, Ross described the Prize as a 'cash reward', observing that he had no qualms about not sharing it with Manson as 'he [Manson] then had a considerable practice'.[17] Ross was particularly aggrieved that the British government had not rewarded him financially and he repeatedly contrasted his position with the French government's recognition of Louis Pasteur.[18]

In the event, Ross's claim to the Prize was disputed. Priority disputes, a normal feature of science and medicine, were particularly bitter in the field of tropical diseases, not least because they were accompanied by inter-imperial rivalries.[19] The Swedish Academy's choice in 1901 was, and remains, controversial, as at least three other men had claims for recognition. Ross had worked only on malaria in birds, while Grassi in Italy had shown mosquito-borne infection of human malaria.[20] The French Alphonse Laveran had identified the malarial parasite in human blood as early as 1880.[21] Above all, there was Manson, who had first propounded the mosquito-malarial theory.

In 1901, Manson supported Ross's priority and disowned suggestions that he should have shared in the Prize. But by this time, relations between them were deteriorating. The first evidence of this occurred soon after Ross's arrival at Liverpool in 1899. In fact, Ross's entire period in Liverpool, from 1899 to 1912, was fraught with insecurity. Ross later wrote of 'secret enemies working against us in London'.[22] Although the Liverpool School was founded earlier, the London School had a larger staff, obtained more research grants, published more and was the centre of British tropical medicine.[23] Its dominance was resented by the staff at Liverpool and elsewhere. David Bruce, who had done pioneering work on Malta fever, and with the British sleeping sickness investigations, objected to Manson's predominating influence.[24] Similarly, G.H.F. Nuttall, then establishing parasitology and tropical medicine at Cambridge, criticised the overt favouritism of the metropolitan medical establishment towards the London School.[25] Ross's position within the medical establishment was not improved, when, after 1898, he began to publish on the practical applications of his research.[26] Indeed, this was to take him outside the realm of scientific and medical debate and into direct confrontation with the colonial administration at all levels, rendering him at a great political disadvantage.

COLONIAL POLICY AND TROPICAL MEDICINE: THE LONDON SCHOOL

The principal motive in founding the London School of Tropical Medicine had been the desire of the Colonial Office to provide for the better training of Colonial Medical Officers and the expansion of their service.[27] Tropical medicine was seen by the Colonial Office as an integral part of its strategy for imperial development. 'Constructive imperialism' centred on the state promotion of railways and research to 'open up' the colonies to private capital and individual initiative.[28] However, trade and capital did not always follow the flag, and the colonial empire was frequently neglected by the British Exchequer.[29] By default, research came to assume a very important place in the rhetoric of colonial development policy. There were three essential roles for research: (i) exploration and discovery; (ii) the prevention of disease; and (iii) the provision of technical advice and services.[30] The work of such metropolitan agencies as Kew Gardens and the Imperial Institute was set alongside that of the London School.[31] Research was not in itself a main vehicle of colonial development: it was a catalyst and adjunct to other forces. But research activity could be used politically to show a metropolitan audience that the Imperial government was doing something progressive in the colonies; and a distant future pay-off could always be promised.

Given the evidence of colonial indebtedness and the scale of imperial responsibilities, British policy held that colonial development would be a very long-term process. It was assumed that the impetus for development would come from Europeans, not from the indigenous populations. With a large time-scale and such assumptions, relatively little was expected from tropical medicine. As long as colonial medical men were trained and serviced the needs of expatriate communities, tropical medical policies could be deemed a success. Mortality and morbidity rates in the colonies had been declining since 1850, so tropical medicine, when established *c.*1900, was working with the grain.[32]

Although designed specifically for Colonial Medical Officers, the courses taught at the London School were also taken by medical missionaries and by overseas medical men.[33] Manson collected able lieutenants, and the School thrived, being widely regarded as the *de facto* medical department of the Colonial Office. The medical problems of the Boer War and the ending of Indian Medical Service training at Netley in 1905 had demonstrated the inadequacy of existing provisions for tropical medicine, and vindicated Manson and the School. Subsequent government grants meant that the School was financially secure. Moreover, in 1905, the London School became linked with University College, London, *via* a shared chair in protozoology. When protozoology and parasitology were taken up in other university biology departments, tropical medicine became contiguous with biological specialisms and not medical ones. In short, it had developed the main features of a 'collegiate controlled' specialism. Meanwhile, the favourable reputation of Manson's School was not hindered by its good relations with the Royal Society. Although medical opposition had at first come from 'traditional' quarters of the profession, and in particular from the Royal College of Physicians and the

Indian Medical Service, more 'modern' sections, including the proponents of experimental medicine and the British Medical Association, became enthusiastic supporters. Ross's Nobel Prize, however controversial, had cast reflected glory upon the whole British scientific and medical community.

ENTREPRENEURS AND TROPICAL MEDICINE: THE LIVERPOOL SCHOOL

The Liverpool School of Tropical Medicine, like its London counterpart, had its origins in Joseph Chamberlain's attempts to interest British medical schools in teaching tropical medicine. To encourage this in Liverpool, Alfred Jones, the leading shipowner, offered £350 p.a. for three years to the medical school of Liverpool. This in turn led to a committee to consider the treatment of malaria in the city which proposed to link teaching, research and treatment at a new School of Tropical Medicine.[34] The first Dean of the School was Professor Rubert Boyce, then Holt Professor of Pathology at the University College of Liverpool and bacteriologist to the Liverpool Corporation.[35]

The School was promoted as an investment in increased colonial trade. When subscriptions were opened, the School received the backing of several leading colonial trading companies. John Holt, whose family chair Boyce held, was anxious, 'to be rid of the dread effects of malaria, which in the past had been the bugbear of our trade, and the vital enemy of European existence'.[36] The link between the Holt family, Boyce and the Corporation is significant. Liverpool had an excellent record in municipal health, and Boyce's arrival promised a firm link between tropical medicine and the most 'modern' trends in British medicine. Through him, the School was seen as a means of extending to the Empire the progressive public health philosophy of the city port.[37]

Liverpool's mercantile interests in the 1900s wished a more vigorous but less restrictive colonial development policy on the part of the British government.[38] They welcomed Chamberlain's 'constructive imperialism' but were disappointed with its limited implementation, and urged the government to do more to promote trade. At the same time, however, they wished less overt political 'interference' in the colonies. In West Africa, in particular, they wanted colonial governments to foster development along African lines. This meant the extension of trade, via native middlemen. In one sense, their policy had its roots in the writings of Mary Kingsley and her respect for indigenous cultures and institutions.[39] But at the same time it offered the quickest and least risky route to improved trade. It was also based on the assumption that native merchants had 'intimate and unprejudiced knowledge of local conditions'.[40] Bernard Porter observes that the defining characteristic of 'Liverpool imperialism' was its rejection of the usual Edwardian generalities about the Empire. Most who thought about empire did so in terms of simple, general moral issues; in Porter's phrase, 'the replacement of one kind of imperial control by another was an unimportant detail — it was all imperialism'.[41] But to Mary Kingsley, and to the businessmen of Liverpool, this 'detail' was vital. Their policy became known as Morelism, after the Liverpool journalist E.D. Morel, who characterized it as 'minimum rule', with commerce as 'the greatest civilizing agent'.[42] In the 1900s Morel wrote a number of articles on Ross, and later Ross contributed a chapter on sanitary matters to one of Morel's most important books, *Affairs of West Africa*.[43] It was clear that in the promotion of commerce and in the promotion of 'minimum rule', tropical public health played a central role.

Ronald Ross arrived in Liverpool when the School opened in April 1899, some six months before the London School began its operations. Ross soon discovered that the 'School' was so in name only, and was close to financial collapse.[44] Initially, the staff consisted only of Ross and one other, and there was no separate building planned. Also, 'survival by subscription' meant that there was no year-to-year stability. For a large, established institution like a voluntary hospital or a medical school, with assets and investment income, this method might be tolerable; but for a small, new School, it was not. Several times Ross was on the verge of leaving or being made redundant, although on each occasion Alfred Jones came to the rescue. Boyce worked very closely with Jones on raising money for the School and at improving its public profile. He abandoned his other posts and concentrated on working at and for the School. If anything, Boyce illustrates the Liverpool style of tropical medical activity more than Ross, as the support of tropical medicine became his sole concern. He 'sometimes told his friends that when he died the word 'cash' would be found written across his heart'.[45]

In his inaugural lecture delivered in June 1899, Ross spoke on the extirpation of the mosquito as the way to solve the problem of malaria.[46] In the same month he wrote to Manson urging that 'We must be first in with the practical side of the mosquito theory or else Grassi will develop it.'[47] From this date we can document Ross's commitment to the practical application of his malarial work. This coincided with his association with Boyce and the Liverpool merchants. Alfred Jones exploited Ross's fame with banquets and public meetings, which he said were to 'work up as much enthusiasm as I can' for tropical medicine.[48] Besides bringing an expected improvement to West African public health, this activity also enhanced Jones's position as a progressive imperialist in Liverpool's business community. Clearly, Ross had joined a group which saw tropical medicine in terms of generating profitable activity in the colonies.

In the early days of the School, two lines of work were suggested. Boyce wanted to build up the teaching of tropical medical officers, while Ross, who won the support of the School's Committee, preferred the strategy of overseas expeditions for field surveys. The first expedition commissioned by the School left for Sierra Leone in October 1899, and eleven others followed before the end of 1903.[49] These ventures became the trade mark of the Liverpool School. First and foremost, they were concerned with investigating and improving sanitary conditions, and each expedition was expected to produce a sanitary report. These activities have been described as 'crusades', but it may be more appropriate to see them as 'entrepreneurial' activities.[50] Each was financed by subscription, and separate accounts were kept and published. Meanwhile, the School promoted itself as a consultancy, and its staff were soon advising authorities in South America, Egypt, France, Belgium and Greece. Eventually, Alfred Jones took so active a role in the School that Ross and his colleagues complained about being treated as his 'employees'. In 1905 Jones even offered the services of Ross and the School to the authorities of New Orleans, following an outbreak of yellow fever; for Ross this was 'advertising', and took entrepreneurial tropical medicine too far.[51]

From the outset, it became clear that the Liverpool School was moving in a direction opposite to its London counterpart. Beginning through Boyce as part of the University's Pathology Department, it became more and more independent, and soon had little connection with the Liverpool medical community. Until the School began its own journal in 1907, its sanitary and other reports were published commercially, and not in the medical literature. Its audience was not primarily scientific or medical, but reflected the interests of merchants, shippers, and colonial investment.

MANSON, ROSS, AND COLONIAL MEDICAL POLICY

Given this institutional background, it is possible to place these 'friendly rivals' in their wider political context. In the first decade of this century, British policy towards its colonial empire was greatly debated. In many respects, debate inevitably centred on the nature, pace, and organization of economic 'development' in the colonies themselves. This debate unavoidably directed attention to the importance of plantations, the degree of necessary British involvement in local administration, and the health and efficiency of native populations. Medical policy was deemed crucial to the future, both in 'opening' up the tropics to Europeans and in improving general public health.

Given the nature of this debate, it was not long before a 'Liverpool view' of colonial development came into conflict with the official view of 'deferred development' favoured by the Colonial Office. Into this conflict between their patrons, Manson and Ross were soon drawn.

The first sign of disagreement between the two men appeared in March 1901, when a deputation from the Chambers of Commerce of Liverpool, London and Manchester, and the Liverpool School urged Chamberlain to appoint 'sanitary commissioners' to inspect and report on the sanitary performance of colonial governments.[52] Ross was in the deputation, and presented a detailed document written by Boyce and himself, arguing for the removal of nuisances and the provision of piped water and building sewers, along with more specific measures directed towards draining ponds and clearing bush. One of the advantages of Boyce's scheme was that it was doubly cost-effective and would bring benefits to both expatriates and natives. Manson did not attend the meeting. Perhaps he knew in advance that Chamberlain would reject the scheme because of its cost;

perhaps he was unwilling to make the whole of colonial policy subsidiary to sanitary policy.[53] In the event, Chamberlain did reject the plan, arguing that it was an unrealistic proposal by scientific experts and that no government dared put its finances in the hands of such experts, 'whatever their scientific acquirement might be'.[54]

Initially, it seems, Manson supported the scheme, telling Ross that 'it can do nothing but good'.[55] Following Chamberlain's rebuff, however, Manson advised Ross to be less ambitious, warning him 'not to begin experiments until he is sure of success'.[56] The key in his warning was the word 'experiments'. To Ross, the mosquito-malarial theory was proven; his deductions on mosquito eradication were sound, and his proposed practical measures, infallible. There was nothing 'experimental' about his programme. Also, the attack on the mosquito was indistinguishable from the support of general public health measures. However, the Colonial Office line, which Manson propounded, was that more laboratory research and trials were needed, and that public health measures would have to await further native education and the funds to pay for several improvements.

Relations between Manson and Ross continued to be cordial through 1902 when Ross was offered lecturing at the London School. In the event, Ross turned the offer into a manœuvre which finally brought him both a chair and tenure at Liverpool until 1912.[57] However, in late 1902 and early 1903, three episodes soured relations between them. These concerned Ross's priority in the mosquito-malarial theory, the reputation of the Liverpool School, and again the promotion of sanitary measures in the colonies.

The question of Ross's priority, disputed at the Nobel elections in 1901, arose again when Manson contributed an introduction to Grassi's new textbook on tropical medicine. Ross complained that Manson's text could be read as endorsing Grassi's behaviour, if not his priority. Manson sought to reassure Ross on both counts.[58] But the well was poisoned and fresh disagreement emerged with news of the discovery of a human trypanosome as the underlying cause of the 'new' African disease of sleeping sickness. In November 1902, Manson and a London colleague, C.W. Daniels, published an article which seemed to attribute priority in the discovery of a human trypanosome to Dr R.M. Forde, of the London School.[59] Joan Smith has observed that 'a major breakthrough in finding . . . one of the causes of the innumerable non-malarial "fevers" of the African coast could only enhance the reputation of the infant School'.[60] But in the same month, Ross, together with Boyce and C.S. Sherrington, rushed letters to the *British Medical Journal* and the *Lancet* vigorously defending a Liverpool man, Dr J.E. Dutton, who had reported finding a human trypanosome while on the School's malaria control expedition to Gambia in 1901.[61]

Ross spoke of reports that were 'calculated to distort' opinion against Liverpool. Manson wrote to Ross strongly criticizing the letters, which were certainly construed by others as a personal attack on Manson.[62] Manson did not, however, reply publicly. Indeed, in his next publication on human trypanosomes in June 1903, he seemed to bow to the Liverpool version of events, saying that it was 'unnecessary to say more on the matter'.[63] By this time, however, the matter had been overtaken by other dramatic events.

In 1901, a major epidemic of sleeping sickness broke out in central and East Africa.[64] The seriousness of the situation led the British commissioner in Uganda to ask the Foreign Office (Uganda had not yet been transferred to the Colonial Office) to approach the Royal Society for assistance in elucidating the cause of the disease and finding measures to control it. The problem created considerable scientific and medical interest, and seemed a golden opportunity for the new tropical medicine. The Royal Society, through its Malarial Research Committee, acted promptly, constituted a new Tropical Disease Committee, and had a three-man research team in the field by June 1902.[65] The First Sleeping Sickness Commission, as it became known, was led by G. Carmichael Low and included Aldo Castellani from the London School and Cuthbert Christy from the Liverpool School. For various reasons the Commission soon collapsed; Christy refused to accept Low's authority and spent some of his time big-game hunting. Low left after three months, and Christy at the end of the year. However, Castellani stayed on and kept the investigations going. In view of the continuing epidemic, and to save face, the Royal Society dispatched a second, more high-powered Commission, led by Sir David Bruce.[66]

Castellani had at first reported the cause of the epidemic as a *Streptococcal* bacterium. By the time Bruce arrived, however, Castellani had turned his attention to trypanosomes instead. Whether Castellani changed his mind independently, or at Bruce's suggestion, or whether Bruce first made the suggestion, was and is, a matter of dispute.[67] Although Manson and Ross were not publicly in the dispute, both supported Castellani. As late as July 1904, long after Bruce had demonstrated to most people's satisfaction that sleeping sickness was a trypanosome disease, Manson was still floating the idea of a 'bacterial cause', implicitly doubting Bruce's work.[68] For his part, Ross offered to write Castellani a testimonial and the two remained friends for many years.[69] Manson and Ross fell out momentarily over sleeping sickness, when in July 1905 Ross asked for a correction in the report appearing in the *Journal of Tropical Medicine*, in which Manson had stated that the First Sleeping Sickness Commission had been 'sent out under the auspices of the London School'.[70] To this Manson agreed, and wrote a letter stating that it had been a Royal Society expedition, and that the London School had only provided two of its three members. Liverpool had, of course, provided the much maligned Christy.[71]

In 1906 the Liverpool School used the continuing sleeping sickness epidemic to urge again its detailed sanitary programmes upon the Colonial Office. The Colonial Office passed them on to the Royal Society because it saw them as 'scientific'; the Royal Society sent them back, saying they were 'administrative'.[72] In Ross's view, the Colonial Office saw the value of tropical medicine and the London School primarily in terms of domestic politics, and not as a vehicle for overseas health policy.[73]

These two simmering differences on questions of reputation and interpretation were soon overshadowed by a third. In 1903 the activities of Liverpool's expedtions, and their implied criticisms of colonial governments, drew a response from the colonial administration. Dr W.T. Prout, the Principal Medical Officer in Sierra Leone, published an article critical of the 'interference' of the Liverpool School's expedition in local sanitary measures.[74] A particular colony, or more usually its principal trading post, would, he said, be offered unsolicited advice from Liverpool experts in how to manage its sanitary affairs. Sometimes this was welcomed, at other times it was not. Certainly the Liverpool School had taken a particular interest in Sierra Leone. From 1901 it had Dr Logan Taylor working in Freetown; and the territory received three expeditions, two led by Ross himself.[75] Taylor found the Principal Medical Officer 'indifferent' to the work of his mosquito brigades, and when Prout went public in 1903, Taylor told Ross that Prout was 'motivated by the jealousy of the Liverpool School'.[76] Ross tried to pursue the matter with the Colonial Office but got nowhere. In the neighbouring colony of Nigeria, Ross and the Liverpool group found an ally in the Governor, William MacGregor. MacGregor, who was medically trained, and Ross became friends and found common cause in bemoaning the inactivity of the Colonial Office on sanitary matters.[77]

Following these episodes, Manson and Ross ceased correspondence. However, they did continue to address one another in public statements. In 1907, for example, Manson announced his opposition to large-scale anti-mosquito and general public health measures in the colonies.[78] He argued that the value of such schemes had not been conclusively demonstrated; and remained wedded to the encouragement of individual health precautions. He also argued that such large schemes as Ross desired were neither economically nor politically possible; here he spoke as a political 'insider', aware of the limitations of the expert and of government priorities. Throughout the decade, Ross and the Liverpool group remained 'outsiders'.[79] They were not, however, to accept defeat easily. In an address on 'The Future of Tropical medicine' in 1909, Ross threw down a challenge to Manson's conception of science. Some tropical medical men, he said,

> were apt to take too haughty a view of their scientific work, to stand above and apart from the throng of men for whom they were working. It was for them to descend, to go personally into the battle, and fight hand in hand in order to save their fellow men from grave and imminent dangers.[80]

In reply, Manson observed that 'The fault was, perhaps not altogether on one side, and the medical men, he thought, failed to convince largely from a lack of articulate expression and eloquence.'[81] He added:

> Circumspection had been forced on [governments] by the mistakes of sanitary advisers . . . if authorities now believed that the most ambitious schemes did not always mean the most rapid progress, they had abundant precedent to justify them.[82]

The division between the two men was now clear. Manson favoured circumspection and steered the London School in that direction. 'Collegiate control' satisfied the Colonial Office. On the other hand, Ross was 'condemned to propaganda and politics', and remained committed to the prevention of malaria through sanitary measures.[83] In *The Prevention of Malaria*, published in 1910, he pursued his novel approach to epidemiology, which he saw as providing mathematical proof of his views.[84] He continued to travel widely, and remained highly valued by patrons of the Liverpool School.

In 1912 the final and possibly their most serious break occurred. That year, Ross left Liverpool, and Manson retired from the London School and his post at the Colonial Office. Manson recommended his former student, W.T. Prout, for a post at the Liverpool School. Manson wrote that if Prout were appointed, 'teaching [in Liverpool] would improve'.[85] Ross took this as a personal affront to his scientific standing, and sued for libel. A dismayed Manson apologized, and paid the small legal fees. The whole affair was kept under wraps, but it ensured that even on his return to London, Ross remained an outsider in the world of medicine and politics.

In the event, he remained so even after Manson's death in 1922. By then Ross appeared deeply frustrated, even vindictive. For example, following the appearance of some laudatory obituaries which gave Manson a prominent place in mosquito-malaria work, Ross wrote to *Nature*, questioning Manson's stature as an experimentalist.[86] This happened at a sensitive time, for Ross was negotiating what he had always wanted: financial and institutional recognition for his work, which was eventually to take the form of the Ross Institute in the suburb of Putney. Five years later, after the appearance of a glowing biography of Manson in 1927, Ross published a pamphlet entitled *Memories of Sir Patrick Manson*, which purported to tell 'the exact truth.'[87] This was a thoroughly nasty publication, full of snide comments dressed up as praise. Why Ross continued to pursue Manson in this way is not clear. Perhaps it had become habitual; certainly by this time Ross was a sick man. Sadly, his own Institute remained isolated, staffed by old friends like Simpson and Castellani. In 1929 he had to endure the opening of the ostentatious London School of Hygiene and Tropical Medicine in Bloomsbury. He had the satisfaction of seeing his name on the façade, but only to one side: Manson's name appeared in the central trio, *Chadwick — Simon — Manson*. With tragic irony, even the Ross Institute was eventually absorbed into the London School soon after Ross's death.[88]

CONCLUSION

Today, Patrick Manson and Ronald Ross are best seen as spokesmen for different colonial medical policies, rooted in different visions of imperial responsibility and representing differing priorities for colonial development. In historical terms, we can no longer speak of a single British tropical medicine, or a single colonial medical policy — there were clearly alternatives. Possibly the institutional and political priorities of London and Liverpool encouraged different kinds of science. In London, tropical medicine became fragmented into specialisms, including protozoology and helminthology, which provided links to biology. The London School remained dominated by its obligations to postgraduate instruction, and by parasitological research, and its practitioners found recognition among their metropolitan scientific peers. Liverpool, on the other hand, developed unique features, like Ross's epidemology, and its audience was not exclusively scientific. The Liverpool School's programme of expeditions and its commitment to practical public health measures in the colonies themselves, continued to reflect the interests of its patrons.

The policy of a disease-specific, research-led approach, directed at individual prevention and treatment, developed by the London School, continued (and perhaps still continues) to dominate tropical medicine. The recipients of such policies were not provided (and in many cases have still not been provided) with the basic public health measures and environmental changes advocated by the Liverpool School. These latter changes, which according to McKeown have been the main long-term determinant of the improvement of health in developed countries, were not given priority in colonial medical policy.[89] With hindsight, Ross may have been correct in his observation that the Empire had done more for tropical medicine than tropical medicine had done for the Empire.

NOTES

An earlier version of this chapter was given to the Society for the Social History of Medicine Colloquium on 'Society and Medicine in Britain' in London in 1977. (See *SSHM Bulletin, 21* (1977), 37–9). This work was greatly helped by the assistance of librarians at the Royal Society, the Liverpool School of Tropical Medicine and the London School of Hygiene and Tropical Medicine, especially Mary Gibson. I would like to thank Roy MacLeod for comments on an earlier draft, and Pat Peck (in Sheffield) and Ruth Bennett and Diane O'Donovan (in Sydney) for deciphering and typing my scripts.

1. The best source on Manson remains P.H. Manson-Bahr and A. Alcock, *The Life and Work of Sir Patrick Manson* (London: Cassell, 1927). A revised version appeared as P.H. Manson-Bahr, *Patrick Manson: The Founder of Tropical Medicine* (London: Nelson, 1962).
2. The two main biographies of Ross are R.L. Megroz, *Ronald Ross: Discoverer and Creator* (London: Allen & Unwin, 1931) and J. Rowland, *The Mosquito Man: The Story of Sir Ronald Ross* (London: Lutterworth Press, 1958). See also: J.G. Crowther, *Six Great Doctors. Harvey, Pasteur, Lister, Pavlov, Ross, Fleming* (London: Hamish Hamilton, 1957). Ross wrote a very full and interesting autobiography: R. Ross, *Memoirs* (London: John Murray, 1923).
3. M. Worboys, 'The emergence of tropical medicine: a study in the establishment of a scientific specialty', in G. Lemaine *et al.* (eds), *Perspectives on the Emergence of Scientific Disciplines* (The Hague: Mouton, 1976), 89–91.
4. R. Johnston and D.Robbins, 'The development of specialities in industrialized

science', *The Sociological Review, 25* (1977), 87–108.

5. O. Temkin, *The Double Face of Janus* (Baltimore: Johns Hopkins University Press, 1977), 436.

6. P.D. Curtin, *The Image of Africa: British Ideas and Action, 1780–1850* (Madison: University of Wisconsin Press, 1964), G. Harrison, *Mosquitoes, Malaria and Man: A History of Hostilities since 1880* (London: John Murray, 1978); D.R. Headrick, *The Tools of Empire: Technology and European Imperialism in the Nineteenth Century* (New York: Oxford University Press, 1981).

7. K. Mellanby, 'Mosquito Manson', *Nature, 270* (24 November 1977), 293; E. Chernin, 'Patrick Manson (1844–1922) and the transmission of filariasis', *American Journal of Tropical Medicine and Hygiene, 26* (1977), 1065–70.

8. This figure is given in P.H. Manson-Bahr, *The History of the School of Tropical Medicine in London, 1899–1949* (London: H.K. Lewis, 1956), 31. The figure would seem to be supported by the fact that, in 1903, overseas membership of the BMA stood at 18 per cent.

9. Manson-Bahr and Alcock, op. cit., n. 1 above.

10. Many of these letters are in the Ross Archives, held in the Library of the London School of Hygiene and Tropical Medicine. An excellent catalogue and index on microfiche has been produced by Mary Gibson of the Library. M. Gibson, *Catalogue of the Ross Archives* (London: LSHTM, 1983).

11. This view is reported by Megroz, op. cit., n. 2 above, 251. Manson's original suggestion was published in the *British Medical Journal* (1893) i, 1306–8.

12. Ross Archives (hereafter RA), 08/035, Ross to T.E. Charles (IMS), 19 December 1898; Ross, op. cit., n. 2 above, 358, Ross to Manson, 15 February 1899. Ross was writing and advising on anti-mosquito measures in 1898; however, there is no evidence that he saw himself promoting or carrying out such measures.

13. RA 02/063, Manson to Ross, 18 January 1899.

14. RA 02/277, Ross to Nuttall, 15 April 1899.

15. Ross, op. cit., n. 2 above, 369.

16. On this controversy see P.H. Manson-Bahr, 'The story of malaria — the drama and the actors', *International Review of Tropical Medicine, 2* (1963), 329–90.

17. In 1908, Laveran was awarded the Nobel Prize for his discovery of the malaria parasite, so honour on one side was satisfied.

18. M. Gibson, 'Sir Ronald Ross and his contemporaries', *Journal of the Royal Society of Medicine, 71* (1978), 611.

19. It could be suggested that there was a 'scramble for African diseases' as well as a scramble for the colonies.

20. R. Ross, *Memories Of Patrick Manson* (London: Harrison & Sons, 1930), 23.

21. As early as November 1901, Ross sought the assistance of Alfred Jones in petitioning the government for a 'reward for his discovery', (RA 12/061). Ross tried again in 1914 (RA 37/097 and 49/218). Ross saw himself as the British Pasteur, and in 1926 finally achieved similar, if less impressive, recognition with the establishment of the Ross Institute in London.

22. Ross, op. cit., n. 2 above, 459.

23. Manson-Bahr, op. cit., n. 8 above, and H.H. Scott, *A History of Tropical Medicine*, 2 vols (London: Edward Arnold, 1939), *passim*.

24. In 1903, Bruce wrote to the Royal Society that Manson was leaking the contents of his letters to the Royal Society. *Archives of the Tropical Diseases Committee*, April 1903. Also, see RA 13/175 for critical remarks on Sambon, Manson's colleague.

25. On Nuttall, see M. Worboys, 'The emergence and early development of parasitology', in K.S. Warren and J.Z. Bowers (eds), *Parasitology: a Global Perspective* (New York: Springer Verlag, 1983).

26. L.J. Bruce-Chwatt, 'Ronald Ross, William Gorgas and malaria eradication', *American Journal of Tropical Medicine and Hygiene, 26* (1977), 1071–9. Bruce-Chwatt notes that Ross's 'conviction of the practical aspects of his work and his relentless battle with the apathy of government are not often stressed by historians' (1071).

27. See R.V. Kubicek, *The Administration of Imperialism: Joseph Chamberlain at the Colonial Office* (Durham, N.C.: Duke University Press, 1969) and R. Hyam, *Elgin and Churchill at the Colonial Office, 1905–1908: Watershed of Empire-Commonwealth* (London: Macmillan, 1968).

28. S.B. Saul, 'The economic significance of constructive imperialism', *Journal of Economic History, 17* (1957), 173–92; and B. Porter, *The Lion's Share: A Short History of British Imperialism, 1850–1983* (London: Longman, 1975), 188–92.

29. A. Beck, *A History of the British Medical Administration of East Africa, 1900–1950* (Cambridge, Mass.: Harvard University Press, 1970), 26–7.

30. On the 'research and constructive imperialism' see M. Worboys, 'Science and British colonial imperialism, 1895–1940' (Unpublished D. Phil. thesis, University of Sussex, 1980), *passim.*

31. Worboys, op. cit., n. 30 above; cf. R. MacLeod, 'On visiting the "moving metropolis": reflections on the architecture of imperial science', *Historical Records of Australian Science, 5* (1982), 1–16.

32. Curtin, op. cit., n. 6 above, 352–3.

33. Manson-Bahr, op. cit., n. 8 above, *passim.*

34. B.H. Maegraith, 'History of the Liverpool School of Tropical Medicine', *Medical History, 16* (1972), 354–68.

35. C.S. Sherrington, 'W.R. Boyce', *Proceedings of Royal Society, B, 84* (1911), iii–x. This obituary stresses Boyce's overriding commitment to the school, to sanitary work in the tropics, and to publicity and fund raising.

36. Quoted in Kubicek, op. cit., no. 27 above, 146.

37. In 1847, Liverpool was the first authority in England to appoint a Medical Officer of Health. See W.M. Frazer, *Duncan of Liverpool* (London: Hamish Hamilton, 1947).

38. B. Porter, *Critics of Empire: British Radical Attitudes to Colonialism in Africa, 1895–1914* (London: Macmillan, 1968), ch. 8. This analysis of Liverpool colonial development policy leans heavily upon Porter's account.

39. M. Kingsley, *West African Studies* (London: Macmillan, 1899).

40. Porter, op. cit., n. 38 above, 251.

41. ibid., 252.

42. E.D. Morel, *Affairs of West Africa* (London: Heinemann, 1902).

43. RA 51/099, 68/004, 68/005, January 1903.

44. RA 02/283, Ross to Manson, 3 June 1899; 49/014, Nuttall to Ross, 23 May 1900; RA 12/062, Ross to Jones, 6 November 1901.

45. Sherrington, op. cit., n. 35 above, viii.

46. R. Ross, 'The possibility of extirpating malaria from certain localities by a new method', *British Medical Journal* (1899) ii, 1–4.

47. RA 02/287, Ross to Manson, 14 June 1899. In April Ross had written of 'bringing the tropics to Liverpool'; RA 02/227, Ross to Nuttall, 16 April 1899.

48. P.N. Davies, *Sir Alfred Jones* (London: Europa Publications, 1978). Also see Liverpool School of Tropical Medicine Archives, TM/16, press cutting books.

49. Maegraith, op. cit., n. 34 above, 358–60.

50. R.E. Dumett, 'The campaign against malaria and the expansion of scientific, medical and sanitary services in British West Africa, 1898–1910', *African Historical Studies* 1 (1968), 164.

51. RA 53/044, 29 October 1911. Ross turned down the opportunity to write Boyce's obituary notice for the Royal Society because he said it would have been too critical.

52. RA 14/180, Pamphlet, *Health and Sanitation in West Africa*. Deputation to Joseph Chamberlain at the Colonial Office, 15 March 1901.

53. *The Times*, 16 March 1901.

54. ibid. Also see RA 14/178. A letter dated 11 July 1901 reports Chamberlain objecting to Ross as an expert on sanitary matters as he was not an 'engineer'.

55. RA 49/067, Manson to Ross, 20 March 1901. Earlier Manson had written to Ross that the backwardness in Africa was due to 'ignorance' of Ross's discovery (RA 49/066, 11 February 1901).

56. RA 49/068, Manson to Ross, 5 May 1901, and 49/073, Manson to Ross, 14 October 1901.

57. RA 12/062-3, Correspondence between Ross and Jones, 6 November 1901 and 8 December 1901.

58. RA 08/104, 08/109 and 08/110.

59. *British Medical Journal* (1903) ii, 1249; *Lancet* (1903).

60. *Journal of Tropical Medicine* (1 November 1902) and *Hospital* (8 November 1902).

61. G. Joan Smith, 'The Liverpool School of Tropical Medicine expedition to Senegambia, 1902, as revealed in the letters of Dr. J.L. Todd', *Annals of Tropical Medicine and Hygiene, 71* (1977), 391–2.

62. RA 13/157, Manson to Ross, 24 November 1902. Also see 13/154, Nuttall to Ross, 29 January 1903.

63. *British Medical Journal*(1903) i, 1249.

64. On the outbreak and the local response see: J.J. McKelvey, *Man against Tsetse: Struggle for Africa* (Ithaca, N.Y.: Cornell University press, 1973); H.G. Goff, 'Sleeping sickness in the Lake Victoria region of British East Africa, 1900–1915', *African Historical Studies*, 2 (1969), 255–68; J.N.P. Davies, 'The cause of sleeping sickness', *East African Medical Journal, 39* (1962), 81–99 and 145–60.

65. J.S.K. Boyd, 'Sleeping sickness: the Castellani-Bruce controversy', *Notes and Records of the Royal Society of London, 28* (1973), 93–110.

66. *Obituary Notices of Fellows of the Royal Society, 1* (1932), 79–85.

67. See Boyd, op. cit., n. 65 above, and A.J. Duggan, 'Bruce and the Africa trypanosomes', *American Journal of Tropical Medicine and Hygiene, 26* (1977), 1080–1.

68. *British Medical Journal*, (1904) ii, 379.

69. RA 47/101–014.

70. *Royal Society Archives*, Tropical Diseases Committee, Minutes of Meeting, 27 July 1905. The article to which Ross objected appeared in *Journal of Tropical Medicine* (15 May 1905), 120–4.

71. ibid., Minutes of meeting, 25 October 1905.

72. Colonial Office 885/9, Royal Society to Colonial Office, 30 May 1906.

73. Ross, op. cit., n. 2 above, 436.

74. *British Medical Journal*, (1903) i, 1349.

75. For detail see Dumett, op. cit., n. 50 above.

76. RA 13/006 and 007; and 13/022 and 13/050.

77. RA 49/180, MacGregor to Ross, 17 April 1901. In September 1902, Ross and MacGregor went to Ismalia and the Ninth (Malarial) Expedition from the Liverpool School.

78. Editorial, *Transactions of the Society for Tropical Medicine, 1* (1907), 1.

79. *Liverpool School of Tropical Medicine, Archives*, TM/15/2, 1 and 2. An appeal talks of 'the Tropical Medicine Movement' in Liverpool (no date, probably 1911).

80. *British Medical Journal* (1909) i, 1545.

81. ibid.

82. ibid.

83. Ross, op. cit., n. 2 above, 485.

84. On this neglected aspect of Ross's work see the interesting paper: P.E.M. Fine,

'Ross's *a priori* pathometry — a perspective', *Proceedings of the Royal Society of Medicine*, *68* (1975), 547–51.

85. RA 34/135, 25 November 1912. Also see Gibson, op. cit., n. 18 above, 617; Prout had been recommended to the Liverpool School in 1907. Boyce and Alfred Jones had promoted his application. RA 32/111, 17 May 1907.

86. Obituaries appeared in: *British Medical Journal* (1922) i, 623–6 and *Lancet* (1922), 767–9; *Nature, 109* (1922), 681–2. For Ross's reply see *Nature, 110* (1922), 38.

87. Ross, op. cit. note 20, *passim*.

88. D. Fisher, 'Rockefeller philanthropy and the British Empire: the creation of the London School of Hygiene and Tropical Medicine', *History of Education, 7* (2) (1978), 142.

89. T. McKeown, *The Modern Rise of Population* (London: Edward Arnold, 1976), 152–63.

2

Imperial health in British India, 1857–1900

Radhika Ramasubban

INTRODUCTION

Among the more important instruments of the British presence in India were those policies of the imperial and colonial governments concerning the investigation, prevention and cure of epidemic diseases. Periodic outbreaks of cholera, enteric fever, malaria, dystentery and diarrhoea, influenza and kala azar endangered the health of European officials — civilian and military — and their families. With the assumption of control by the Crown from the East India Company in 1857, the army in India came to constitute the largest single concentration of British troops outside the United Kingdom — one-third of all British forces. High rates of illness and death from epidemic diseases threatened the security of this force and prompted health measures across the subcontinent. To the extent that large-scale epidemics affected Britain's international trade, the living conditions of the general population assumed increasing importance too. But the army occupied a centre-stage position in evolving a colonial health policy that would make British India liveable for the British.

There were other factors, however, which directed the evolution of imperial public health policy in India. The choice and transfer of technologies for disease control were influenced by prevailing scientific theories and their vicissitudes in the metropolis; by international pressures acting on the movement of men and materials; by the political, economic and military ambitions of the imperial government; by local response; by the success of local populations in impressing their points of view upon the Government of India, and by the organizations and institutions responsible for the operation of British medical policy throughout India.

THE ARMY AND SANITARY REFORM

Death and invaliding from epidemic diseases haunted the East India Company's European troops in India from the early nineteenth century. In the 1860s, when the British made their first significant health intervention, the death-rate in the

British army on the subcontinent was 69 per mille, while an estimated 84 per mille were constantly in hospital.[1] 'In round numbers, the whole British army went three times to hospital every year.'[2] Recruits entering India were reduced to less than half their original number in eight years. Of the total number of British deaths in the army in the first half of the nineteenth century, only 6 per cent were due to military conflict. The rest were caused by four major diseases — fevers, causing 40 per cent of all deaths and three-quarters of all hospital admissions; dysentery and diarrhoea; liver diseases; and cholera, the greatest killer, particularly when the troops were on the march.[3] The diseases which killed European soldiers were endemic to the country. The general population, too, died from them in large numbers, although perceptive observers noted that what among the population had, before 1817, been only occasional localized outbreaks, now took the form of regular and widespread epidemics.[4] This was particularly the case with cholera which, spread by marching troops, seemed to have 'engrafted itself on the soil',[5] and with epidemic malaria, which accompanied the creation of large-scale irrigation, road and railway building works.[6]

The responsibility for European health in India had been entrusted as early as 1764 to the Indian Medical Service instituted by the British East India Company. Indian Medical Service officers headed military and civilian hospitals (the latter in the presidency towns of Bombay, Calcutta, and Madras), accompanied Company ships and marched with armies on expeditions. As the need for medically trained personnel grew, medical colleges were established for the training of subordinate staff: the Calcutta and Madras Colleges were founded in 1835 and the Bombay and Lahore Colleges in 1845 and 1860. The high rates of mortality in the army in India engaged the serious attention of the British. Although Indian Medical Service practice was almost exclusively hospital based, a sanitary perspective in these matters was introduced in 1835 by an Indian Medical Service officer, Sir James Ranald Martin. Following his proposal, all Indian Medical Service officers were required to report on the climate, medical topography and sanitary statistics of the districts, stations and cantonments under their care, and to provide a basis for better selection of sites for camps and for the formulation of guidelines for sanitary improvements in barracks, hospitals, transport ships, and camps.[7]

Several factors influenced the timing of the first significant health intervention in the 1860s. One was the threat to British military power posed by the mutiny of 1857. With this came a general concern in England for the health of British troops at home and abroad, promoted by the recent experience of the Crimean War. The East India Company's army had relied on Indian soldiers (for every European soldier there were eight Indians). Following the mutiny, the British army serving in India was drawn into the Imperial British Army and European troops were increased to about a third of the Indian army's total strength. What had earlier been a ratio of 39,500:311,038 was brought to 65,000:205,000 by 1864. The European strength increased to 72,573 in 1887, with 80,000 recruits as the target.[8] The problem of acclimizating such large numbers to Indian conditions and ensuring their health, therefore, assumed great importance. The short service system was introduced with the Crown take-over,[9] accompanied by a younger age for recruitment. Observation revealed high mortality rates among these younger recruits, large numbers of whom succumbed to disease within the first two years of arrival. Given the need to fill the vacancies caused by mortality, invaliding and the return of men finishing their terms, an average of 10,000 recruits was required annually to maintain the level of 80,000 men. Considering the voluntary character of the army, this proved difficult. The costs would be prohibitive, as invalided men were a 'total loss to the service as much as the men who die[d]', as they had to be supported.[10]

Under these circumstances the causes of mortality and morbidity had to be tackled, and there were strong arguments put forward by British sanitarians — 'with the mercantile Briton's spirit'[11] — that money spent on sanitation would show visible gains with immediate effect in money terms. While, earlier, the 'hopeless Indian climate' had been lamented, there were now compelling arguments to focus attention on those local conditions which had to be 'preventible and prevented' for 'only at such a price could India be held by a British force'.[12] The unilateral military orientation of health policy in British India was also facilitated by the imperial colonization policy. Apart from European civilian officials and their families, who were of paramount importance, the size of the rest of the European community in India was very small and limited to 'upper ranks', mainly planters and merchants employing Indian labour.[13] During the latter half of the nineteenth century, the total European population in India amounted to about 0.06 per cent of the population of British India and, of this, more than a third was accounted for by British troops alone.[14] For this small minority came a health policy different from that developing in the contemporary settler colonies of Australia, Canada and South Africa.

A Royal Commission was appointed in 1859 to enquire into the sanitary state of the army in India. In the absence of scientific knowledge about the specific causes of epidemic diseases, the Commission could only conclude that they 'appear, disappear and reappear in different periods and at different degrees of intensity but always occur among populations exposed to certain unhealthy conditions'.[15] The conditions which tempered the intensity and frequency of disease were well known: proper drainage, improved cultivation, better housing and ventilation, better methods of sewage disposal and a better water supply. And there was proof that attention to such measures worked, as this had led to a fall in mortality in England.

The initiation of sanitary reform in the army was in keeping with the prevalent understanding of disease in England, which supported belief in quarantine and environmental control as the main instruments of combating disease.[16] Accordingly, the physical placement of the European civil and military population in India was henceforth based, as far as possible, on the principles of metropolitan sanitary science. Using criteria of soil, water, air and elevation, the Royal Sanitary Commission laid down elaborate norms for the creation and development of distinct areas of European residence, and the 'cantonment', 'civil lines', 'civil station' and 'hill station', regulated by legislation, developed into a colonial mode of health and sanitation based on the principle of social and physical segregation. From the time of the Royal Commission's report of 1863, the location and layout of European civil and military areas were decided by criteria of health set by the prevailing medical scientific theories of miasma and environmental control rather than by political and strategic criteria. Most of the troops were located at 'hill stations' or on elevated ground. In cases where strategic stations were unhealthy, only small forces were posted there, to be reinforced at short notice. According to the Cantonments Manual of 1909,

> It should be carefully borne in mind that the cardinal principle underlying the administration of cantonments in India is that the cantonments exist primarily for the health of British troops and to considerations affecting the well-being and efficiency of the garrison, all other matters must give place.[17]

That death-rates could come down under improved sanitary conditions was clear from the fact that the same diseases which accounted for a mortality rate of 69 per 1000 among the British soldiers took a relatively lower toll of British army officers and civil servants and their families in India (the respective mortality rates were 38 in 1000 and 20 in 1000). This was attributed to better planning of bungalows, better water supply and drainage, and periodic holidays in the hills. The *ad hoc* selection of army stations amidst marsh lands, the absence of proper drainage and water supply and, significantly, ill-ventilated and overcrowded barracks, were identified as the factors which encouraged disease among the troops. A striking anomaly was that mortality among the Indian troops, when they lived with their families while in permanent military stations, was only 20 per 1000, the same as for European civil servants. When they moved into barracks, they died with the same rapidity and from the same diseases as British soldiers. Clearly, therefore, better adaptation to the local climate did not render them disease-proof. Finally, army mortality rates did not vary between stations, which were spread over every variety of climatic conditions. The tropical climate, therefore — although known to deteriorate health over a long period of time — was clearly not an all-important factor. Sanitary measures, when combined with improved diet (particularly controlled consumption of meat and liquor),[18] clothing suited to the climate, and small-pox vaccination, could safeguard the health of British troops. In the words of the Royal Commission, 'apart from the question of humanity, the introduction of an efficient system of hygiene in India is of essential importance to the interests of the Empire'.[19]

Cantonment acts, regulations and codes were issued, modelled on Public Health Acts in Britain.[20] The Military Cantonments Act XXII of 1864 was the first comprehensive legislation. This instituted sanitary police under the overall charge of medical officers, and sanctioned the registration of deaths and the recording of observations in the interests of public health.[21]

Three Sanitary Commissions were set up in 1864 for the presidencies of Bengal, Bombay and Madras, to effect the transfer of technologies which had a successful record of controlling disease in England and which could be applied to Indian conditions. This technology consisted of regular statistical reports on the origin and spread of epidemics and on measures taken to combat them. Each Commission comprised one civil member, the others being drawn from the military engineering, medical and sanitary branches of the army.[22] A system of army medical statistics for British India was instituted, uniform with that in use in Britain, and medical officers coming to India henceforth took a course in military hygiene at Netley beforehand.

The premier cadre among the medical officers now coming to India were members of the Army Medical Department (later renamed the Royal Army Medical Corps), deputed for the medical and sanitary care of British troops serving in India. Officers of the Army Medical Department were employed as executive medical officers of British station hospitals, in staff appointments and on specialist duties. The position of Director of Medical Services was, until almost the end of British rule, always occupied by an Army Medical Department officer, although in theory Indian Medical Service officers were also eligible for this appointment. The Indian Medical Service, the other important arm of the medical services, now became exclusively responsible for the health of the Indian troops. Although primarily a military service, those Indian Medical Service officers who were in excess of peacetime requirements were lent to the civil government for employment in civil departments, and were liable to recall in the event of war. Civil work encompassed presidency and district headquarters hospitals, the health of the police and inmates of jails and lunatic asylums, the health of ports and shipping, official patients and private practice and, under the new dispensation — vital statistics, vaccination and general sanitation.[23]

While segregation was an effective tool, full improvement in the health of European troops could not be brought about by neglecting sanitary precautions in adjacent Indian areas, particularly in the large and unplanned cities, where grossly unsanitary conditions prevailed. Nor was contact with the local populations at these sites avoidable. Servants and tradesmen from the Indian areas serviced the cantonments and civil lines, and Indian soldiers frequented the towns and bazaars. European fears of miasma emanating from the Indian quarters had led to the construction of walls between European and Indian locations, both military and civilian. The perception of the 'native' population as a secondary source of infection required the sanitary machine to encompass them, particularly for an understanding and prevention of the 'more obvious causes of disease' in their midst.[24] The Royal Sanitary Commission voiced concern for the health of the Indian troops and recommended that cantonment planning should also be extended to 'native lines'. And in a despatch to the Government of India in 1863, the Secretary of State for India pointed out,

The determination of the effects of local causes on the mortality of the native population, besides its intrinsic value in connection with the welfare of the people of India, cannot fail to have an important bearing on the health of the Europeans resident among them.[25]

The Sanitary Commissions, which were purely investigative and advisory bodies, were also asked to collect and analyse medical statistics and to recommend measures to improve general public health. A good number of municipalities came to be constituted, the registration of births and deaths was introduced, and vaccinators were appointed.

Within two years of their institution, however, the Sanitary Commissions were wound up. The army's sanitary perspective was beginning to take concrete shape: sanitary improvements in barracks, hospitals and stations had begun, promoted by legislation. To investigate the conditions of the general population and its interface with the army, a Sanitary Commissioner was appointed, between 1866 and 1867, to each of the presidencies of Bengal, Bombay and Madras and to the provinces — Punjab, Burma, United Provinces and Central Provinces of British India.[26] The Bengal Sanitary Commissioner became the Sanitary Commissioner to the Government of India, as its adviser on sanitary matters. This position was reserved for the Indian Medical Service but was subordinate to the Director of Medical Services, who was the supreme executive authority. The provincial Sanitary Commissioners, also drawn from the Indian Medical Service, were again only advisers, with no executive powers. Their duty was to tour their respective provinces looking into the prevailing sanitary conditions, investigating major epidemics, supervising the work of vaccinators, and preparing annual reports. These reports, with those of the Army Medical Department and Indian Medical Service, were compiled into a comprehensive annual report by the Sanitary Commissioner to the Government of India, and formed the basis for imperial vital statistics and disease control.

THE CONSOLIDATION OF SANITARY REFORM

The investigative tradition was an integral part of the sanitary movement concurrently taking place in England. Regular statistical reports were seen as essential to any systematic public health control, and since the establishment of the office of the Registrar-General of Births, Deaths and Marriages in 1836, the steady accumulation of statistical evidence had generated a demand for further research into the causes of epidemic diseases.[27] Following this tradition, the Government of India appointed in 1861 its first systematic enquiry into a major epidemic of cholera which swept through northern India in 1861, even as the Royal Commission's enquiry was under way. This epidemic starkly exposed the poor state of knowledge regarding disease conditions in the country, for if disease had to be prevented it had to be sought out, not waited for. The facts highlighted by the Cholera Enquiry (Strachey) Commission were followed up in the annual sanitary reports.[28]

Of all diseases, cholera played the key role in shaping colonial health policy in the latter half of the nineteenth century. The impact of the 1861 epidemic was not confined to India alone. It was followed by another epidemic in 1865, which spread from Egypt and across Europe to England. Cholera had been responsible for initiating the early public health era in Britain. The 1861 epidemic proved the final and most powerful spur to sanitary legislation in England — the Sanitary Act of 1866, which embodied the important principle of compulsion by a central authority.

This epidemic also gave rise to four international sanitary conferences — held by European countries in 1866, 1874, 1875 and 1885 — which attempted to work out acceptable quarantine measures, to systematize existing knowledge about disease, and to recommend measures for prevention.[29] As the 1861 epidemic had begun in India, the first conference, at Constantinople, placed India at the top of its agenda.

The Constantinople conference of 1866 put the British government into a quandary by pronouncing India the 'natural home' of cholera. In the absence of agreed knowledge about the cause and mode of infection, the conference surmised that the spread of cholera epidemics was due to rapid movements of groups of people and their personal effects, animals, merchandise, and the ships and railways carrying people, and with them disease, across great distances. Influencing the intensity of an epidemic and its persistence were local insanitary conditions — overcrowding, lack of ventilation, contaminated water and food, absence of drainage, and miasma from porous soil impregnated with organic matter. The conference pronounced that, in the case of India, the movement of pilgrims and large congregations at fairs and festivals was the single and 'most powerful of all the causes which conduce to the development and propagation of epidemics of cholera'.[30] In the opinion of the conference, when the pilgrims congregated, the cholera spread among them and when they dispersed they carried the contagion over long distances. While quarantine at seaports was one unavoidable measure of prevention, 'in accordance with the principles now admitted regarding the transmissibility of cholera and its mode of propagation', the effectiveness of quarantine would require that it be accompanied by the combating of the disease at its 'primary sources'.[31] The conference stressed the need for stricter implementation of rigorous and lengthy quarantine, for both sea and land movements, greater cleanliness, and the disinfection of ships, houses, and merchandise, and care to avoid overcrowding. The Government of India appointed a committee to look into the recommendations of the conference.[32] In turn, this committee recommended preventive sanitary and curative arrangements at pilgrim centres and on pilgrim routes. It also reiterated that the only far-reaching solution to the spread of cholera was a complete system of sanitation and town planning in cities, towns, and villages, along with military cantonments.

The international arrangements outlined for quarantine, and recommendations regarding the pilgrims, were particulary irksome to Britain and its government in India. Quarantine at seaports, which had from the first cholera epidemic in

Europe in 1831–2 been the only, admittedly inadequate, preventive measure, was resented by Great Britain, which had the largest international maritime trade as well as the most frequent troop and naval movements to and from its colonies. In the face of stricter quarantine restrictions imposed by the Constantinople conference, and international pressures to control cholera within India and its spread abroad, Britain instituted its own investigations into the scientific foundations of quarantine policy. There was much disagreement about whether local conditions of soil, air, and water, rather than contagion, carried through people and their effects, caused the spread of epidemics, and whether cholera could be prevented through sanitary improvements rather than through quarantine. Medical opinion in England supported such a strategy. A deputation of leading medical men to the president of the Privy Council in 1867 observed that there was 'a strong argument as to the necessity for a comprehensive investigation of the whole subject'.

> No country is so deeply concerned in the right solution of this difficult question of State medicine as Great Britain with her colonies. Besides the magnitude of her commercial relations with every part of the world, the interests of her army and navy, scattered as they are over the face of the globe and liable to be subjugated, by the operation of quarantine regulations, to serious inconveniences, in moving from one place or station to another, demand such an enquiry at the present time.
>
> It is moreover, confidently believed that the well-considered expression of opinion by this country, after a searching investigation, could not fail to have a great influence with most Continental States, as well as with all our colonies, and would eventually lead to the adoption of a more judicious system of defence against the introduction of foreign disease than is at present generally relied upon.[33]

In 1868, at the suggestion of the Army Medical School, two medical officers — T.R. Lewis and D.D. Cunningham of the Army Medical Department and Indian Medical Service respectively — were sent to Germany after completing the course at Netley, for further training in research. On their return to India, they were appointed special assistants to the Sanitary Commissioner with the Indian government. They launched a special enquiry, sanctioned by the Secretaries of State for War and India, into the mode of origin and spread of cholera in India.[34]

Even as the scientific investigations got under way, practical sanitary measures were intensified in all cantonments, smaller military stations, jails, and hospitals, such as drainage improvement, checking of water sources, abandonment of infected areas and the location of European troops in the hills as far as possible. Infected cases were isolated and barracks and hospitals fumigated. The prohibitions upon soldiers going into Indian cities or cholera-affected areas were more strictly enforced and 'sanitary cordons' (suggested by the Constantinople conference) were erected around cantonments to prevent persons residing in nearby villages and localities, and those suspected of carrying cholera, from entering the area.[35] The simultaneous resort to sanitation and quarantines, to clean-ups and isolation, was in keeping with sanitary practice in Europe, given the confusion regarding the aetiology and transmission of cholera.

It was the contagionist focus of the Constantinople conference on the rapid movements of large groups of people — especially pilgrims — which was problematic for the Indian sanitary establishment, which was now compelled to look into this large and complex issue. The immediate response to these international pressures was the framing of new rules for marching troops which, with their high vulnerability to cholera attacks, had been the principal agency for the spread of cholera through the regions occupied by the British in the first half of the nineteenth century. The rules pertaining to railway travel included provision of good drinking water and wholesome meals at halting stations, isolation of the troops from the native towns and bazaars *en route* and at their destination, thirty-minute stops every four hours, and travel for not more than twelve hours at a stretch.[36]

The line of investigation followed by Lewis and Cunningham, which came to dominate the Indian sanitary establishment's thinking, rejected the prevailing contagionist theories of cholera causation and transmission. Following the approach of the German scientist, Pettenkoffer, the 'Indian' theory was that cholera was related to the soil, its moisture content and variations in the level of subsoil water, which in turn was determined by climate, i.e. seasonal fluctuations in rainfall and humidity. The cholera poison from choleraic discharges developed neither in the water nor in the human body but, rather, the special *nidus* in which it multiplied was alluvial soil containing organic matter and salts and which, being moist and porous, reacted with the air and developed into infecting matter. This matter rose from the ground by means of water and the air contained in its interstices, and penetrated through the respiratory and probably the alimentary passages as well.

This analysis argued for the importance of segregation from the sources of noxious air, and of obtaining water from 'pure' sources, far from human habitations. Above all, it argued that 'locality' — characterised by soil, water and climate — was the determining factor in an epidemic, and that sanitary improvements were, therefore, the only protection against cholera. The use of asphalt for paving barracks and cantonment grounds (thereby trapping down the air emanating from porous soil), greater attention to drainage, the qualitative examination of water-supply sources in military and civil stations for organic matter and sewage, and reporting of defects and their remedy by the executive officers on the spot — all these were seen as more effective than belief in the communicability of the disease through humans and, therefore, than belief in quarantine.[37]

By the early 1870s, systematic statistics about cholera mortality were accumulating with the regular publication of annual sanitary reports. Despite the daily registration of climate and subsoil fluctuations in numerous stations all over British India, meant to aid military authorities in estimating the probable course of epidemics, another major epidemic swept across northern India in 1872 and again in 1875. Mortality was high again in the years 1881 and 1882.[38] In deference to international regulations, an infrastructure was set up for port health. By the Native Passenger Act of 1870, all pilgrim ships sailing to the Red Sea were more strictly supervised and required to hold a bill of health and a certificate to 'show that they are not overcrowded and that they are properly provisioned'. In 1882, Medical Boards were appointed at the chief ports of British India to report on whether cholera was epidemic or not at these ports, and bills of health to outgoing ships were based on these reports.[39]

Aiding efforts in the direction of sanitation was the differentiation of enteric fever within the omnibus category of 'fevers'. Whereas enteric fever was formerly returned as 'remittent' or 'continued' fever, from 1871 it came to be recorded separately on post-mortem examinations, although admission cases continued to be entered as remittent or malarial fever, due mainly to difficulties in recognition.

Enteric fever was the most fatal of all the diseases to which the European soldier was prone. Although also called 'Bengal remittent fever', since its incidence was highest in that presidency, it was present throughout India and in every station and cantonment. The Madras and Bombay presidencies, too, showed a rise in deaths from enteric fever, although not as steep as in Bengal.[40] That it was enteric fever which dominated the fever profile became clearer as accuracy in differential diagnosis improved. The recorded death-rate from enteric fever in Bengal rose from 1.62 in 1872 to 5.70 in 1886 to 6.78 per mille in 1894, while the rest of the 'fevers' — intermittent, remittent and simple/continued — declined from 1.78 to 0.99 to 0.41 per mille in the same period. The all-India death-rate from enteric fever peaked at 9.01 in 1872 and 10.17 in 1898.[41]

The general rise in the incidence of enteric fever deaths, however, was not a function of improved diagnosis alone. The greater incidence among European troops was also attributable to the demographic profile. A larger proportion of younger men now comprised the force in India. And, under the short service system, those serving in India for two years and under during the period 1871–87 accounted for about one-third (32.3 per cent) of the total strength of the European army. In the decade 1877–87, the deaths per mille for those under 25 years of age registered an increase from 2.45 to 5.37. The increase in death-rate in the age group 25 to 29, for this period, was of a relatively lower order (rising from 1.55 to 2.63). The death-rate for those in the age group 30 years and above in fact registered a decline, coming down to 0.68 from its previous level of 0.99. The decreasing death-rate due to enteric fever against rising age compares with the incidence of enteric fever by duration of stay. While the deaths per mille of recruits in their first two years of residence in India rose from 3.31 in 1877 to 7.31 in 1887, the rise in the death-rate among those in their third to sixth year of stay was of a much lower order (1.35 in 1877 to 2.37 in 1887). For those in their seventh to tenth year of residence, the death-rate actually registered a slight decline (0.90 to 0.82 between 1877 and 1887).[42] The high positive correlation between the incidence of enteric fever and young age or shorter duration of stay in India could, perhaps, be explained in terms of development of natural immunity with extended stay and rising age.

In 1874, a special enquiry was launched into enteric fever among European troops in the presidency of Bengal. The aim was to discover whether local insanitary conditions caused enteric fever.[43] Investigations revealed that surface drainage was universally defective, barracks were improperly constructed and close to 'native cities' where insanitary conditions prevailed, and soldiers consumed impure water from tanks while visiting 'native bazaars'.[44] The commission stressed that the continuing vulnerability of the young European soldier's health could only be overcome by greater attention to practical sanitary measures. Although it was now known that a variety of micro-organisms 'in their evolution in the human body disturb functional activity, lessen vital power and may ultimately annihilate motion', what was still unknown was the 'act or process by which the minutest and lowliest of created organisms, destroy the highest'.[45] Under the circumstances, what had been done in England ought to be repeated in India, since the enteric fever of England and that of India were one and the same. Practical sanitarians in England, in the absence of knowledge regarding the single or exact cause of enteric fever, had nevertheless eradicated the disease through general sanitary reform. The case for a more comprehensive and meticulous sanitation policy covering all stations and cantonments was now irrefutable.

By the end of the century, under the combined impact of segregation and sanitary measures, the death-rate among the British troops in India fell to 14.62 per mille, a saving in life 'equal to a British regiment per annum'.[46] In the following decade (1900–9) it was 9.91 per mille, and declined further to 7.12 per mille between 1920 and 1925. Cholera death-rates declined from 3.029 and 3.22 per mille in the 1860s and 1870s, respectively, to 1.11 in the last decade of the century. From the early years of the twentieth century its severity reduced, and, barring 1900, 1902 and 1908 when the mortality ratio was 1.45, 1.06 and 1.10, the cholera mortality ratio per thousand of strength never exceeded 1.0. The death-rate from enteric fever, which was an average of 6.42 in the years 1886 to 1902, started declining from 1903, and although the average during the decade 1900–9 was 3.8, from the start of the second decade of the century mortality never exceeded 1.0. The mortality for bowel complaints — the third most important disease afflicting European troops — which was 0.90, 1.60 and 0.89 during the 1860s, 1870s, and 1880s respectively, fell to 0.49 by the turn of the century and in the 1920s had fallen to 0.03 per mille.[47]

THE GENERAL POPULATION AND THE PILGRIM QUESTION

Cholera, which had spurred sanitary reform in the British army, was also the focus for extending medical administration to the general population. The international pronouncement on Indian pilgrim congregations turned the government's attention towards pilgrim centres and pilgrim routes, and the annual sanitary reports began to carry features on the major fairs and festivals in different parts of the country. At one of the biggest fairs in 1867 — the Kumbh Mela, held once in twelve years in northern India — some *ad hoc* sanitary arrangements were made as a test case and temporary hospitals were set up for isolation of infectious cases. These proved successful in curbing cholera on the fair grounds, but when the pilgrims dispersed they seemed to carry the cholera back to their villages, and to create foci of the disease in regions through which they travelled. If cholera were indeed caused by filth at fair sites, then such filth was known to have always existed in northern India. Yet epidemics were not known to be a regular occurrence causing huge mortality before the consolidation of British rule in the region.[48]

The contradictory data which accumulated around pilgrim movements only served to make the question more complex. The puzzling mode of cholera transmission and the fear of invasion by the disease into army and European enclaves led the government to resort to sanitary cordons around pilgrim encampments, land quarantine along pilgrim routes, and the prohibition of pilgrims from entering the neighbourhood of military stations.[49] Notwithstanding the policy of segregation of the enclave population and containment of the disease within 'native areas', the anti-contagionist stand of the Indian sanitary establishment raised for the government the unpalatable option of providing for an extensive public health machinery on an enduring basis, not only for pilgrim centres but also for the general population. The officials who sought Indian opinion on the matter of sanitary measures at pilgrim centres found that people were willing to submit to any measures calculated to promote their health. The first experiment at the 1867 Kumbh Mela had impressed pilgrims.[50] The MacKenzie Committee, appointed by the Madras government to look into the question of pilgrim control in that presidency, cited the Kumbh Mela experiment and urged the government to undertake such measures as were likely to demonstrate the desirability of sanitation, and to act as an incentive for the general population to adopt voluntarily modern sanitary principles in their towns and villages.[51]

Even as the question of finding the resources for curative and preventive measures at fair sites was being posed, doubts were expressed as to whether improving the salubrity of these centres might not actually have the effect of attracting greater numbers, and thus aggravating the problem of pilgrim control.[52] The railways added a dimension to the public health problem well beyond the confines of the pilgrim centres. The absence of rapid communications had hitherto kept disease strains localized. With the railways, this isolation broke down. The conditions of railway travel also facilitated the spread of disease. Pilgrims were stuffed into overcrowded third-class carriages and dirty goods wagons with no ventilation, lighting, drinking water or sanitary arrangements. Because allowing pilgrims to climb in and out at stations would cause delays, doors were fastened from the outside and not opened for hours at a stretch. For years, no provision existed for clean accommodation, drinking water or meals at halting stations. Death from suffocation and disease, cholera, smallpox, malaria, dysentery, and diarrhoea, and conditions conducive to tuberculosis, became more frequent as pilgrim traffic increased. The spread of communications also meant that pilgrims now poured into holy places in much larger numbers and in constant streams, overburdening local accommodation. All this further aggravated the problems of sanitation.[53]

The pilgrim question continued to fester through the late nineteenth century. Cholera in the army had almost disappeared, and the spread of cholera beyond the country's borders was being kept in check through port health regulations. But epidemics continued to rage among the general population. It was only in the second decade of the twentieth century that the Government of India ordered an exhaustive review of the pilgrim situation. The Pilgrim Enquiry Committees[54] found that even fifty years after the introduction of the railway system into India, the facilities were appalling. The *ad hoc* arrangements made by the government at the large pilgrim centres were inadequate. Hospital care, where it existed, was unsatisfactory and did not reflect recent advances in knowledge about cholera, or the use of bacteriological examination to prevent 'carriers' spreading the disease. Nor was there any organization for the compulsory notification of infection. Detailed and carefully investigated reports of the origin and spread of epidemics and of measures taken to combat them were lacking. Whatever limited recording and reporting was done was 'inaccurate and careless', as the Sanitary Inspectors upon whom this task fell were poorly qualified.[55] In the absence of accumulation of accurate knowledge, remedial measures could only be based on surmise. If this was the case with the largest festivals, the smaller ones escaped attention altogether, and these constituted as great a danger as the large ones as *foci* for the spread of epidemics.

There were clearly identifiable areas where effective government intervention was essential if the complex linkages between disease at pilgrim centres and in the country at large were to be snapped. Apart from checking the worst abuses of railway travel, these included the compulsory notification of cholera; the enforcement of legal power to ensure the treatment of cases; compulsory vaccination against smallpox; more skilled sanitary and scientific officers to tour the provinces for a steady accumulation of information; the provision of filtered and piped water supplies to overcome the pollution of irrigation canals and rivers through the traditional practice of washing and defecating close to the water sources; and the extension of hospital facilities.[56]

But sanitary reforms were expensive where they concerned a large and complex population. Further, such reforms and their administration required personnel qualified in medicine and sanitation to be intensively deployed among the general population, as well as effective legislation backed by enforcing agencies. Such a huge commitment of funds and personnel was not the brief of a colonial government. The focus on pilgrims and pilgrim centres permitted the assertion that compulsory measures would offend people's religious sensibilities and be construed as interference in their customs.[57] To quote Kiernan 'practically any government action outside the sphere of revenue sacred to British needs, could be construed as interference with religion'.[58]

The bogey of interference in the religion and customs of the people was not new, but was more self-consciously applied after the Mutiny. Eighteenth-century East India Company officials, many of whom recognized in India a superior civilization, had been replaced in the early nineteenth century by administrators who saw their mission as 'civilizing' and 'modernizing' Indian society. Indian society was seen as a *tabula rasa*, waiting to be impressed in a western mould. The civilizing influence would be western social and economic institutions, especially education, and western religion, i.e. Christianity. After the Mutiny, however, the enthusiasm for remaking Indian society declined. Theories of racial exclusiveness came to the fore as Britain established itself as the governing power and as the European establishment in the country perfected the mechanisms of physical and social segregation.[59]

Outside the feeble intervention represented by the pilgrim problem, the actual exercise of responsibility for public health was left entirely to the concerned local bodies in the various administrative units — the country was divided into provinces which were further subdivided into districts. There were municipalities for the larger towns, created on the English model through Municipal Acts for the various provinces between 1871 and 1874. District Boards were set up for the rural and semi-urban areas from 1881, again on the elective principle but often headed by the District Collector, and required to raise their own resources through the levy of local cesses. In addition to other developmental responsibilities for the areas under their jurisdiction, these bodies were expected to provide for drainage, water supply and general sanitation and maintenance of hospitals and dispensaries, on the advice of the District Civil Surgeon and the Deputy Sanitary Commissioner.

These local bodies made no impact on sanitation. There was no regulation compelling municipalities to employ medical officers of health, with the result that they largely employed only Sanitary Inspectors, who, too, were untrained. The District Local Boards employed no public health staff at all, apart from vaccinators who were poorly paid and ill-educated. The local authorities also showed a distinct preference for expending their resources on communications, especially roads, schools, and dispensaries, symbols of civilization and of British rule. Their ineffectiveness led, between 1888 and 1893, to the formation of a Sanitary Board for each province, composed of administrative and public works officers in addition to the Sanitary Commissioner and the Inspector General of Civil Hospitals. The function of these Boards was to provide a fillip to municipalities and district boards through technical advice on sanitary works, backed by funds contributed by the provincial government.[60]

But the weakness of the basic investigative and executive structures was a fundamental one.[61] The district-level fulcrum on which the Sanitary Boards rested was the Civil Surgeon (an Indian Medical Service officer). In addition to his primary responsibilities — which included his regular medical duties, the medico-legal work of the district, medical charge of the jails and, more perfunctorily, inspection of outlying dispensaries — he was expected to be the adviser on sanitation in the municipalities of the district. His own lack of experience or of any formal training in sanitation was compounded by a lack of authority to enforce his recommendations. Overseeing several districts were the Deputy Sanitary Commissioners of each province. These officials, who were Indian Medical Service officers, were the former Superintendents of Vaccination who, in 1881, were given composite responsibility for supervising general sanitation as well as vaccination and vital statistics.[62] Upon them rested the entire burden of investigating the province. But they (and, indeed, even the Sanitary Commissioners themselves) had no executive or disciplinary authority over the civil surgeons or local governments. The Deputy Sanitary Commissioners were a hopelessly small number even for their investigative functions. In Bengal, for instance, one temporary and four permanent officials were expected to oversee a population of about 71 million. Madras, with a population of 35.5 million, had three Deputy Sanitary Commissioners, while the Central Provinces and Assam, with populations of 13.5 million and 5 million respectively, had none.[63]

The Deputy Sanitary Commissioners were also poorly motivated. Ever since the institution of this cadre, it proved very difficult to attract competent and interested men to the department. Sanitary experts were not recruited into the Sanitary Department, nor was there a requirement that entrants should acquire formal training in public health and general hygiene in the course of their career. The Department was also unpopular because, for positions other than that of provincial Sanitary Commissioner, its salaries were lower than the civil surgeoncies, which afforded the opportunity for private practice and, in the presidency towns, the prestige of attachment to medical colleges and teaching hospitals. For the Indian Medical Service men coming to India, the primary attraction was the civil surgeoncies. The 'best' among them refused to come into the Sanitary Department; the 'most capable' men left it, relegated as they were to being an unconnected link in a weak and nebulous structure lacking a coherent and decisive policy; and even among the most ordinary few who came to it against their will and remained discontented, the Department was a stepping stone to a civil surgeoncy.

At the other end of the scale were the executive agencies described earlier, with their meagre and generally untrained public health staff, where the onus of registration of deaths by cause rested with the village *chowkidar* (watchman), and the tackling of epidemics was the responsibility of the district revenue subordinate officials. Until the end of British rule, this structure remained essentially unchanged, and no provision came to exist for central legislative or executive control.[64]

In the wake of the Pilgrim Enquiry Committees in the second decade of the twentieth century, some remedial measures came to be focused on the pilgrim problem. The conditions of pilgrim movements were regulated. Conveying pilgrims in closed airtight wagons meant for goods was discouraged, eating houses at railway stations were licensed, and provision was made for drinking water and toilets at stations. At pilgrim centres, special efforts were made to check and periodically cleanse water sources (wells, tanks) and ensure general cleanliness.[65] But the neglect of public health measures among the general population, accompanied by an intensification of trade and commerce and the growth of population in seaport towns, as well as repeated famines, the increasing impoverishment of the rural areas and the flow of migrants into the cities in search of work,[66] produced a plague epidemic in 1896. This was followed by successive epidemics which spread the disease to large parts of the country and which by 1918 had taken a toll of almost 10.5 million lives.[67] The plague entered Bombay from Hong Kong, conveyed by rats on ships. It was striking that all the plague deaths occurred among the Indian population. Between November 1896 and April 1897 in Bombay, only one 'pure European' and eight 'domiciled Europeans' died of plague. In the following four months, between December 1897 and April 1898, the death toll among the latter group fell to four.[68] The absence of accurate vital statistics made it difficult to estimate the death-rates among the Indian population, but 70 per cent of the cases admitted into hospital died in the immediate aftermath of the first outbreak.[69]

The plague, like cholera before it, invited international condemnation of the British government in India. But, unlike cholera, it prompted quick and decisive action. An epidemic of such proportions in an important commercial seaport town which caused the flight of skilled labour from the city and held out the possibility of considerable trade dislocation if the disease spread to other Indian ports by railway, was quite a different problem to the cholera outbreaks in pilgrim centres. Two pieces of legislation were passed — the Births, Deaths and Marriages Registration Act of 1896 and the Epidemic Diseases Act of 1897. The granting of legal status to vital registration and the notification of three diseases — plague, cholera and smallpox — was long overdue. But they were also in response to an International Sanitary Conference which met in Venice in 1897. The Conference drew up a list of susceptible articles prohibited from export out of infected ports, and required that an infected country should notify all cases of plague and conduct thorough medical examinations of all passengers boarding ships.[70]

Backed by the Epidemic Diseases Act, a plague committee, set up and charged with 'keep[ing] down the death rate while preventing panic and trade dislocation and lessen[ing] the risk of a third epidemic', undertook compulsory measures to combat the plague. This followed the new medical policy of the Indian government. The irrefutability of contagion, reinforced by germ theory advances, had come to be accepted in India from about the last decade of the nineteenth century. The old enthusiasm for fumigation and isolation — which were selectively employed in the case of troops in an earlier era — now came to be revived where the public health was concerned, in the belief that all sorts of bacteria could be destroyed in this manner. Police cordons conducted house-to-house searches, deaths were reported, the sick were isolated, dilapidated houses were vacated and disinfected and the occupants removed to camps, rural migrants were detained, and at railway stations passengers and their luggage were disinfected. Check points were instituted at major railway stations and at entry points on the borders of provinces and regions. And precautions were particularly stringent to prevent infected persons from entering the vicinity of large ports like Calcutta.[71]

This first direct intervention in public health, where earlier *laissez-faire* was the watchword, was not only violent and insensitive but, although unappreciated at the time, was also to prove scientifically inaccurate.[72] The single most important factor contributing to bubonic plague was insanitation, which created conditions for rats and rat fleas. And overcrowding and squalor among the teeming poor in cities like Bombay were appalling.[73] Deliverance from the public protests generated in Bombay by the plague measures, and from the panic among rulers and ruled alike, came from the new bacteriological science. Waldemar Haffkine, a Russian emigré research worker from the Pasteur Institute in Paris, whose successful anti-cholera vaccine trials in Bengal from 1893 had led the government to institute compulsory vaccination for troops and civil servants,[74] was called upon for help, and by January 1897 he had developed an anti-plague vaccine which proved to have a success rate of 80-90 per cent. Haffkine personally conducted the inoculation programmes and made efforts to popularize vaccination, and urged government to exempt inoculated persons from compulsory measures and detention camps. After 1898 the politically unwise compulsory measures were given up. But public health policy continued to vacillate.

Although Haffkine had been formally taken into government service in a non-pensionable capacity since 1897, he was still regarded as an outsider, and his initiative was resented by the authorities who saw it as an undue concern for their Indian subjects and as an interference in their public health policy. The growing popularity of inoculation also required more money, men, and technical and administrative facilities to be put into the anti-plague measures, and the Government of India found Haffkine's repeated requests irksome.[75] The British Army Medical Department on its part saw his authoritative handling of the epidemic and his apparent command over the new scientific knowledge as a threat to their professional monopoly in India. This was the first large-scale impact in India of the germ theory's potential.

The Government of India at this time was not sufficiently aware of the importance of the new scientific advances. It had, in fact, ignored the path-breaking discovery of the mode of transmission in malaria by Ronald Ross in 1897. Ross had worked on this problem under the colonial government's very nose while in the Indian Medical Service. Some of the Indian princes were quick to respond. Forming a committee which made an offer in 1899 to the Government of India to finance an all-India medical research institute, they made it a condition that Haffkine be appointed Director.

In an era when scientific rivalry was an integral part of the national rivalries among the European powers, the leadership of the new science could not be left in the hands of a foreigner, nor applied to civilian ends. Its role in relation to the army had to be worked out first. The sponsoring of a research institute — even if fully funded — by Indian princes clashed with the prevailing attitude towards Indian princes and Indians in general which had strong racist overtones — what Salisbury, then Prime Minister of Britain, referred to as 'the damned nigger attitude'.[76] The Government of India suspended Haffkine from all research and administrative responsibilities on trumped-up charges of negligence and administrative ineffectiveness,[77] and in this manner the 'princes' offer' was permanently dropped.[78] The leadership of the Bombay Plague Research Laboratory was taken by a Royal Army Medical Corps official. It followed that only those with both medical and military training would be appointed to head research laboratories.[79] The undermining of Haffkine's contribution found its ultimate expression in the end of the inoculation drives. The efficacy of his vaccine was not given proper testing; inoculation, being 'only a personal prophylactic measure', no longer remained at the centre of the anti-epidemic campaign.[80] Deaths from plague continued unabated, at an average of 500,000 every year from the beginning of 1898 until 1918. In fact, in the ten years from 1898 to 1908, there were an estimated 20,000 deaths a week. In 1904 alone, about 1.5 million deaths from plague were recorded.[81]

The plague epidemic, which precipitated the deterioration in public health conditions that was to continue through the early decades of the twentieth century[82] — accentuated by the 1918 influenza epidemic, and resulting in the first negative growth rate returned by the 1921 census — demonstrated the continuing reluctance of the government to move in the direction of extended public health measures. Like smallpox vaccination before it, plague inoculation foundered on the rocks of inaction, justified as caution in reducing the pace of sanitary reform for fear of pressurising public opinion.[83]

This was, in fact, quite contrary to the native Indian response. The result of the inoculation drives — the first major attempt at epidemic control — was a growing desire for sanitary reform among the general population. Representations were made by Indians requesting the government to take the initiative in maintaining the struggle against plague, and in widening the scope of sanitary reform.[84]

But the prospect of a large-scale and expensive intervention was an alarming one for a colonial government. In the opinion of the Sanitary Department, the living conditions of the general population had gone 'beyond the influence of sanitary effort',[85] and the government followed the route of leaving the field to the curative efforts of the private medical profession. In a despatch of 1900, the Secretary of State for India reiterated that it was in the best interests of the people of India that the spread of an independent Indian medical profession be encouraged 'which alone can adequately supply the needs of the people'.[86] The historical option of tackling the problem of public health through wide-ranging and enduring preventive sanitary measures — as was done in western countries — was thus lost.[87]

NOTES

This paper is part of a continuing study on the origins of modern medical science in India under colonial rule. Some of this work has been published earlier in ***Public Health and***

Medical Research in India: Their Origins Under the Impact of British Colonial Policy (Stockholm: SAREC, 1982). By a happy coincidence, the main points made in this publication have also been expressed independently in a later publication by David Arnold, 'Medical priorities and practice in nineteenth-century British India', *South Asia Research, 5* (2) (1985) 167–83. I am grateful to Professor Charles Cooper for the many discussions from which I have benefited in the course of my work on this study, and to Professor Roy MacLeod, Dr Milton Lewis and Dr Michael Worboys for their comments on earlier drafts.

1. *Report of the Commissioners Appointed to Enquire into the Sanitary State of the Army in India* (henceforth *Royal Sanitary Commission Report*), *Parliamentary Papers*, vols 1 and 11, 1863. (Cmd 3184), xix.

2. Florence Nightingale, 'Life or death in India' and 'Life or death by irrigation, 1874', *Annual Report of the Sanitary Commissioner with the Government of India* (henceforth *Annual Sanitary Report*), 1873–74, Appendix 49.

3. The other important cause of invalidity was the high rate of venereal disease which, at any one time, hospitalized one-third of the European troops. Venereal disease rates among Indian soldiers were low. As concern for the health of the British soldier increased, ways were sought to combat this seemingly intractable problem. For a fuller treatment of the subject see Kenneth Ballhatchet, *Race, Sex and Class Under the Raj: Imperial Attitudes and Policies and their Critics* (London: Weidenfeld & Nicholson, 1980).

4. Nightingale, op. cit., n. 2 above; 'Report on the Hardwar cholera of 1867' by John Murray, Inspector General of Hospitals, Upper Provinces. India Office Records (hereafter IOR) V/26/844/1, *Proceedings of the Sanitary Commissioner for Madras*, Appendix B.

5. Cf. *Royal Sanitary Commission Report*, n. 1 above, 31.

6. Cf. Nightingale, op. cit., n. 2 above; *Report of the (Baker) Committee*, 1845 (Calcutta, 1847); also, Leela Visaria and Pravin Visaria, 'Population (1757–1947)', in Dharma Kumar (ed.), *The Cambridge Economic History of India* (Cambridge: Cambridge University Press, 1982), vol. 2; and Ira Klein, 'Death in India, 1871–1921', *Journal of Asian Studies, 32* (4) (1973), 639–59. See also a recent article by Ira Klein which, while highlighting the linkages between famine relief policy and the developmental ethos in the second half of the nineteenth century, argues that while famines took a considerable and dramatic toll of human life in this period, it was the continuous occurrence of epidemics which was the single most important cause of high mortality among the Indian population in the latter part of the nineteenth century. Ira Klein, 'When the rains failed: famine, relief, and mortality in British India', *Indian Economic and Social History Review, XXI* (2) (1984), 185–214.

7. Martin, a veteran of twenty-two years military service in Bengal and later Physician to the Council of India, was an ardent advocate of sanitary reform, and served on the Royal Sanitary Commission. Cf. J.R. Martin, 'Suggestions on the hygiene of camps and cantonments' and 'Medical arrangements for field services and sanitary precautions necessary in camps, barracks and hospitals', in *Royal Sanitary Commission Report*, n. 1 above.

8. *Imperial Gazetteer of India* (Oxford: Clarendon Press, 1909), vol. IV, ch. XI.

9. ibid. The system was premised on the belief that the spirit and traditions of the British army could be preserved only by the return of regiments to England.

10. Cf. Nightingale, op. cit., n. 2 above, 49. A Government of India despatch (no. 459 of 1864, Military Department) to the Secretary of State for India challenged the accuracy of the Royal Commission's death-rate estimates, warning that it was dangerous to sound so alarming as no soldiers would then volunteer for recruitment. *Royal Sanitary Commission Report*, n. 1 above.

11. ibid., 50.

12. ibid., 49.

13. *Select Committee* [on] European Colonization and Settlement in India, First Report, 1857–1858 (261), vii, Part I, 1, 159; Second Report, 1857–1858 (326), vii, Part I, 165; Third Report, 1857–1858 (415), vii, Part I, 373; Fourth Report, 1857–1858 (461), vii, Part II, 1.

14. *Imperial Gazetteer of India* (Oxford: Clarendon Press, 1909), vol. 1, ch. IX.

15. *Royal Sanitary Commission Report*, n. 1 above.

16. Cf. B.L. Hutchins, *The Public Health Agitation, 1833–48* (London: A.C. Fifield, 1909); C. Fraser Brockington, *A Short History of Public Health* (London: J. & A. Churchill, 1956); C. Fraser Brockington, *Public Health in the Nineteenth Century* (Edinburgh and London: E. & S. Livingstone, 1965); Jeanne L. Brand, *Doctors and the State: The British Medical Profession and Government Action in Public Health, 1870–1912* (Baltimore: Johns Hopkins University Press, 1965).

17. A.D. King, *Colonial Urban Development* (London: Routledge & Kegan Paul, 1976), 118.

18. Even in barracks, Indian soldiers were found to have less dysentery and liver disease than European soldiers. *Royal Sanitary Commission Report*, n. 1 above.

19. ibid., 166.

20. The British public health legislation then in force included the Public Health Act, 1848; the Nuisance Removal Act and Disease Prevention Act, 1855; and the Local Government Act, 1858. Cf. Fraser Brockington, *Public Health in the Nineteenth Century*, n. 16 above.

21. *Gazette of India* (2 March 1864), 84–6.

22. ibid.

23. Government of India, *The Army in India and its Evolution* (Calcutta: Government Printer, 1924), ch. XIII; *Imperial Gazetteer of India*, n. 8 above, ch. XIV. In 1861, the IMS strength was 819, of which 326 belonged to the military reserve. D.G. Crawford, *A History of the Indian Medical Service, 1600–1913*, 2 vols (London: W. Thacker, 1914), vol. 1.

24. *Royal Sanitary Commission Report*, n. 1 above, 78.

25. Military Despatch no. 297, 1863. Supplement to *Gazette of India* (2 March 1864), 140.

26. *Imperial Gazetteer of India*, n. 8 above, ch. XIV.

27. R.H. Shryock, *The Development of Modern Medicine: An Interpretation of the Social and Scientific Factors Involved* (London: Gollancz, 1948).

28. *Report of the Commissioners Appointed to Enquire into the Cholera Epidemic in Northern India* (Cholera (Strachey) Commission), 1861–62, (Calcutta, 1864).

29. While earlier conferences gave priority to cholera, subsequent meetings had broader interests. Western nations were developing national health systems, and since epidemic control transcended national action, the need for international organization was unanimously realized. The 1874 conference proposed to set up a permanent international council to check epidemics. This became a reality in the early twentieth century — the International Office of Public Health in Paris. Shryock, op. cit., n. 27 above, 199.

30. Quoted by the Cholera Committee, 1867, 'appointed to report upon the arrangements which should be made to give practical effect in the Madras Presidency to the recommendations and suggestions of the International Sanitary Conference', *Report of the Cholera Committee* (Madras, 1868), 3.

31. ibid.

32. *Proceedings of the Sanitary Commissioner for Madras*, Report of the MacKenzie Committee, 'Report and Order of the Madras Government Regarding the Control of Pilgrims in the Madras Presidency, 1868'.

33. Memorial on Quarantine, quoted in *Report of the Cholera Committee*, 1867, n. 30 above, 46–9.

34. *Annual Sanitary Report*, 1868, 26.

35. *Annual Sanitary Report*, 1875, 17–18.

36. *Report of the Cholera Committee*, 1867, n. 30 above, 35.

37. 'A report on the microscopic objects found in cholera evacuation', *Annual Sanitary Report*, 1869; T.R. Lewis and D.D. Cunningham, 'Cholera in relation to certain physical phenomena: a contribution towards the special enquiry sanctioned by the Right Hon. the Secretaries of State for War and for India', *Annual Sanitary Report*, 1876, Appendix A; also *Annual Sanitary Reports* of 1872 and 1875; W. Center, 'Memorandum on Indian waters and water analysis', *Annual Sanitary Report*, 1882, Appendix A. Cf. a recent paper by John Chandler Hume which highlights the controversial reception in Indian sanitary circles of Cunningham's theory. John Chandler Hume, Jr, 'Colonialism and sanitary medicine: the development of preventive health policy in the Punjab, 1860–1900', *Modern Asian Studies, 20* (4) (1986), 703–24.

38. *Annual Sanitary Reports* for the relevant years.

39. *Annual Sanitary Report*, 1884.

40. *Annual Sanitary Report*, 1887 and 1894.

41. *Annual Sanitary Report*, 1872 and 1898.

42. *Annual Sanitary Report*, 1887, 29.

43. *Annual Sanitary Report*, 1875, 72.

44. *Annual Sanitary Report*, 1875, 71–3; 1887, 21.

45. *Annual Sanitary Report*, 1887, 25.

46. *Annual Sanitary Report*, 1900, 121.

47. Calculated from the *Annual Sanitary Reports* for the relevant years, 1900–29.

48. Murray, op. cit., n. 4 above.

49. MacKenzie, op. cit., n. 32 above.

50. 'Report by Assistant Surgeon Cutcliffe on sanitary measures at Hardwar', cited in MacKenzie, op. cit., n. 32 above.

51. ibid.

52. ibid.

53. *Report of the United Provinces Pilgrim* [Robertson] Committee, 1913 (Simla, 1916); *Report of the Bihar and Orissa Pilgrim [Robertson] Committee*, 1913 (Simla, 1915); *Report of the Madras Pilgrim* [*Clemesha*] Committee, 1915 (Simla, 1916); *Report of the Bombay Pilgrim* [*Clemesha*] *Committee*, 1916 (Simla, 1916). The railway companies justified their use of goods wagons on the theory that Indians liked to travel in droves and, therefore, in goods wagons, and would feel 'insecure' in passenger carriages (*United Provinces Pilgrim Commitee Report*, 1913, 45–9). However, the Committee found the opposite view among passengers, who expressed their preference for carriages, and who protested at being charged third-class fares and made to travel in goods wagons (49). Under these circumstances it was difficult for the Pilgrim Committees to raise the issue of a sanitary tax, which could otherwise have been levied by an extra charge on railway tickets.

54. The Committees found that in most places, what passed for hospitals were merely dilapidated thatch or matting huts where the sole permanent staff was a watchman. In others, the location was in remote desolate wastelands outside the towns and without accommodation for the staff or patients' relatives. It was not surprising, therefore, that nobody wished to avail of such 'facilities' (*Report of the Madras Pilgrim Committee*, 1915, 18; *Report of the United Provinces Pilgrim Committee*, 1913, 23).

55. *Report of the Madras Pilgrim Committee*, n. 53 above, 13.

56. The policy was wanting in these major respects as late as 1920. Cf. *Report of the Madras Pilgrim Committee*, n. 53 above.

57. Mackenzie, op. cit., n. 32 above, 8.

58. V.G. Kiernan, *The Lords of Human Kind: European Attitudes towards the Outside World in the Imperial Age* (London: Weidenfeld & Nicholson, 1969), 38.

59. Some references may be cited here: F.G. Hutchins, *The Illusion of Permanence: British Imperialism in India* (Princeton: Princeton University Press, 1967); Eric Stokes, *The English Utilitarians in India* (Oxford: Oxford University Press, 1959); John Strachey, *The End of Empire* (London: Gollancz, 1961); David Dilks, *Curzon in India* (London: Hart-Davis, 1969), vol. 1. Also see a more recent study by David Arnold, 'Cholera and colonialism in British India', *Past and Present*, no. 113 (1986), 118–51. Also by the same author, 'Medical priorities and practice in nineteenth century British India', *South Asia Research, 5* (2) (1985), 167–83.

60. *Imperial Gazetteer of India*, n. 8 above, vol. IV, ch. IX.

61. This discussion is based largely upon C.A. Bentley, 'Note to the Indian Sanitary Services', IOR L/E/7/992, Appendix II.

62. The Vaccination Boards were amalgamated with the Sanitary Department on the premise that insanitary conditions, such as bad drainage and polluted drinking water, were the chief causes of smallpox. Cf. *Annual Sanitary Report*, 1881. For an earlier discussion of smallpox, see the *Report of the Bengal Smallpox (Lamb) Commission* (Calcutta, 1850).

63. The population figures are from the 1891 Census. The total population of British India was 221,239,515 and the distribution over the provinces was as follows:

Bengal	32.2%
Bombay	8.5%
Madras	16.1%
United Provinces	21.2%
Central Provinces (including Berar)	6.1%
Punjab	8.5%
Assam	2.4%
Burma	3.4%

Source: Imperial Gazetteer of India, vol. 1 (Oxford: Clarendon Press, 1909).

64. Bentley, op. cit., n. 61 above.

65. ibid.

66. D.R. Gadgil, *The Industrial Evolution of India in Recent Times* (Oxford: Oxford University Press, 4th edn, 1942). The Great Famine which broke out in 1896–7, and took particularly acute form in the Bombay presidency, its worst period extending up to 1905, was also responsible for the flow of migrants into Bombay from the surrounding countryside. In three months alone — April, May, and June of 1897 — up to 300,000 migrants came to Bombay in search of work. Cf. *Report of the Bombay Plague Committee* 'appointed by Government Resolution no. 1204/720 on the Plague in Bombay, July 1897–April 1898' (Bombay, 1898).

67. IOR L/E/7/1134, File 3656, Norman White, 'The prevalence of epidemic disease and port health in the Far East', 1923.

68. *Report of the Bombay Plague Committee*, n. 66 above, Table F. 5.

69. *Report of the Plague Research (Lyons) Committee* (Bombay, 1897), 8.

70. *History and Proceedings of the Bengal Plague [Risley] Commission, 1896–1898* (Calcutta, 1899).

71. *Report of the Bombay Plague Committee*, n. 66 above, 59

72. The elucidation of the 'rat flea' theory — i.e. the transmission of the disease from rat to man through the rat flea — was the contribution of a British Plague Research Commission, which conducted comprehensive investigations between 1905 and 1913. This comprised bacteriologists from the Lister Institute in London, and selected members of the

Indian Medical Service, who were directed by an Advisory Committee consisting of representatives of the Royal Society and the Lister Institute, together with the nominees of the Secretary of State for India. Their discovery was 'one of the most comprehensive, compact and successful pieces of scientific investigation ever undertaken by Englishmen'. As German and Russian Commissions had failed, this considerably enhanced Britain's prestige in the great power rivalries that characterized the early twentieth century. For elaboration, cf. R. Ramasubban, *Public Health and Medical Research in India: Their Origins under the Impact of British Colonial Policy* (Stockholm: SAREC, 1982).

73. *Report of the Bombay Plague Committee*, no. 66 above. The Bengal Plague Commission found the same conditions in Calcutta: op. cit., n. 70 above. For a detailed discussion of Bombay, see Ira Klein, 'Urban development and death: Bombay City, 1870–1914', *Modern Asian Studies, 20* (4) (1986), 725–54.

74. Edyth Lutzker and Carol Jachnowitz, 'The curious history of Waldemar Haffkine', *Commentary* (June 1980), 61–4.

75. IOR L/E/7/431, R and S 1719/1901.

76. Dilks, op. cit., n. 59 above, 240.

77. Haffkine left India in disgrace and spent the next few years taking his case to the scientific community in Europe. He was never officially exonerated by the colonial government, but after India's independence the Bombay Laboratory was renamed the Haffkine Institute. Ronald Ross, who had also been slighted by the government of India, ardently advocated Haffkine's case through the 'letters' columns of *Nature* (cf. especially 1907).

78. IOR L/E/7/431, R and S 2096/1904, R. Harvey, DG–IMS, 'Note on the bacteriological requirements of India' (2 May 1899).

79. IOR L/E/7/431, R and S 2096/1904, Amthill, Governor General in Council to Broderick, Secretary of State for India (18 August 1904).

80. *Report of the Punjab Plague [Meredith[Committee* (Simla, 1910).

81. Lovat Fraser, *India Under Curzon and After* (London: Heinemann, 1911).

82. After 1918, plague death-rates fell a little; the combined mortality of four plague epidemics between 1918 and 1922 was only 402,295. But there followed an increase and an average of 100,000 annual deaths occurred until 1930, when the rate again dropped to an average of 50,000 deaths annually until 1935. H.H. Scott, *A History of Tropical Medicine* (London: Edward Arnold, 1939), vol. II, 714–15.

83. *Report of the Punjab Pilgrim Committee*, 1910.

84. ibid., 1–2.

85. *Annual Sanitary Report*, 1900–1, 123.

86. IOR L/E/7/431, R and S 1127/1900. Some of the vicissitudes of this process, its direction and ethos moulded by the Indian Medical Service and by metropolitan organizations like the General Medical Council, have been discussed by Roger Jefferey, 'Recognizing India's doctors: the institutionalization of medical dependency, 1918–39', *Modern Asian Studies, 13* (2) (1979), 301–26.

87. Colonial health policy came to be focused on the production of known vaccines and on bacteriological and pathological investigations, as a sounder scientific basis for army health, as well as upon research into tropical diseases in military laboratories, accompanied by contributions to research centres in the metropolis, notably the London School of Tropical Medicine. These aspects are discussed in Ramasubban, op. cit., n. 72 above.

3

European medicine in the Cook Islands

Raeburn Lange

INTRODUCTION

The incorporation of the Cook Islands into the western-based structure of Christian adherence and the international network of economic relationships long preceded the establishment of foreign political control over this far-flung group of fifteen small islands in the South Pacific. When a British Protectorate was set up in 1888, followed by New Zealand annexation in 1901, the islands had professed a national Christian allegiance for more than half a century, and the global economy had impinged on Cook Islands life at a great many points in the period since about 1830. The role of nineteenth-century missionaries and traders as agents of change, though pre-colonial, is too important to be ignored. The ideological, economic, and political power they exerted is not to be compared, however, with the ever more pervasive ascendancy enjoyed by the colonial administration set up just before the twentieth century began.

This essay is an examination of colonial medicine in a small corner of the imperial world during the colonial period from 1888 to the late 1940s. Although control by the New Zealand Government was not relinquished until 1965,[1] this study ends with the middle of the twentieth century, when the introduction of antibiotics greatly changed the value of colonial medicine and its place in the life of the Cook Islands people. In the late 1940s, also, the precise nature of colonial administration was altered (a Legislative Council was set up in 1946), and the pace of economic and social change accelerated. In the area of medicine and in the wider environmental context, the late 1940s saw the end of an era, even if the period of colonial rule had two crucial decades still to run.

THE PRE-COLONIAL PERIOD

European medicine was introduced to the Cook Islands as one of many cultural innovations brought by British Protestant missionaries. First arriving in the group in 1827, the London Missionary Society workers were for many years the most important carriers of the new technological, organizational, and intellectual possibilities of the post-contact era. Non-missionary foreign residents were few in number until the final quarter of the century, although whalers and traders made frequent short visits to some of the islands in the southern part of the group. European visitors and residents, both missionary and commercial, were able to introduce the Cook Islanders to many foreign items that were quickly seen to be of value, and a money economy based on cash crops, and linking islanders with the outside commercial world, was inaugurated.[2]

Although the missionaries' conscious purpose was evangelism, they did of course carry with them their British conviction of the superiority of western social, technological, and economic values and practices. They did not, however, envisage the introduction of foreign political power. Their vision was of an indigenous Christian state, enjoying the benefits of European civilization but excluding the evils of a large resident community of foreign planters and traders who might follow an unchristian lifestyle and wield an undesirable political influence. In the coming of European missionaries, and in their introduction of European medicine, there was no thought of the usefulness of medical innovation in any imperialism other than the expansion of the Christian gospel and a vaguely defined 'Christian civilization'.

Significant though they were as the first carriers of European medicine to the Cook Islands, the first generation of missionaries had an ambivalent perception of medicine, a perception that was scarcely more 'scientific' than the ancient Cook Islands view of health and ill health. They took it for granted that illness and other physical adversity was part of the destiny of all mankind, and indeed discerned in this the omnipotence of God, who was able to control and overrule the operation of evil. On occasions God would permit disease and disaster to occur, or even send it, but always in order to further his own beneficent purposes. John Williams interpreted a particular epidemic as 'a timely interposition of an all-wise and overruling Providence'.[3] This is the meaning the missionaries endeavoured to see in all the epidemiological and climatic disasters of their first decades in the Cook Islands. Few of them escaped serious illness in their own families. Far from the medical aid available in Sydney or Auckland, they felt sickness and death as an ever-present possibility, and it is not surprising that the missionaries developed to the full their emotional commitment to the doctrine of divinely sanctioned affliction. Nor is it surprising that they often displayed little real interest in the physical identity and character of the diseases that 'humanly speaking' were responsible for illness and death.[4]

Dysentery, influenza, measles, whooping cough, mumps, tuberculosis — the catalogue of epidemic diseases striking the Cook Islands in the middle decades of the nineteenth century is long and depressing.[5] These visitations took an alarming toll of life and health, especially on Rarotonga, and were largely responsible for a fall in the island's population from nearly 20,000 in the 1820s to fewer than 10,000 at the end of the century.[6] Disease and depopulation severely challenged the missionaries' and islanders' emotional and theological attitude to affliction. As the years passed, however, the continuing (though lessening) ravages of introduced disease were seen by the people as part of normal experience, in the same way that ancient endemic diseases like yaws and filariasis were perceived. The people's view of life was modified to accommodate *maki-mate*, periods when distressingly destructive illness prevailed. It is significant that the people's new Christian understanding of illness was not dissimilar to their traditional integration of health and ill health into the religious dimension of life.[7]

The missionaries' theological stance towards suffering and illness by no means precluded an active and practical response to the plight of the sick. From the beginning of their residence in the Cook Islands, the missionaries found themselves strenuously engaged in medical work. Confronted with an unnamed epidemic not many months after he settled on Rarotonga in 1827, Charles Pitman went out every day for nearly six weeks, dispensing purgatives until supplies were exhausted and then resorting to bleeding where this was considered 'prudent'. He believed that many deaths could have been avoided if enough medicine had been available.[8] In the years to come the missionaries spent a good deal of their time administering drugs, performing the ancient but not yet discredited therapy of bloodletting, seeing to the comfort and nutrition of the sick, and giving spiritual advice to the ill and dying. Medicines were dispensed without charge, administered either on systematic rounds of the homes of the sick or distributed from the mission itself, often at set times in the morning and evening.

Medical therapy in the first part of the nineteenth century relied heavily on drugs with a purgative or emetic action, and it was these drugs that the missionaries used most. Among the purgatives they ordered from London were jalap, colocynth, rhubarb, castor oil, Epsom salts (magnesium sulphate), calomel (mercurous chloride), and grey powder (mercury and chalk). Ipecacuanha, bluestone (copper sulphate), and tartar emetic (antimony potassium tartrate) were used as emetics. Opium-based analgesics found a place too: examples are paregoric (camphorated tincture of opium, used against diarrhoea) and opium tincture (opium powder and laudanum). Among other supplies were peppermint; alum; nitric acid; solutions and compounds of potassium, iodine, and arsenic; spirits of hartshorn (aqueous solution of ammonia); basilicon ointment (a resinous preparation); and opodeldoc (a soap liniment). Blistering materials (powders, plasters, and salves) were applied externally for internal disease.

There were never enough medicines to meet the needs of the missionaries and the island populations they sought to serve with these supplies. Furthermore, the missionaries were always acutely conscious of their lack of training for the medical work they found so necessary. Apart from George Gill, who was given some instruction before leaving London, and E.R.W. Krause, whose education had included some medical training at the University of Berlin,[9] the nineteenth-century Cook Islands missionaries were all self-taught, relying heavily on trial and error, accumulated experience, and books.

Preventive action was less prominent than curative work in missionary medicine, largely because this aspect of medical work in the western world was little developed until the latter part of the nineteenth century. In seeking to exclude foreign diseases the missionaries were handicapped by the very limited contemporary understanding of infective processes. They had some awareness of contagion, as Williams showed during the Rarotonga epidemic of 1830, when he 'did not think it prudent' to enter affected dwellings 'lest, by any means, I should convey the disease with me' to 'a new and populous group of islands [Samoa]'; he did not hesitate, however, to meet and talk with many of the victims in the open air, before sailing off to other islands.[10] From the medieval period onward Europeans had indeed developed the practice of quarantine without any clear knowledge of how infection was transmitted. This hazy recognition of contagion was responsible in the Cook Islands for occasional gestures towards limiting contact between the shore and ships with sick men on board. Smallpox vaccination, one of the first effective preventive measures developed by medical science, was employed by the missionaries on at least two occasions (1841 and 1867).[11] But until well into the nineteenth century they did not generally recognize that epidemic sickness originated in contact with visiting ships. On Rarotonga in 1830, Pitman found it 'was not an easy thing to persuade them' that ships did not bring disease.[12]

Although knowledge of ways by which new diseases entered a community was uncertain, there was even less knowledge of the role of environmental factors in the transmission of disease. It is not surprising that for many years the missionaries made few comments on prevailing practices of sanitation and few attempts to improve them. Admittedly their consistent efforts to alter the housing preferences of their flock were motivated by a belief that the new styles were healthier, and no doubt the people learned a certain amount from the mission households' own domestic example, but there appears to have been little or no specific instruction in these matters.

Not until the English sanitary reform movement (inspired to a large extent by pre-bacteriological objections to 'miasmatic' effluvia from an insanitary environment) got under way in the second half of the century, and the germ theory became widely accepted in the latter third of the century, did the missionaries in the Cook Islands begin to take a real interest in sanitary education. W.N. Lawrence, for instance, spent a good deal of his time in the late 1880s urging the people of Aitutaki to adopt healthier lifestyles.[13] The missionaries began to adopt the practice of conducting regular house-to-house tours of inspection. About 1870, James Chalmers and his wife began to make such rounds on Rarotonga, accompanied by the district pastor and his wife, with the aim of encouraging clean and tidy dwellings (as well as of engaging in spiritual discussion).[14] It is not stated where the idea originated, but it could well be that the mission was simply taking over the traditional custom of regular inspection of local agricultural activities by the *ariki* (chief).[15] Known as *tutaka*, these tours of inspection became a regular part of missionary practice. Pastoral care was often a reason for conducting *tutaka*, but recognition was increasingly made of their potential for encouraging clean-ups of houses and surroundings and providing the opportunity for sanitary advice and instruction.[16]

Giving attention to medical matters, especially on the curative side, was a service the missionaries were happy to provide. Having seen a medical need, they found it impossible to refuse to attempt to alleviate it, despite their consciousness of being poorly prepared for the task. Medical work was seen as a humanitarian adjunct to their real work; it was felt to be 'perfectly compatible with the higher duties of our station'.[17]

European medicine met with a mixed response. There appeared to be a readiness to try therapeutic innovations, and the missionaries were never short of patients. The people were able to assimilate something of the slowly developing European understanding of infective and environmental factors in disease. The Cook Islanders had long been aware of how foreign disease was imported, and their alertness was no doubt reinforced by the growing European recognition of the dangers of contagion. But it would be wrong to suppose that the missionaries were completely satisfied with their flock's attitude to medical treatment or environmental sanitation. The explanation is not merely a simple resistance to innovation, or, more positively, a continuing adherence to ancient attitudes and practices rooted in a strongly persisting Polynesian culture. It is plain that the new approach to sickness and its treatment was not as diametrically different from the ancient Polynesian approach as might appear at first sight.[18] Furthermore, the new remedies were seen eventually to be little more effective than the old. The missionaries were not expert in these treatments, but even in the hands of trained physicians early-nineteenth-century medicine could often avail little. Not until the century was nearly over were significant advances made in European therapeutic and preventive medicine, and few of these made much impact on missionary practice.

The advent of new medical technology had little effect on the diseases the Cook Islanders had long learned to live with. When disastrous new diseases arrived these, too, were scarcely touched by European medicine, and after the first traumatic decades the people learned to accept these also.

THE ADVENT OF COLONIAL GOVERNMENT

In 1888, in response to overtures from New Zealand, where aspirations for political power in the Pacific had long been expressed, a British Protectorate was established over the southern Cook Islands. In 1890, F.J. Moss, a former New Zealand parliamentarian and a man of wide Pacific experience, was sent to Rarotonga as British Resident. The British Governor in New Zealand believed that the 'principal if not the only interest' of the New Zealand Government in supplying and paying for the British Resident was to foster New Zealand's trade interests in the Cook Islands.[19] Certainly it was hoped in New Zealand that the export trade in fruit and copra could be built up and that there would be an increasingly profitable involvement of New Zealand firms in the group's economy. But the New Zealand Premier asserted that his country was also motivated by a concern to forestall French expansion and by a desire to enhance the welfare of the islands' inhabitants.[20] The Resident himself was indeed eager to promote social advancement: upon taking up his duties he told the chiefs and people that his object would be 'to aid you in governing justly and wisely for the promotion of your own welfare and the welfare of your children, and for the advancement in civilisation and prosperity of your fertile and beautiful islands'.[21] Although apprehensive that increased European settlement might be facilitated and that power might slip from the grasp of the ruling missionary-influenced chiefs, the missionaries acclaimed the Protectorate and expressed hopes that liquor control would be improved and that 'by wise legislation and tender regard for these weaker races' the new guardians would 'save our natives from otherwise speedy destruction'.[22]

During his term of office (1890–8), Moss endeavoured to guide the Islands' authorities in a federal system of responsible self-government, and to step up the pace of social and economic development. In 1898, however, he was replaced by W.E. Gudgeon, a forceful administrator with military and judicial experience among the New Zealand Maori. It was clear that changes were in the offing, and in 1900 the British Government agreed to the annexation of both the northern and southern groups by New Zealand. Gudgeon became Resident Commissioner. Once again the welfare of the Cook Islanders was stated to be a major consideration in the assumption of power by an external authority. New Zealand's good record in 'looking after native races' had long been advanced as an argument for closer control of the Pacific Islands,[23] and Seddon (the Premier) again told the Governor in 1900 that as well as preserving British imperial interests and New Zealand's commercial interests, annexation would ensure that 'the care and civilisation of the natives would be duly attended to'.[24]

From Gudgeon's appointment until the constitutional changes of 1946, executive control over legislation, justice, expenditure, and other aspects of government steadily increased. The administration of the group was effectively in the hands of successive Resident Commissioners appointed by and responsible to the New Zealand Government. European purchase or leasing of land never proved possible on a large scale, so a system of plantations worked by local labour never developed, and the population of European residents remained small. Care of the Cook Islanders' physical welfare was included in the responsibilities of the colonial administration, always as a benevolent and avowedly disinterested humanitarianism, but clearly also as part of New Zealand's hopes that an energetic, self-reliant and civilized people would participate in and contribute to the expected commercial development of the group.

A HEALTH SERVICE ESTABLISHED

In keeping with his own interest in Pacific culture and society, and with the New Zealand Government's professed desire to safeguard and enhance the welfare of its new Polynesian charges, Moss kept the matter of health and disease before him throughout his term of office. He shared the conventional belief that like other Pacific peoples the Cook Islanders were dying out, though he was not certain that the trend was continuing and on occasions expressed some hope that depopulation had ceased. He could see a number of reasons for population decline in the group, and felt that remedial action on a broad front (the encouragement of economic development and modern education as well as medical services) could and should be taken.[25]

After his first exploratory tour of the southern group in 1891, Moss felt that the government proposals attracting most interest were English-language schools, the exclusion of foreign disease, and the provision of hospitals.[26] His first priority was the improvement of the quarantine laws, and he quickly became convinced that existing curative and preventive medical services were inadequate. In 1893 he began to explore means of providing a doctor for Rarotonga, in the belief that a medical officer could deal with 'the large amount of disease' and might also, 'by instilling a knowledge of hygiene among the people, arrest the gradual decrease of the population'.[27] Within the next few years Moss was able to set up a government-supported private medical practice and a small hospital, both on Rarotonga. These particular arrangements were changed after an acrimonious wrangle among the official and commercial residents of Rarotonga, and Moss's successor Gudgeon was less hopeful that population decline could be arrested.[28] But a long-lasting pattern had been established: the colonial government would place considerable importance on providing a professionally qualified and hospital-based curative service available to European residents but understood (as the missionaries' medical activities had been) as primarily for the benefit of the Cook Islanders. This understanding was enshrined in the comprehensive Cook Islands Act (1915), which included clauses stating that government medical services were available for all persons, free of charge (again the missionary tradition) except for Europeans.[29]

After 1900, the government medical service was run by qualified doctors recruited in Great Britain, Australia, and New Zealand. Usually there were two such Medical Officers, one based on Rarotonga where the hospital was situated and the European population largest, and the other an Assistant who would make periodic visits to the outer islands to attend to their Polynesian populations. It was recognized that such visits were difficult to arrange and unsatisfactorily brief and superficial, and in fact the proper servicing of the outer islands by European doctors never proved feasible. Untrained volunteers (traders, missionaries, and government agents) assisted with dispensing, but eventually it was found that resident European nurses provided a better answer to the problem.[30] The first Island Nurse was appointed in 1918 to Aitutaki.

The idea of training Cook Islanders as medical workers among their own people was only slowly taken up, although it eventually led to an almost entirely locally staffed health service. Nurses were trained from 1917, and often stationed on the outer islands. A more ambitious approach to the employment of local people in the health service was later inaugurated by S.M. Lambert, an American doctor who directed the Rockefeller Foundation's health programmes in the Pacific. Lambert had been impressed by the Native Medical Practitioners (NMPs) trained by the Fiji Government since 1888, and in the 1920s was enthusiastically advocating the emulation of the Fiji system by other Pacific groups and the establishment of a central institution for their training. The production of carefully instructed Pacific Islanders who would be 'doctors' to all intents and purposes would 'cause a profound change in health conditions'. Lambert believed that here was 'the answer to many Pacific Island medical problems', especially in a far-flung group like the Cooks.[31]

The New Zealand administrators' response was very favourable,[32] and Cook Islands trainees were regularly sent to Suva (Fiji) after the reorganized Central Medical School opened its doors in 1928. Within the limits imposed by the relatively small number of NMP candidates sent to Suva in the succeeding decades, the occasional official inclination to undervalue their services, and the often inadequate facilities given them, the Medical Department was well served by its Suva-trained personnel. Quite apart from their appeal as indigenous practitioners, the NMPs could be paid much less and be far more flexibly deployed than European medical officers. They constituted a valuable answer to the dilemma of Outer Islands medical provision and formed the backbone of a health service that after the Second World War was to move more and more into the hands of Cook Islanders.

Although curative in emphasis, the government medical service was not entirely hospital-based. The Medical Officers made domiciliary visits on Rarotonga, and, particularly in the earlier years, visited the villages on stated days to be available for consultation. Later a more usual practice was to call in to houses displaying a piece of white cloth which denoted sickness within. In the late 1920s a district nursing programme was set up in the villages, in close co-operation with the women's child-welfare committees that flourished in these years. On the outer islands the work of nurses and NMPs was even less institutional in character.

Preventive and environmental health was recognized as part of the responsibility of the Administration and its Medical Officers, although the doctors varied in the degree of interest they displayed in matters not strictly clinical. A large part of the responsibility for the inspection and enforcement of public health fell to the Island Councils, village health committees, and *Au Vaine* (women's committees), and no initiatives in this field could be taken without the active co-operation of bodies such as these. The people participated willingly, for instance, in the ambitious programme of village 'soil sanitation' carried out in the 1930s to combat intestinal parasitism,[33] although the enthusiasm undoubtedly evident during the installation of the system was not carried over into its subsequent maintenance.

The medical service became increasingly expensive. As the number of staff grew, as the hospital expanded in size and sophistication, and as more costly therapeutic and preventive programmes were instituted, so the annual spending on health rose. Total expenditure reached £8,504 in 1926/7. The depression of the 1930s brought a cutback and then stagnation, but medical expenditure was growing again by the end of that decade. The rate of increase quickened after the War, so that the expenditure of 1944/5 was doubled in 1946/7 (to £25,295).[34] It was not to be expected that local revenue could keep pace with the increased cost of the medical service. The original intention had been that customs duties would support New Zealand's limited expenditure in the Cook Islands, but government revenue from this and other sources grew only slowly. The value of exports and imports did begin to rise significantly in the first decade of the century, and continued, with fluctuations during the First World War and the depression of the 1930s, to grow throughout the period, but the economic potential confidently seen in the late nineteenth century was never realized. Locally generated government revenue was soon overtaken by expenditure.[35]

Inevitably the burden of government services fell more and more heavily on New Zealand, and in this annual expenditure the costs of the medical service (together with those of the education system) were very prominent. In this context the long-expressed conviction that it was New Zealand's disinterested duty to provide health care was reiterated ever more forcefully. 'By the annexation of these Islands,' urged the Resident Commissioner in 1915, 'we have made ourselves responsible for the health of their Native inhabitants.'[36] The moral case for increased New Zealand aid for the group's educational and medical services was successfully pleaded in these years by Maui Pomare, the minister responsible for the Cook Islands, and in the 1930s the obligation of trusteeship and guardianship was an effective argument in the recommendation of his successor, Sir Apirana Ngata, that the financial outlay on these services should not be reduced to the extent that the economic depression seemed to demand.[37]

THE EFFECTIVENESS OF COLONIAL MEDICINE

The health service brought to the Cook Islanders in the twentieth century was not one they themselves designed or created. But they used it, and as time went on they provided more and more of its operational staff. It was clear, however, that western medicine was not utilized as fully as it might have been, and there sometimes appeared to be a curious resistance to self-evidently beneficial public health reforms. Furthermore, there remained a persistent adherence to the non-scientific Polynesian system of medicine that had its roots in pre-European days. There were many reasons for this, including the logistic inadequacy of the official medical service, the inability of some European medical personnel to inspire the people's confidence, the existence of cultural obstacles to full use of the hospital and other curative services, and a deep commitment to the superiority of 'Maori medicine' for certain conditions of ill health. Even the putative technological superiority of western medicine was in many ways an illusion. Evidence that it was superior accumulated only slowly. The treatment of yaws after the First World

War was the first spectacular demonstration of therapeutic efficacy, and the startling successes of penicillin and other antibiotics did not come until the end of the period. In their misgivings about the new system, the Cook Islanders were more than a little justified.

Viral infections

Infectious disease brought from outside, the cause of so much illness and mortality in the nineteenth century, was still a real risk thereafter. In keeping with the importance Europeans were giving to quarantine and reflecting a new awareness of the dangers faced by isolated populations, an attempt to exclude infections was the first strategy employed against disease in the group by the new governing authorities after 1888. Moss had seen to the institution of quarantine measures even before providing curative services,[38] and this approach was in harmony with the Cook Islanders' long-standing and well-founded awareness of how some of their diseases had arrived on their shores.

Quarantine measures were sometimes successful, sometimes not. They were first put into operation in 1898 against measles, which by then was recognized as very likely to do considerable damage among island populations. In subsequent influenza, chicken-pox, and whooping cough epidemics, considerable morbidity and mortality was experienced, indicating that port health procedures were either neglected or ineffectual. By the 1940s, however, the declining susceptibility of the Cook Islanders to viral infections, in the southern group at least, was approaching that of the population of Australia and New Zealand. Exposed comparatively frequently now to infectious diseases that a hundred years before had taken a great toll of life, most Cook Islands populations by the 1940s were immunologically well equipped and at risk only if very young, in a state of debilitation already, or given inadequate nursing.

Leprosy

In contrast to the declining destructiveness of introduced viral infections, another foreign disease established itself in the Cook Islands many years after the time of early European contacts and did its greatest damage in the twentieth century. Leprosy (Hansen's disease) was not widely known to exist in the group until 1890, although the infection had arrived some years before that. The first evidence of leprosy in the Cook Islands is found in W.W. Gill's report of a mission visit to the northern group in 1871.[39]

An early informal system of segregation in the northern group and later on Aitutaki was put on a firmer footing by the Administration shortly after 1900, but no therapy was available until after 1912 when Antileprol was first administered. Made from oil of chaulmoogra (a plant traditionally used in Indian and

Chinese medicine), the capsules were used after this as an oral medication when available, and were thought to be effective in some cases.[40] A further advance in treatment was brought by the Chief Medical Officer on his return from England in 1921. He and his staff began to administer injections of a chaulmoogra derivative (ethyl esters of the oil) to the patients on their various isolation islets. A distinct improvement was noted in some, but none was cured.[41] With indications of further spread it was increasingly being recognized that the problem of endemic leprosy was proving too much for the Cook Islands, and a new approach was rather suddenly taken in the mid-1920s: an agreement was reached with the Fiji Government that all Cook Islands leprosy cases and suspects should be admitted to the big leprosy establishment on the island of Makogai. In all, 280 Cook Islands cases were admitted to Makogai between 1926 and 1953, when it was decided not to send any more.

Chaulmoogra, the first leprosy treatment to have any effect at all, was the only curative possibility right through the period under study. It appeared to be only occasionally useful however, and was quickly abandoned after 1947 when the vastly superior sulphone drugs (especially Dapsone) became available. But an explosive outbreak on Aitutaki in the mid-1950s was to demonstrate anew the continuing gravity of the problem.[42] Before then, in the absence of an effective therapy and a precise knowledge of how the disease spread, and in a situation where finance and personnel were always in short supply, leprosy had proved an intractable problem indeed for those responsible for its control in the Cook Islands.

Tuberculosis

An even greater health problem than leprosy, and one evident much earlier, was tuberculosis. It is impossible to document its introduction, but the disease was inescapably prevalent by the late nineteenth century. A naval surgeon wrote in 1893 that tuberculosis was more prevalent on Rarotonga than in any other place he had visited, and was the principal cause of death there.[43] The precise extent of the infection in the Cook Islands could not be measured until scientific procedures (tuberculin testing and radiographical surveys) were developed towards the middle of the twentieth century, but the seriousness of the tuberculosis problem was officially recognized long before that. Even though medical science was beginning to come to grips with tuberculosis at the end of the nineteenth century, for many years yet the disease seemed scarcely amenable to treatment or control. Gestures were made towards isolation and treatment in the 1920s and 30s, but only in 1945 was a sanatorium opened. As a Wellington official commented, it was 'not unjust' that New Zealand should make a substantial grant for the project, since tuberculosis was an introduced disease.[44] The campaign against this infection had hardly begun by 1945, and many of the economic, social, and cultural factors in the prevalence and spread of the disease continued to operate, but a base had been set up for the subsequent struggle to control and defeat the insidious bacillus.

Intestinal parasitism

Infestation by worms was recognized as a Cook Islands health problem only in the late nineteenth century, although the whipworm (*Trichuris trichiura*) and hookworm (*Necator americanus*) had probably been brought in by the original Polynesian settlers.[45] *Ascaris lumbricoides*, a roundworm, was most likely introduced some time in the nineteenth century.[46] Surveys in the 1920s demonstrated the extent of worm infestation,[47] and a mass treatment programme for hookworm was begun at the instigation of Dr S.M. Lambert. Only a few years before in Fiji, he had pioneered the use of carbon tetrachloride (and later the even more effective tetrachlorethylene) as a replacement for the hazardous and vastly less effective oil of chenopodium previously used, and this is what was used in the Cook Islands.[48] Complete coverage of the population could not always be achieved, but with spasmodic treatments being offered, both to individuals and whole populations, and with the completion of a latrine installation programme in the southern group (1932–5), the life-cycles of intestinal parasites were disrupted to such an extent that an appreciable diminution in the infection rate for hookworm (if not for *Ascaris*) was soon observed. Pockets of hookworm infection remained, but nowhere were the infestations heavy, and it was clear that *Necator* was one disease agent that had been severely hindered in its activities before the end of the period.

Enteric diseases

Epidemics of acute enteric disease continued to occur in this period. Unsatisfactory water-supplies and sanitation were probably often implicated in outbreaks of dysentery and gastroenteritis. Typhoid fever and related salmonelloses were associated with a poor sanitary situation. But by the 1930s, TAB vaccine was available for preventive inoculation in times of danger, and typhoid cases had become less common by the end of the period.[49]

Yaws

An infection seriously afflicting the Cook Islanders long before the advent of Europeans greatly expanded their complement of diseases, yaws did not survive the middle of the twentieth century as a major medical problem. When the present century began, however, yaws was not only undefeated but also not even recognized as a disease in its own right. The condition identified by this name had long been known in Africa, Asia, and America, but very little was understood of its aetiology until the early twentieth century. Its existence in the Pacific was not recognized until the late nineteenth century, although because of the misidentification of yaws as 'syphilis', some indication of its prevalence was left in the historical record. Administrators and doctors continued to refer to the ravages of 'syphilis' until the First World War. Yaws was not identified until the arrival in 1912 of a new Assistant Medical Officer with Scottish postgraduate qualifications in tropical medicine.[50] After the war, medical opinion no longer clung to the identification of this endemic treponemal infection as venereal syphilis.

Recognition of the true identity of yaws changed many an attitude to the disease, but no new approaches in treatment were needed. 'Syphilis' in the Cook Islands had probably already been treated with neoarsphenamine, which Ehrlich had developed in 1912 from his 'salvarsan' of 1909. By the 1920s the neoarsphenamine treatment used for syphilis was available (in the form of intravenous NAB injections) for the large-scale treatment of yaws. The results were impressive, and systematic courses of injections were given on Rarotonga and on the outer islands when possible. After the development of Bicreol (a bismuth compound that could be injected intramuscularly), the net could be thrown much wider than with the expensive NAB injections. By 1926 the Administration could declare that yaws (except in tertiary cases) was no longer a serious problem.[51] But a continuing programme of NAB and Bicreol injections was annually reported in the 1930s and 40s. Although these metal injections were superseded after the Second World War by the more permanently effective and less toxic penicillin, yaws was well on the way to elimination even before the War.

Filariasis

Another important disease only tardily appreciated by European medicine was filariasis. Long present in the Cook Islands, although not well delineated in the documentary evidence for the group's past health conditions, this infection was scarcely recognized until the late nineteenth century. Nothing was understood of its aetiology or of its connection with elephantiasis. Only with the work of Wucherer in Brazil (1868), Lewis in India (1872), and Bancroft in Queensland (1878) was the role of the filarial worm and its larvae recognized; the mosquito was shown to be the vector by Manson in 1877.[52] It was not until 1911 that Manson-Bahr demonstrated the distinctiveness of the eastern Pacific vector, and even then much remained to be discovered about the aetiology and clinical nature of the disease. The first indication in the Cook Islands of any scientific interest in the disease and its vector is found in the reports of the new Assistant Medical Officer Maclurkin in 1912. Having read about Manson-Bahr's recent work on Fiji filariasis, and benefiting no doubt from his junior's up-to-date knowledge, the Chief Medical Officer (Baldwin) began attempting to convince the Administration and the people of the need for mosquito control.[53]

Quantitative study of filarial disease in the 1920s showed that the rate of infection was considerable.[54] In the inter-war years many filarial abscesses were dressed and treated, but no preventive therapy was known. Mosquito control operations were fitfully carried out. The affliction of many Second World War troops with filariasis stimulated a new scientific interest in the disease, and preventive measures were stepped up by the Cook Islands Administration after the war. It was clear later, however, that the more energetic control programme had resulted in little change in the prevalence of microfilaraemia and elephantiasis since the first study in 1925.[55] Vector control had proved very difficult, and European medicine made little impact on filariasis until Hetrazan (diethylcarbamazine) became available as a treatment in the 1950s.

Non-communicable and degenerative diseases

Some conditions left almost no trace even in twentieth-century Cook Islands historical evidence. Before the middle of the century no information was recorded about hypertension, coronary disease, or cancer. Later studies of obesity and hypertension[56] demonstrated their prevalence and supported the hypothesis that environmental factors were more important than genetic susceptibility. If the hypothesis is correct, the movement (observable on all the Cook Islands but varying in rapidity and extent) away from the ancient Polynesian subsistence diet and livelihood resulted in a much greater incidence of coronary and cerebrovascular and probably other degenerative disease among the mid-twentieth-century Cook Islanders than among their forebears. Contact with the outside world was of course partly responsible for this, but western medicine was ill-equipped to meet the need or even recognize it during most of the colonial period.

By the time of the First World War, extinction of the Cook Islanders was still sometimes predicted. Attention to the people's health was by then being proposed increasingly often, however, as the only means to their physical salvation. 'I believe they can be made healthy,' declared the Chief Medical Officer in 1912, 'and I desire to do what I can to preserve what I believe to be a race worth preserving.'[57] Only in 1916 did the census results bring forward a confident assertion that the population was 'holding its own' and 'no longer diminishing'.[58] By 1926 it could be proclaimed by the Minister (Pomare, who twenty years before had boldly written of having 'not the slightest doubt that, given fair opportunities for sanitary reforms and medical attendance, a few years' time will find the Natives healthy, prosperous and numerous'),[59] that the Cook Islanders were indeed 'healthy, increasing in numbers, happy and prosperous'.[60] From that time on there was no doubt that depopulation had ceased; in time, fears of overpopulation began to be expressed.

Population statistics for the early part of the twentieth century are not very reliable, but it seems that the group's Polynesian population nearly doubled within the first half of the century, from 8,173 in the 1902 census to 14,288 in the 1945 census, with an acceleration of annual growth after 1916 and a period of maximum growth between 1926 and 1936.[61] Analysis of fertility and mortality patterns and their role in population trends is limited by the poor quality of the data,[62] but the outlines of a falling death-rate and rising birth-rate can be charted. As the annual total of births and deaths drew apart, and in the absence of large-scale emigration until the very end of the period, the population of the Cook Islands increased. But it is not clear precisely how far the birth-rate rose above that of the pre-colonial period, or how much the death-rate declined.

Nor is there sufficient information for it to be known exactly what determined these trends. The official view in the 1930s was that the fall in mortality was due to New Zealand's provision of medical services and the successful onslaught on disease.[63] But better preventive and curative services cannot have been more than part of the reason for a declining death-rate. The waning susceptibility of the people to some of the infectious diseases that had affected them so savagely in the nineteenth century was surely an important factor in the decrease of mortality. But these and other diseases continued to flourish in the mid-century Cook Islands, bringing death to some of the people, disfigurement and disablement to others, and varyingly tolerable states of ill health to a great many more. Only a few of the many diseases old and new had successfully been denied their accustomed place in the Cook Islands' epidemiological picture by 1946, when over twelve decades of close European contact and five decades of colonial medical activity had passed.

CONCLUSION

New Zealand's motivation for establishing a colonial presence in the Cook Islands was largely commercial. But it was never possible to rule the islands without regard to the physical welfare of the indigenous inhabitants. Even in pre-colonial days, scarcely understanding their share in the unwitting culpability of the invading foreigners who had introduced dangerous new infections to a long-isolated population, the missionaries had established a tradition of humanitarian concern. After the advent of colonialism the new administrators and their policy-making superiors back in New Zealand felt a strong commitment to a benevolent guardianship of the people under their care. At this time there was little recognition that contact with the outside world had promoted changes in the people's lifestyle (for example in diet, settlement patterns, and modes of housing) that sometimes deleteriously affected their health. But, paternalistic and often uncomprehending though it was, this trusteeship included at times a recognition that the people must be directly involved in measures concerned with their health and welfare. This awareness reflected New Zealand's recent experience with Maori health reform and the continuing influence of Maori leaders who had participated in it before entering politics.

Unlike medical services in other more inhospitable colonies plagued by diseases dangerous to visitors and new residents, European medicine in the Cook Islands was never intended primarily for the foreign population. Nor was attention given to the indigenous people's health by New Zealand's colonial policy-makers principally as a financial investment. The idea of promoting a healthy island race in order to ensure the colony's greater profitability to New Zealand was not entirely absent, but it was never in the forefront. In fact the ever-increasing burden of providing a medical service was accepted as a government obligation even when the financial costs of running the colony seemed to outweigh the commercial value of New Zealand's relationship with the group.

It was only towards the end of New Zealand's formal colonial power in the Cook Islands that effective ways of combating many of the group's health problems became available. Until then, administrators and medical personnel were unable to do more than attempt to provide a hospital-based and treatment-oriented service, although efforts were made at times to extend the medical service into the community and to confront environmental and social factors in the prevalence of some diseases. With hindsight we can perceive the limitations of European medicine introduced into a non-European environment and culture. But it is just as clear that many of the assumptions and methods of European medicine, including the idea that the people's health was a government responsibility, became firmly established despite their limited effectiveness and restricted scope. Like other introduced aspects of western culture, they have lived on as strongly persisting features of post-colonial life in the Cook Islands. The many-faceted legacy of foreign contact and control is a reminder that colonialism is an elusive and complex phenomenon.

NOTES

1. In that year the Cook Islands became an internally self-governing territory in free association with New Zealand. Foreign relations and defence were retained as the responsibility of New Zealand, in consultation with the Cook Islands government.
2. For a survey of nineteenth-century Cook Islands history, see Richard Gilson, *The Cook Islands 1820–1950* (Wellington: Victoria University Press, 1980), 20–56.
3. John Williams, *A Narrative of Missionary Enterprises in the South Sea Islands* (London: John Snow, 1837), 83.
4. The phrase was used in commenting on the effectiveness of a medicine used by the mission, (London Missionary Society (hereafter LMS) Archives, South Seas Letters (hereafter SSL), Charles Pitman to LMS, 2 July and 17 August 1830), and in reporting a missionary's death on Raiatea (LMS Archives, *South Seas Journals* (hereafter *SSJ*), C. Barff and A. Buzacott, item 104, [1834?]. Items in the LMS Archives were consulted on microfilms held in the Hocken Library, University of Otago, Dunedin, New Zealand.
5. See R.T. Lange, 'Plagues and pestilence in Polynesia: the nineteenth century Cook Islands experience', *Bulletin of the History of Medicine, 58* (1984), 325–46.
6. Precision in nineteenth-century Cook Islands population statistics is not possible. For a detailed discussion see R.T. Lange, 'A history of health and ill-health in the Cook

Islands' (Unpublished PhD thesis, University of Otago, 1982), 24–6, 145–56, Appendix I.

7. The history of Cook Islands attitudes to health is further discussed in R.T. Lange, 'Changes in Rarotongan attitudes toward health and disease: historical factors in the development of a mid-twentieth-century understanding', *Pacific Studies, 10* (1) (1986), 29–53.

8. LMS Archives (SSL), Pitman to LMS, 6 November 1827; Journal of Charles Pitman (Hocken Library, Microfilm 184), 9 July 1927.

9. *LMS Archives* (SSL), G. Gill to LMS, 7 February 1846: SSL, Application Papers, Krause.

10. Williams, op. cit., n. 3 above, 282.

11. *LMS Archives* (SSL), W. Gill, returns for 1841: A. Buzacott, *Mission Life in the Islands of the Pacific* (London: John Snow, 1866), 108; SSL, W.W. Gill to LMS, 30 March 1867.

12. Pitman, *Journal*, 2 February 1830.

13. *LMS Archives* (SSL), Lawrence to LMS, 27 September and 30 November 1888.

14. *LMS Archives* South Seas Reports (SSR), Chalmers, 23 December 1872.

15. This is the view of Pupuke Robati and Leonie Martin, 'Tutaka in the Cooks', *South Pacific Bulletin, X* (1960), 53–5.

16. *LMS Archives* (SSL), Lawrence to LMS, 16 May 1887: SSR, G.A. Harris, 14 December 1888; SSL, Harris to LMS, 13 January 1891, 11 January 1892.

17. William Ellis, *Polynesian Researches*, 3 vols (London: Henry G. Bohn, rev. edn, 1859), vol. III, 44–6.

18. Further discussion of this point will be found in Margaret Mackenzie, 'Cultural and social aspects of pre-school children's health in Rarotonga, Cook Islands' (Unpublished PhD thesis, University of Chicago, 1973), ch. 3; Dorothy Shineberg, ' "He can but die": missionary medicine in pre-Christian Tonga', in Neil Gunson (ed.), *The Changing Pacific: Essays in Honour of H.E. Maude* (Melbourne: Oxford University Press, 1978), 285–96; Lange, op. cit., n.6 above, 169–81, 201–4.

19. New Zealand, *Appendices to the Journal of the House of Representatives* (hereafter *AJHR*), 1894, A-1, no. 21, 20. See also material in *Governor's Papers* (National Archives, Wellington), G.11/1. The advent of colonial government is described in W.P. Morrell, *Britain in the Pacific Islands* (London: Oxford University Press, 1960), 283–96; Gilson, op. cit., n. 2. above, 57–109.

20. *AJHR*, 1894, A-1A, no. 37, 3.

21. *AJHR*, 1891, A-3A, 2.

22. *LMS Archives* (SSL), Lawrence to LMS, 27 September, 30 November; Harris to LMS, 3 November; J.J.K. Hutchin to LMS, 15 November 1888; SSR. Lawrence, 2 January 1889.

23. Extract from *Fiji Times*, 21 July 1900, *AJHR*, 1900, A-3A, 1. See also Angus Ross, *New Zealand's Aspirations in the Pacific in the Nineteenth Century* (London: Oxford University Press, 1964).

24. Seddon to Ranfurly, 16 April 1900, *AJHR*, 1901, A-1, 6. See also *New Zealand Parliamentary Debates*, 114, 1900, 388–426.

25. *AJHR*, 1891, A-3, 20; 1892, A-3, 10, 35.

26. *AJHR*, 1891, A-3A, 3.

27. *AJHR*, 1894, A-1, no. 26, 25.

28. *AJHR*, 1902, A-3, 55.

29. Section 42 (1) and (2), Cook Islands Act, *Statutes of the Dominion of New Zealand*, 1915.

30. The experience of New Zealand with resident nurses in Maori districts was probably influential here. See R.T. Lange, 'The revival of a dying race: a study of Maori health reform, 1900–1918, and its nineteenth century background' (Unpublished MA thesis, University of Auckland, 1972), 237–40.

31. S.M. Lambert, 'Medical conditions in the South Pacific', *Medical Journal of Australia* (22 September 1928) (2), 363; *AJHR*, 1926, A-3, 32, 40. For Lambert's advocacy of the NMP system and his role in the establishment of the Central Medical School, see his *A Doctor in Paradise* (London: J.M. Dent, 1942).

32. It is noteworthy that the Chief Medical Officer in the Cook Islands (E.P. Ellison) and two of the New Zealand Cabinet Ministers directly involved (Maui Pomare and Apirana Ngata) all had a strong background in the Young Maori Party in New Zealand.

33. *AJHR*, 1932, A-3, 3; 1934, A-3, 5, 10; 1935, A-3, 3, 11, 12.

34. Expenditure doubled again by 1951/2 and again by 1957/8. By 1964, the eve of independence, it had reached £208,297. All statistics are from *AJHR*, 1900–64.

35. For commerce and government revenue, see Gilson, op. cit., n. 2 above, 79–82, 136–68, 186–91, Appendices 1–3.

36. *AJHR*, 1915, A-3, 7.

37. *AJHR*, 1932, A-3, 1–4; 1934, A-3, 3; Health Department Archives, National Archives, Wellington, correspondence between Secretary of Cook Islands Department, Minister for the Cook Islands, and Director-General of Health, August and September 1935, H.170/337 (11952). See also Gilson, op. cit., n. 2 above, 166–8.

38. *AJHR*, 1891, A-3, 36; 1891, A-3A, 6, 13, 19; 1892, A-3, 15.

39. *LMS Archives* (SSL), Gill to LMS, 18 August 1871.

40. Cook Islands Archives, Rarotonga, Cook Islands Administration file 258, Duncan to Resident Commissioner, 21 January 1914; file 252, Baldwin to Platts, 18 January 1916. See also papers on file 254/1.

41. Cook Islands Archives, file 6/1, Trotter to Resident Commissioner, 6 February 1921; *AJHR*, 1922, A-3, 9; 1923, A-3, 5; 1924, A-3, 5.

42. N.R. Sloan, *Leprosy in Western Samoa and the Cook Islands* (Noumea: South Pacific Commission, 1954).

43. O.W. Andrews, *AJHR*, 1894, A-3, 18, 19–20.

44. Cook Islands Archives, file 6/1/2, Acting Secretary to Minister, 1 June 1944, and other papers on the file.

45. Lambert, op. cit., n. 31 above, 373; P.A. Buxton, *Researches in Polynesia and Melanesia*, 2 vols (London: London School of Hygiene and Tropical Medicine, 1928), vol. II, 93.

46. Buxton, op. cit., n. 45 above; S.M. Lambert, 'Health survey of the Cook Islands, with special reference to hookworm disease', *AJHR*, 1926, A-3, 39.

47. *AJHR*, 1924, A-3, 5; 1925, A-3, 5; 1926, A-3, 36–39; A. McKenzie, 'Observations on filariasis, yaws, and intestinal helminthic infections in the Cook Islands', *Transactions of the Royal Society of Tropical Medicine and Hygiene, XIX* (1925), 144–5; Lambert, *A Doctor in Paradise*, n. 31 above, 266.

48. Lambert, *A Doctor in Paradise*, n. 31 above, 14, 140–50; *AJHR*, 1926, A-3, 7, 37–39.

49. Island Territories Archives, National Archives, Wellington, IT 101/1/11, E.P. Ellison Report, 1930–1; *AJHR*, 1932, A-3, 7; 1936, A-3, 4; 1937, A-3, 2; 1938, A-3, 3, 6; 1946, A-3, 16.

50. A.R. Maclurkin, *AJHR*, 1913, A-3, 23.

51. *AJHR*, 1926, A-3, 7, 34–35; 1927, A-3, 7.

52. Wesley W. Spink, *Infectious Diseases: Prevention and Treatment in the Nineteenth and Twentieth Centuries* (Minneapolis: University of Minnesota Press, 1978), 383–4.

53. *AJHR*, 1913, A-3, 23–26; Cook Islands Archives, file 258, Baldwin to MacCormick, 4 June 1912.

54. McKenzie, op. cit., n. 47 above; S.M. Lambert, *AJHR*, 1926, A-3, 34, 35.

55. D.D. McCarthy, 'Filariasis in the Cook Islands', *New Zealand Medical Journal, LVIII* (1959), 739.

56. Medical Research Council of New Zealand, *The Health of Two Groups of Cook Islands Maoris* (Wellington: Department of Health, 1966); Ian A.M. Prior, 'The price of civilization', *Nutrition Today* (1971), 2–11.

57. Baldwin, *AJHR*, 1912, A-3, 10. See also *AJHR*, 1911, A-3A, 11–12 (Stout); 1914, A-3, 29 (Maclurkin); 1915, A-3, 6 (Northcroft).

58. *AJHR*, 1917, A-3, 3.

59. *AJHR*, 1906, H-31, 69.

60. *AJHR*, 1926, A-3, 1.

61. See Appendix II in Lange, op. cit., n. 6 above. Population growth continued until the 1970s, the largest figure (21,323) being recorded in the 1971 census.

62. Analysis of some aspects of Cook Islands demographical data since 1890 will be found in P.H. Curson, 'Birth, death, and migration: elements of population change in Rarotonga 1890–1926', *New Zealand Geographer, XXIX* (1973), 51–65; Norma McArthur, *Island Populations of the Pacific* (Canberra: Australian National University Press, 1968), 191–230; Lange, op. cit., n. 6 above, 352–5.

63. *AJHR*, 1936, A-3, 2–3.

4

Medicine and German colonial expansion in the Pacific: the Caroline, Mariana, and Marshall Islands

Wolfgang U. Eckart

INTRODUCTION

Before 1920, Germany was in possession of a colonial empire in Africa, China, and in the southwestern Pacific covering in total an area of about 1,140,000 square miles. Its colonial population numbered just under 14 millions. Compared with the other colonial powers, Germany entered the 'scramble' for overseas possessions quite late, when she hoisted flags in her African territories, including Togo, the Cameroons, German East Africa, and German South-West Africa, in 1884/5. In Asia and in the Pacific, with the exception of New Guinea (which was annexed in 1884), she arrived even later. The Marshall Islands became German in October 1885; Kiau-chou, a small spot on the Chinese shore, was occupied in 1897; the Caroline and Mariana Islands were bought from Spain in 1899; and finally four Samoan Islands came into German possession following agreements with the United States in 1900.

The so-called German *Schutzgebiete* (Protectorates) in the Pacific were divided into two large administrative areas: the western included the northern part of New Guinea (*Kaiser-Wilhelmsland*), the Bismarck Archipelago, Bougainville and Buka, the Caroline, Marianne (except Guam), Palau, and the Marshall Islands. The eastern area was Polynesian, and included the Samoan Islands of Savaii, Upolu, Manono, and Apolima. This colonial empire in the Pacific covered an area of nearly 95,000 square miles, and at the outbreak of the First World War its population numbered more than 600,000, though its German population never exceeded 1,350. Seen from an economic perspective, Germany's Pacific possessions experienced a notable forward development; but this contributed principally to imperial profits, and the islands never became self-supporting. The main export commodities were copra, caoutchouc, and phosphate, which secured good prices on the international market.

As in Africa and China, the Treaty of Versailles in 1919 deprived the *Kaiserreich* of all its Pacific colonies, which were converted into 'mandated territories' and placed under the administration of the Allied Powers. Thus Nauru, with its valuable phosphate deposits, was placed under the administration of Great

Britain, Australia, and New Zealand; German New Guinea, the Bismarck Archipelago, and the Solomon Islands, under that of the Commonwealth of Australia; and German Samoa, under that of New Zealand; whilst German Pacific possessions north of the Equator were placed under Japanese mandate.

During and after the negotiations at the Versailles Peace Conference, Germany was denounced as a country unworthy of remaining a colonial power. Her 'failure in the domain of colonial civilization' was 'so evident that the Allied and Associated Powers' could 'not give her a second chance nor abandon thirteen or fourteen million natives once more to a fate from which the War had delivered them'. The objections of the German delegates to the Peace Conference were brushed away. In Germany this accusation was called the *Koloniale Schuldlüge* ('colonial guilt lie'), and until 1945 Germany defended herself against this accusation, referring especially to her colonial medical services and their contribution to the material well-being of Germany's Pacific islanders.

In considering whether this defence was well grounded, it is instructive to look at these medical services. Although much has been written on Germany's colonial activities in the Pacific, little is known about the particular medical dimension of these activities. This arises because many archives were destroyed or scattered during and after the two world wars. Another reason is the regrettable lack of German interest in the history of colonial medicine. Much work remains to be done reconstructing the imperial medical situation in the former German *Schutzgebiete* in Africa and in the Pacific. This paper cannot survey the medical system in all the German possessions[1] but, following an overall view of German imperial medical administration, it will focus instead on three examples of that administration in action — in the Caroline, Mariana, and Marshall Islands — and will discuss the characteristic aspects of German colonial medicine in the Pacific area.[2]

GERMAN IMPERIAL MEDICAL ADMINISTRATION

Between 1884 and 1914, exactly 510 German physicians were sent out to Germany's *Schutzgebiete* in Africa and in the Pacific, and to her Chinese *Pachtgebiet*, Kiau-chou. Most (380) served as *Stabsärzte* (surgeon-majors) in the colonial *Schutztruppe* (Protectorate troops) in Togo, the Cameroons, and *Deutsch-Südwestafrika*, or as *Marinestabsärzte* in Kiau-chou. Only 130 worked as *Kaiserliche Regierungsärzte* (government physicians) under the *Kolonialabteilung des Auswärtigen Amtes*, founded in 1890, and the *Reichskolonialamt* which succeeded the *Kolonialabteilung* in 1907. The establishment of the *Reichskolonialamt* was the result of a serious political crisis set off by the South-West African war (1904–7), and which led to new elections ('*Hottentotten-Wahlen*'), and to a change in the structure of Germany's central colonial administration.

It is extremely difficult to find biographical information about the colonial physicians, but most had a military background. Especially in Africa they were

Map 4.1 German positions in the Pacific Ocean

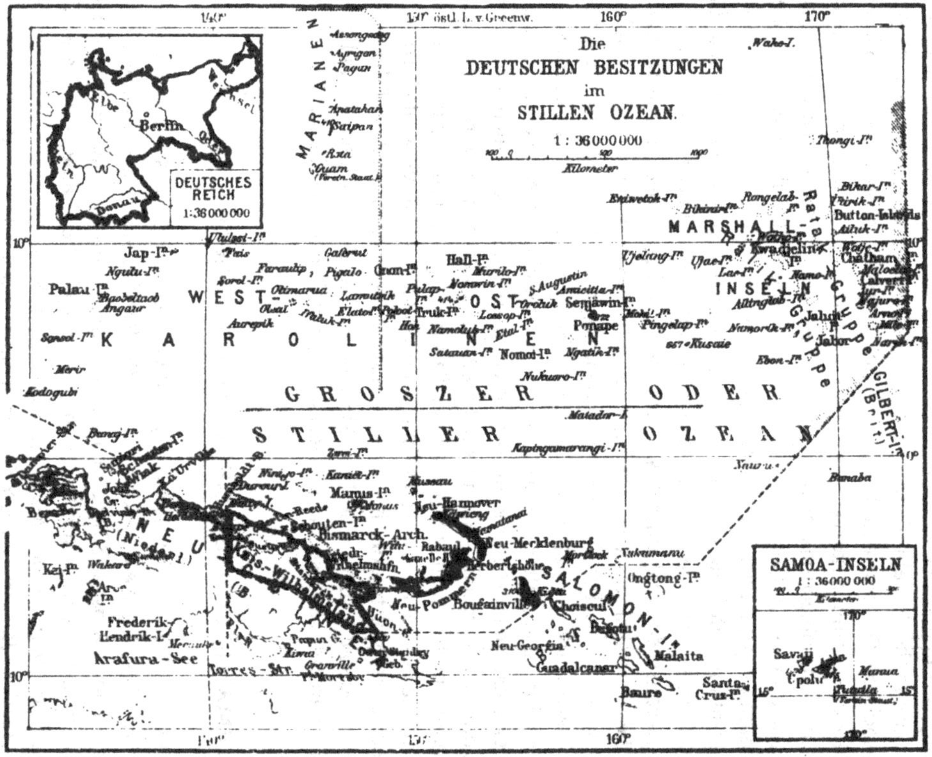

Source: Alwin Wünsche, *Die deutschen Kolonien*, Leipzig: R. Voigtländers Verlag, 1912: 234.

frequently transferred from the *Schutztruppe* and appointed to civil *Regierungsärzte*. In these cases the *Kommando der Schutztruppe* and the *Kolonialabteilung/ Reichskolonialamt* worked closely together. Each colonial physician, regardless of whether he was ordered to the *Schutzgebiete* as *Stabsarzt* or as *Regierungsarzt*, underwent a special training in tropical medicine which, before 1901, took place in the *Kaiserliches Gesundheitsamt* in Berlin. This required about two weeks and was organized by the *Medizinalreferat* (founded in 1899) of the *Oberkommando der Schutztruppe* or of the *Kolonialabteilung* in connection with the *Kaiserliches Gesundheitsamt*. After the foundation of the *Institut für Schiffs- und Tropenkrankheiten* in Hamburg in 1901, Germany's colonial physicians, whether in a civilian or a military capacity, had to be trained there in courses on tropical medicine by Bernhard Nocht, director of the Institute from 1901 to 1930. The courses in Hamburg took three months and concentrated especially on the 'classical' tropical diseases, such as malaria and sleeping sickness, but also gave training in conducting independent medical research into tropical diseases in general. Originally, the Hamburg institute had been designed in 1899 by Robert Koch and Paul Kohlstock, who was head of the medical department of the *Oberkommando der Schutztruppen* at that time. Koch and Kohlstock were planning to have the institute built in Berlin as a colonial medical school; but at the same time a similar project was already in the blueprint stage at Hamburg, where the *Senat der Hansestadt* wanted to build such an institution in the harbour area. Against Koch, Kohlstock, and the *Reichstag*, Hamburg finally succeeded with its plan. Parallel to the courses in Hamburg, colonial physicians could also participate in additional training programmes held by the *Reichsgesundheitsamt* and (since 1905) by the department of tropical diseases and tropical hygiene of the *Institut für Infektionskrankheiten (Robert Koch Institut)* in Berlin.[3]

In the *Schutzgebiete*, Germany's *Stabsärzte der Schutztruppe* were chiefly responsible for German and native military personnel; nevertheless, they could also be ordered to care for civilians, and especially for the colonial civil servants (*Kolonialbeamte*), but normally not for natives, except in German East Africa where most of the German physicians belonged to the *Schutztruppe*. Germany's *Regierungsärzte* were put under the command of the local *Medizinalreferat der Schutzgebietsverwaltung* and were immediately responsible to the colonial Governor. In no case did they form a 'race apart' but were closely integrated into the colonial establishment. They had to give quarterly sanitary reports to the Governor which, together with his comments, were sent to Berlin. *Regierungsärzte* were responsible for the government hospitals; they had to travel through the *Schutzgebiet* to organize vaccination campaigns and to give reports on the state of public health. They also had to accompany expeditions and were members of special *Seuchenkommissionen* which were occasionally installed to fight major epidemics. In Africa the German *Regierungsärzte*, especially military physicians, frequently circulated among different *Schutzgebiete*. In the Pacific we only find a 'micro'-circulation of that kind. Physicians circulated among different islands, but were never sent to Africa. Most of Germany's *Regierungsärzte* returned home during or after the First World War. But it is not clear whether they all returned. Some of them undoubtedly served as German *Stabsärzte* on the European or Near Eastern battlefields of the First World War. But some former colonial doctors were later found in the Hamburg *Institut für Schiffs- und Tropenkrankheiten*; some of them published colonial reminiscences and remained impenitent representatives of German colonial policy.[4]

Apart from a few officers, leading native *Polizeitruppen*, there were no German contingents of the *Schutztruppe* in the Pacific; thus we do not find German *Schutztruppenärzte*, but only civil *Regierungsärzte*. Between 1884 and 1914, a total of 32 of the 130 *Regierungsärzte* were sent to the Pacific, most of them to Kaiser-Wilhelmsland (German New Guinea). While in Kaiser-Wilhelmsland Germany's health policy can be compared to her colonial health policies in Africa, in the Carolines, the Marianas, and the Marshalls there were important differences. Because of the vast distances between islands, the German physicians were isolated and unable to provide all with equal medical care. Moreover, particular ethnic and economical factors arose which were to be of great significance to the history of German colonial medicine in these islands.

THE CAROLINE ISLANDS: A CHAIN OF MEDICAL FAILURES

Sold to Germany by Spain in 1899,[5] the Caroline Islands formed the largest German possession in the Pacific.Extending over nearly 2,000 miles, the Carolines included more than 900 islands, and (in 1900) about 35,000 native inhabitants.[6] Because of its vast extent, the Carolines had to be governed by western and eastern administrations, seated at Yap and Ponape respectively.

Some two years after the establishment of German administration, two *Kaiserliche Regierungsärzte* at a time were stationed in the archipelago — one on Yap, the other on Ponape. Both positions were filled continuously by German doctors (Table 4.1) to 1914, and the climatic as well as the sanitary conditions of the islands between 1899 and 1914[7] are documented in many reports to Berlin.

Table 4.1: German *Regierungsärzte* on the Caroline islands, 1901–1914

Western Carolines (Yap)		*Eastern Carolines (Ponape)*	
1902–7	Dr Born	1901–7	Dr Max Girschner
1907–10	Dr Buse	1907–9	Dr Paul Schnee
1910–11	Dr Mayer	1909–14	Dr Max Girschner
1911–14	Dr Buse		

Source: Medizinal-Berichte über die Deutschen Schutzgebiete, 1903/4–1911/12 (Berlin: Mittler & Sohn, 1905–15); *Reichs-Medicinal-Kalender für Deutschland, 1901–1914* (Leipzig; Georg Thieme, 1901–14).

Besides their duties in the old Spanish hospitals on Yap and Ponape, the *Regierungsärzte* travelled to the many islands regularly, but were not able to explore the whole territory medically and demographically, nor were they able to care for the total population adequately.[8] None the less, their medical reports give a clear idea of the major health hazards facing the native population, and especially of the alarming threat posed by epidemics. In Ponape, more than 2,000 people had died from dysentery, influenza, and smallpox under Spanish administration between 1843 and 1854. Under German administration on Tsis, Tobi, and Truk nearly 600 people died from imported epidemics between 1902 and 1909. One of these was a whooping-cough epidemic, brought to Tobi by the German research vessel *Peiho*; there more than 300 islanders died.[9]

Other threats were posed by natural disasters, for instance the typhoons of 1905 and 1907, which nearly destroyed whole stands of palm- and bread-trees in the Eastern Carolines. Not only the most important sector of the islands' economy, based on single-crop farming, but also the staple food of the native population was swept away. Famine and hundreds of cases of 'pseudo-beriberi' caused by malnutrition followed. In 1905, about 120 islanders died on Pingelap and Olol, and more than 200 on Satanan, Lukunor, and Etol in 1907. The colonial administration of the Eastern Carolines immediately initiated remedial measures, but also took political advantage of the islanders' distress by disarming them. At that time, Dr Max Girschner, *Regierungsarzt* of the Eastern Carolines, was also deputy *Bezirksamtmann* (District Senior Clerk).[10]

Another major health hazard confronting the native population arose from the reckless resettlements enforced by the colonial administration between 1905 and 1908. In 1905, more than 460 people from Pinegelap and Olol were deported to Saipan, Ponape, and Truk; two years later, 1,500 Mortlock islanders were brought to Ponape; and only one year later, 629 of them were sent from Ponape to Saipan. Under the cloak of an emergency measure, these resettlements were intended to put the islanders to regular work, and to deprive the local chiefs of their power by taking their subjects away from them. With the deportees, diseases were brought to new places. Thus, not only people but also epidemics travelled criss-cross through Micronesia. Dysentery ('*Ruhr*'), brought to the Mortlock islands by native police forces from New Guinea in 1906, was carried to Ponape in 1907, and to Saipan where it caused a big dysentery epidemic only one year later.[11]

Today it is very difficult to understand why Germany's colonial physicians never examined these factors when discussing the causes of the extinction of the native population in Germany's Pacific territories. Probably such reasoning could have lead only to a general critique of German colonial imperialism in the Pacific, and thereby to self-criticism that — at least for colonial officials — was unthinkable before 1914. At the time, Germany's *Regierungsärzte* had to look for other factors. Using Yap as an example for the whole archipelago, it is possible to see how they and other officials observed and interpreted what was called the *Aussterbe-Mechanismus*[12] (mechanism of extinction) of the native population of the Caroline Islands.

When German doctors began their medical services in the Carolines, there seemed to be no doubt that the native population of the Western Carolines, and Yap in particular, was declining rapidly.[13] As one ship's doctor, a Dr Sunder, who occasionally visited the islands, reported:

> Die Bevölkerung ist nach den Aufzeichnungen der spanischen Missionare, bestätigt durch zahlreiche verlassene Hausstätten und geringe Kinderzahl in stetigem Rückgang begriffen. Tuberkulose, Syphilis, Gonorrhoe wirken, unterstützt durch Sitten und sociale Verhältnisse, hin auf den Untergang der braunen Bevölkerung Yaps. Schade, wenn dieses nette, liebenswürdige, arbeitswillige, an Kultur hochstehende Völkchen in Kurzem nur noch der Vergangenheit angehören würde.[14]

This report was sent to *Bezirksamtmann* Arno Senfft (1864–1909), a typical imperial German government official. Senfft was born in Weimar, on 28 March 1864. After making his way up in the Saxon (*Großherzogtum Sachsen-Weimar*) and Württemberg (*KönigreichWürttemberg*) civil service, he, highly bemedalled, entered the German colonial service in 1899, and was ordered to hoist the *Kaiserreich*'s flag on the Caroline Islands. Together with the governor of German New Guinea he took possession of Sonsorol (6 March 1901), Merir, Pulo Ana (7 March 1901), Tobi, and Helen Reef (12 April 1901). Senfft became *Bezirksamtmann* of Yap in 1901. In 1907 he was entitled *Vizegouverneur* (Vice-Governor), and made himself a name as a political expert on Pacific affairs in the *Kolonialabteilung des Auswärtigen Amtes*. His most important articles on 'Germany in the Pacific' were published between 1903 and 1905. In 1909, Senfft travelled to Hong Kong, in an unknown capacity, and died there, of unknown causes, on 16 March 1909.[15]

Senfft must have been an ambitious and difficult superior, frequently holding opinions different from his experts. In explaining the declining population of Yap, he held other reasons responsible. In Senfft's opinion, the 'lax morals of the Yap' hindered reproduction and reduced fertility. But Senfft was hopeful that under the influence of German administration, and by the care of an experienced, philanthropic German physician, both lax morals and the public health could be improved.[16]

One year later, in 1902, a Dr Born, exactly the type of physician Senfft had been looking for, arrived on Yap. And indeed, Born's first medical report reflected the impetuous philanthropic enthusiasm that would motivate him for the next five years.[17] During these years, Born (about whom little is known) was not only government physician but also deputy *Bezirksamtmann*, and could combine medical expertise with political authority to win the allegiance of influential native chiefs. Born successfully demonstrated the effectiveness of his medicine *ad oculos*[18] of the chiefs, winning important support among the tribes, and instituted a programme of basic medical education. Each tribe had to delegate one young man to be instructed by the government physician; these men were then sent back to their tribes to establish small medical stations. Thus, Born supplied a large number of islands with a basic medical service, and could concentrate upon the larger problem, the decline in population.[19] Soon, Born found three major causes of this fatal fact: widespread prostitution, occurring in the meeting-houses (Bäwai) of each village; a large number of 'disgusting skin diseases', most of them in the genital region; and alcoholism, throughout the population.[20]

In his report to Berlin, Born elaborated upon these factors. The younger and good-looking women in the 'Bäwai-houses', being at the peak of their fertility, were careful not to become pregnant. Men preferred to have their sex lives in the Bäwai-houses rather than at home. Fewer children would be the inevitable consequence.[21] Of course this European explanation did not quite meet all the facts. One important fact omitted, was that the impressive number of syphilis infections (affecting about 50 per cent of the population) may well have been the main reason for sterility on a large scale.[22] This fact also underlay Born's second explanation: most of the 'disgusting skin diseases' were syphilitic or caused by other VD infections.[23] Born's third explanation might also have been well founded. Although the colonial administration had tried to fight alcoholism by strict prohibition,[24] the problem persisted. In all, the situation did not differ very much from that under the Spanish administration, which Born described with disgust:

> Ganze Ortschaften, Männer, Frauen, Kinder betrunken war . . . nichts Seltenes! Mord, Diebstahl, Brandstiftung im trunkenen Zustande waren an der Tagesordnung. Die Mütter fütterten die Kinder mit Schnaps; der Alkohol beherrschte die ganze Insel und die Bevölkerung nahm rapide ab.[25]

Table 4.2: Decline of population on Yap, 1900–1912

Year	*Counted population*		*Decline of population*
1900	7,464		– (= 0,00%)
1907	6,624		– 840 (= 11,20%)
1912	6,269		– 355 (= 5,30%)
Average:	6,785	(1907–1912)	– 595 (= 8,25%)

Source: Ludwig Külz, Zur Biologie und Pathologie des Nachwuchses bei den Naturvölkern der deutschen Schutzgebiete', *Beihefte zum Archiv für Schiffs- und Tropenhygiene, 23* (3) (1919), 118–20.

Although Born's explanations of the decline in population were obviously not correct in all details, most of his recommendations — viz. the reduction of prostitution, rewards for families with three or more children, a determined fight against infectious diseases, and the rigid enforcement of prohibition — carry conviction. Unfortunately, his campaign would require medical personnel and, of course, money. It is not surprising that neither the colonial Governor nor the *Kolonialabteilung des Auswärtigen Amtes* in Berlin granted the physician's demands. Enthusiastic about Germany's overwhelming successes in the field of bacteriology, the colonial department of the foreign ministry staked everything on this card — which meant neglecting everything other than bacteriology — and persuaded Born to do the same. During the following years a disappointed Born concentrated exclusively on the fight against infectious diseases, especially tuberculosis.[26] This he finally held responsible for the population's continuing decline between 1900 and 1907 (Table 4.2).

In 1907, Born left the archipelago. His successor, Dr Buse (again, about whom little is known), confirmed the importance of tuberculosis among other infectious diseases in his first medical report to Berlin:

> Bei den Japleuten ist die Vererbung der Tuberkulose von den Eltern auf die Kinder, die Übertragung durch Hausinfektion stets deutlich gewesen. Die Frage der starken Abnahme der Japbevölkerung scheint mir dahingehend beantwortet werden zu müssen, daß dem Tuberkelbazillus ein großer Teil zur Last fällt.[27]

Buse's attitude towards the decline in population did not change until 1914. A Dr J. Mayer, who was Dr Buse's locum tenens for a short time (1910/11), did not send detailed reports to Berlin. Thus, Born's multi-causal explanation and his programme of reform were buried indefinitely.

Late in 1913, the *Reichskolonialamt* sent a demographic expedition to its possessions in the Pacific, to establish reasons for population decline.[28] The results of this expedition, led by Dr Ludwig Külz, were not published until 1920 and appeared too late to change things in the Pacific under German rule. None the less, they completely confirmed Born's theories and recommendations.[29] In the meantime, however, the Carolines had been given to the Japanese. The 'careful service and maintenance' of the native population 'whose last hour had come' had been 'interrupted suddenly'; as Külz interpreted the situation: 'Die Japaner haben unser Erbe angetreten, und es ist kaum eine leise Hoffnung möglich, daß in dem mühsamen Fürsorgewerk die neuen Herren in den alten Bahnen der Deutschen wandeln werden.'[30] Of course, this presentiment (1919) was already part of post-war German colonial revisionism. The Japanese were to be accused of defectiveness in colonial administration even before they could install their administration in the Carolines. In fact, the islanders were not better off under the Japanese. The 'new masters' did not care for the health situation of the native population and concentrated upon Japanese settlements. In this sense, Külz was correct; the Japanese did not 'walk in the old paths laid down by the Germans' who had never thought of larger settlements in the islands. With regard to what Külz looked upon as the 'arduous welfare work' of the 'old masters' he was wrong; such had never been set up.

THE MARIANA ISLANDS: WOULD THE CHAMORROS DIE OUT?

The Marianas, or Ladrone Islands, form a chain of fifteen islands lying in the western Pacific between latitude 13°N. and 21°N., and longitude 144°E. and 146°E.; with a total land area of 450 square miles. The northern islands are volcanoes; the southern islands are extinct volcanoes covered with coral limestone. The islands were annexed by Spain in 1564, but a century passed before colonization was attempted. A period of ruthless wars against the natives (the Chamorro, a people of mixed Micronesian, Filipino and Spanish descent) followed. In 1898, after the Spanish-American war, the southernmost island, Guam, was ceded to America, and in 1899 the remaining islands were sold to Germany. Under German administration, copra, trepang, tortoiseshell, and nacre were exported to the mother country. A few weeks after Germany had taken over the islands, she established a *Bezirksamt* on Saipan, the main island of the group, to take up colonial administration. However, this post was never filled. From 1899 to 1906 the Marianas were administered by the *Bezirksamtmänner* of Ponape, Eastern Carolines (Dr Albert Hahl, 1899–1902; Viktor Berg, 1902–6); after 1906, together with the Palau Islands, they were administered by the *Bezirksamtmänner* of Yap, Western Carolines (Arno Senfft, 1899–1909; Rudolf Karolowa, 1909; Georg Fritz, 1909–10; Dr Hermann Kersting, 1910–11; Dr Baumert, 1911–14). In 1911 the total population of Saipan amounted to *c.* 2,500 natives, 22 Europeans (15 Germans, 7 Spaniards), and 38 Japanese.[31]

Undoubtedly, the Marianas were one of the most neglected groups of German islands in the Pacific; in 1906, they were economically still at a stage of a 'colonial experiment', with unproductive plantations, fierce typhoons, and a population that did not rise above 3,000 before 1914. It is not surprising that the absence of medical care during the first years of German administration was a true reflection of the islands' insignificance to colonial government. None the less, in 1900, the German *Bezirksamtmann* in the Eastern Carolines, Viktor Berg, alarmed by reports of a high morbidity among native workers, applied for a government physician for the Marianas, to be based in Saipan.[32] His petition was not accepted until 1909. In the meantime, the Marianas were visited only sporadically by German doctors. Continuous medical care was entrusted to an unskilled German male nurse. From 1903 to 1914 three German physicians visited the Marianas, but only two of them stayed there for more than a few months (Table 4.3).

The first German physician to reach Saipan on a tour was Dr Max Girschner, who was originally stationed as the government physician in Ponape, the capital of the Eastern Carolines. Girschner stayed in Saipan for only four months (26 October 1903–29 February 1904), but his report on the health of the indigenous population was alarming. He was especially shocked by the high infant mortality, mostly caused by navel infections, syphilis and infant framboesia.[33] A longer stay in the Marianas and an intensive educational campaign would have helped. But Girschner, in a hurry to leave these unpleasant islands, had his own methods. He tried to improve poor childbirth hygiene by arbitrary interference with the

Table 4.3: German Regierungsärzte on the Mariana Islands, 1903–1914

1903/4	Dr Max Girschner (visitation tour)
1905/6	Dr Max Girschner (visitation tours)
1909/11	Dr Paul Schnee
1912/14	Dr J. Mayer

Source: Medizinal-Berichte über die Deutschen Schutzgebiete, 1903/4–1911/12 (Berlin: Mittler & Sohn, 1905–1915); *Reichs-Medicinal-Kalender für Deutschland, 1901–1914* (Leipzig: Georg Thieme, 1901–14.

traditional system of midwifery. Old midwives were replaced by a small group of younger women, trained in the fundamentals of western obstetrics, and the German male nurse was ordered to be present at every delivery. Girschner then left the islands. There is no evidence that anything changed after his departure.[34]

A similar fate befell his attempt to cure the large number of people infected with syphilis or framboesia by the administration of potassium iodide and calomel. After a short time Girschner ran out of both drugs, and the condition of his patients was worse than it had been before.[35] A final link in the chain of his medical failures was the small island hospital Girschner opened on Saipan. This wooden construction had not a single glass window, and ether-narcosises and operations had to take place in semi-darkness because continuous winds forced the shutters closed. Under these conditions the sterilization of surgical instruments, to say nothing of microscopy, was impossible.[36]

The only successful colonial medical measure was a vaccination campaign against smallpox, carried out not by the government physician but by the male nurse on his own initiative between 1901 and 1905.[37] More than 1,500 people were vaccinated, and up to 1914, in contrast to other islands, no case of smallpox was reported on the Marianas.

After 1904 there were two other medical visitations to the Marianas (1905 and 1906), but these were confined to medical observation. Only a few notes on the results of these tours have ever been published. Even the colonial records in Berlin are silent. Obviously, the health of the Mariana Islands was not considered important enough to be documented.

It is therefore not clear, why, in 1909, a government physician was eventually stationed on Saipan. Dr Paul Schnee arrived on the island in July, and immediately demanded the reconstruction of the old, dilapidated hospital.[38] It is doubtful that his request was granted, because his first report from the island was also the last. Nevertheless, this report is interesting because it reflects the new European ideas of racial hygiene (*Rassenhygiene*) applied to the alarming reports of decreasing population in the colonial Pacific. In 1910, Schnee reported to Berlin that:

> Die Chamorros [major population on the Marianas] sind offenbar eine degenerierende Rasse. Wohl infolge der *Inzucht* werden die Kinder in der Weise kleiner, daß es sogar den Eingeborenen schon auffällt. Die Kinder sind dabei

> auch schlecht entwickelt, besonders die Knaben. Jene der Karoliner [there was always a small group of workers from the Carolines on the Marianas] machen einen kräftigeren Eindruck und entwickeln sich in der Pubertätszeit zu kräftigen Gestalten. . . . So erfreulich es an und für sich ist, daß hier viele Kinder geboren werden, so kann ich darin schließlich nur eine ungesunde Überproduktion erblicken, die durch Erschöpfung der Mütter wieder die Rasse schädigt. Leider verschmähen die geistig hochstehenden Chamorros eine Verbindung mit den kräftigen Karolinern durchaus.[39]

Although prompt measures should have been initiated by the *Regierungsarzt* to save the indigenous population from extinction, nothing happened. Instead, Dr Schnee lost himself in such a wealth of detailed exotic medical impressions of the Marianas that even the important facts of his report to Berlin were overlooked. In a counted population of 2855, there were 448 people suffering from grave eye diseases, 351 from framboesia, 160 from chronic skin diseases, and 180 from dysentery.[40] Thus, nearly 45 per cent of the population was seriously ill, a fact that should have alarmed Berlin. But Berlin did not react to this report in any way.

The last *Regierungsarzt* on the Marianas was Dr J. Mayer who had already served as government physician on the Carolines in 1910/11. Mayer's reports, assuming such were sent to Berlin, have never been published, and cannot be found in the files of the *Reichskolonialamt*. We know only his name and the fact that he was on the Marianas from the *Reichs-Medicinal-Kalender*. However, it is unlikely that things changed dramatically during the two years of his service on the Marianas.The 'degenerating race' on a group of Pacific islands so unimaginably far away from Germany, whose prosperity was repeatedly nipped in the bud by typhoons of the most severe kind, could not look forward to a concerned medical policy from its self-appointed mother country.

THE MARSHALL ISLANDS: A STORY OF COPRA AND LEPROSY

The Marshall Islands in the western Pacific, forming two chains from northwest to southeast, and comprising only thirty-two atolls with a total land area of 65 square miles, were Germany's smallest colonial territory.[41] In 1885 she annexed the islands, unclaimed to this date, making Jaluit atoll the administrative centre. Until 1906 the Marshalls remained an autonomous administrative district; after 1906, they were attached to the Governor of German New Guinea.[42] In general, the state of health on the Marshall Islands was similar to that on the neighbouring Marianas and Carolines. Periodical and dangerous waves of influenza, imported regularly by mail boats or merchant ships; dysentery, brought by Chinese workers; skin diseases, and, of course, syphilis, affected many. A few cases of leprosy could be quarantined and had no influence on the general health. Tuberculosis was rare.

From 1894 German government physicians were stationed on Jaluit and, after 1906, also on Nauru. On this latter island they also worked for the Pacific Phosphate Company, which maintained the only hospital on the island.[43] This fact, of course, was not without consequences: while, on Jaluit, medical care was free,[44] the native people of Nauru had to pay for it by an onerous copra tax (*Kopra-Steuer*) amounting to 15000 lbs per annum, which was nearly half the average crop of the smaller islands. This practice was not abolished until 1912.[45]

Table 4.4: German *Regierungsärzte* on the Marshall Islands, 1894–1912

Jaluit		*Nauru*	
1894–9	Dr Schwabe	1906–7	Dr Walbaum
1899–1903	Dr Bartels	1907–14	Dr Adolf Müller
1903–8	Dr Schwabe		
1908–9	Dr Liesegang		
1909–12	Dr Born		
1912–?	Dr Braunert		

Source: Medizinal-Berichte über die Deutschen Schutzgebiete, 1903/4–1911/12 (Berlin: Mittler & Sohn, 1905–1915); *Reichs-Medicinal-Kalender für Deutschland, 1901–1914* (Leipzig: Georg Thieme, 1901–14).

Between 1894 and 1914 a total of seven German *Regierungsärzte* were stationed in the Marshalls. Five of them worked on Jaluit, two on Nauru (Table 4.4). As one of the most remarkable government physicians of the Marshalls, Dr Born must be mentioned. We know him already from the Caroline Islands, from which he moved to Jaluit in 1907. In his new location, Born not only concentrated upon the health situation on the Marshalls; he also observed the British medical system on the neighbouring Gilbert and Ellice Islands, where Dr Alexander Robertson was working as a medical officer. There must have been good relations between Born and his British colleague. They visited each other frequently and it seems as if they were on friendly terms. Obviously, the health situation on the Gilbert and Ellice Islands was quite similar to that of the Marshalls. Robertson was especially confronted with a large number of cases of framboesia tropica, but only a few cases of leprosy and elephantiasis were reported; among the regularly imported 'European' diseases, tuberculosis, bronchitis, pneumonia, syphilis, and gonorrhoea were widespread. Robertson and Born undoubtedly exchanged experiences in the treatment of diseases, and in surgery. Once, Robertson was allowed to perform a difficult operation on one of Born's patients. The German *Regierungsarzt* was especially impressed by the medical education of Robertson's native assistants, whom he had observed during stays on Butari-tari and Tawara, where his colleague was responsible for the administration of two government hospitals. Robertson's assistants received their basic education at the British government school on Fiji. After their return to the Gilberts, they were trained medically by the government physician and then sent back to their home islands.

Encouraged by his experience of medical education on Yap, but also influenced by his British colleague's example, Born initiated a similar project of medical education on the Marshalls, thereby providing a great number of islands with basic medical care.[46] The foundation of the first hospital on Jaluit (1911) was his work, too.[47] In 1912 Born died of typhoid fever in the islands. His successor on Jaluit was a Dr Braunert, about whom, again, nothing is known but his name. In retrospect, Born's effect upon the native population was overshadowed by the influence of the most important chartered company in the islands, the Jaluit-Gesellschaft. In 1902, Irving M. Channon, sent to the Marshall Islands by the American Board of Commissioners for Foreign Missions in Massachusetts (the 'Boston Mission'), characterized the Jaluit-Gesellschaft as a 'soulless corporation', solely concerned with the exploitation of native and foreign workers. In his opinion, the colonial administration of the Marshall Islands was totally in the hands of the company.[48] Channon was perfectly accurate in describing the uncompromising capitalistic methods of exploitation — including increases in copra taxes and pay cuts at the same time — used by the company.[49] Four years earlier, Channon would have noticed that even this withering description was an understatement.

Around 1895, officials of the company and Dr Gustav Schwabe, one of Born's three predecessors (see Table 4.4), had discovered isolated cases of leprosy in the archipelago.[50] It seemed advisable to put those cases under quarantine on a small island. However, since most of the islands were owned and exploited by the Jaluit-Gesellschaft, the company would have been obliged to bear the cost of quarantine measures. So a plan was devised to shift all costs to the public. All islands were levied with additional leprosy copra taxes to amortize the worth of the island of Killi (fixed at 25,000 marks), which was so unproductive as to be chosen as a proper place for the quarantine ward.[51] All after-costs were to be shifted to the *Reich* by the 'generous donation' of the island to the colonial government.[52] The native population of the Marshall Islands would have been forced to meet substantial additonal taxes (see Table 4.5).

Each pound, the company calculated, would yield four *Pfennige*. Thus, the forced raising of the copra production would bring in an additional annual profit of about 11,450 marks, enough to amortize the 'worthless' island within two and a half years.[53] Soothing the outraged population of the archipelago would be the government's task:

> Der zur Durchführung dieser Maßregel zu erlassenden Verordnung sollte unserer Ansicht nach eine Einleitung vorausgesetzt werden, welche einerseits die Notwendigkeit der Isolierung andererseits die humane Fürsorge der Regierung betont, damit dadurch die bestehenden Vorurteile abgeschwächt und die Abneigung der Eingeborene thunlichst überwunden werde.[54]

Obviously, the *Kolonialabteilung* was sceptical about such a Greek gift.[55] But what could be done? The government physician, Dr Bartels at that time, was asked

Table 4.5: Additional leprosy copra taxes on the Marshall islands

Island	*Old copra tax* (lbs)	*Additional leprosy copra tax* (lbs)
Ebon	60,000	20,000
Namurik	25,000	9,000
Jaluit	30,000	16,000
Ailinglab and northern Raliks	40,000	16,000
Mille	40,000	10,000
Arno	50,000	16,000
Majeru	50,000	14,000
Maloelab and Aur	25,000	9,000
Mejit	10,000	2,500
Total:	320,000	112,500

Source Zentrales Staatsarchiv der DDR (GDR) Potsdam, R. Kol. Amt 10.10, no. 5784, Jaluit-Gesellschaft to *Kolonialabteilung des Auswärtigen Amtes*, Hamburg, 3 November 1898.

for an expert medical opinion. Bartels did not hesitate, and his opinion was scathing. Seen from the medical as well as from the political point of view, he wrote, the company's plan was impracticable. Neither regular medical visitations nor the nourishment of the sick on Killi would be possible:

> Wer aber soll für ihre Nahrung sorgen? Sie selbst sind nicht imstande, und noch viel weniger ihre schwer erkrankten Leidensgenossen, die Kokosnüsse von den Bäumen zu holen, von der Haut zu befreien und zu schaben, Fische zu fangen u.s.w. Soll nun eine Anzahl gesunder Kanaker zu diesem Zwecke mit isoliert werden, um ebenfalls lepros zu werden? Oder soll der Krankenwärter auf die Kokospalmen klettern? Das würde so ziemlich seine einzige Beschäftigung sein, die ihn vor dem Trunk oder dem Wahnsinn retten könnte; denn zur Pflege ist er theils entbehrlich, theils außerstande.[56]

An additional leprosy copra tax, Bartels wrote, would only increase the hostility of the natives against the colonial government. Once again, they would say, the Germans want to take more money from us than we are able to give. Instead of the company's plan, Bartels suggested the erection of a quarantine ward, surrounded by two barbed-wire obstacles, on Jaluit.[57] The government agreed. A camp of this kind was installed on Jaluit and remained until 1910. The old plan of a quarantine island was realized in 1911, but not by the Jaluit-Gesellschaft. Dr Born humanized the leprosy quarantine by isolating his patients on a small island near Jaluit, where he induced the government to finance a leprosy station.

Thus, the company was thwarted by the intervention of government physicians. None the less, up to 1914, the Jaluit-Gesellschaft would continue to be responsible for the bad health among native and foreign workers from China and Melanesia on Nauru, the phosphate island, for years to come. In 1905 the German Government granted a mining concession to the Jaluit-Gesellschaft to excavate phosphate on Nauru for ninety-four years; this concession was immediately transferred to the British Pacific Phosphate Company Ltd (PPC) which amalgamated with the Jaluit-Gesellschaft in 1906. The British company was allowed to keep its name and to appear independent, but it had to pay immense royalties to the Jaluit-Gesellschaft and was in fact an appendage of the German company, which was intent on being the only independent company on the Marshall Islands. Malnutrition and terrible hygienic conditions in the working camps of the Pacific Phosphate Company caused epidemics and many deaths year after year (Table 4.6).

Table 4.6: Epidemics among foreign and native workers on Nauru, 1908/9–1909/10

Epidemic	1908/9 fallen sick with	1908/9 died of	1909/10 fallen sick with	1909/10 died of
Beriberi	217	66	702	51
Dysentery	196	23	132	2
Typhus	30	7	1	1
Influenza	674	2	421	–
Total:	1117	98	1256	54

Source: Medizinal-Berichte über die Deutschen Schutzgebiete, 1908/9–1909/10 (Berlin: Mittler & Sohn, 1910/11).

In 1907, *Regierungsarzt* Dr Walbaum, who was stationed on Nauru after 1906 and also had to serve the company there, dared to air his grievances in a report to Berlin:

> Einer besonderen Besprechung bedürfen die Gesundheitsverhältnisse unter den Arbeitern der Pacific Phosphate Company. Dass sie seit der Ankunft der [chinesischen] Kulis von vornherein recht ungünstige waren, wurde bereits im letzten Berichte erwähnt. Zu einem Teile sind daran jedenfalls die äusseren Verhältnisse schuld. . . . Nachdem im Mai infolge polizeilichen Einschreitens ein Teil der verabreichten Nahrungsmittel als ekelhaft und gesundheitsschädlich von der Ausgabe ausgeschlossen ist, ist es bez. der Verpflegung vielleicht etwas besser geworden. Zu Wasch- und Trinkzwecken steht dem Gros der Arbeiter nur das minderwertige, brackige Wasser aus einigen Wasserlöchern zur Verfügung, und nur zum Kochen wird ihnen Regen-resp. Condensorwasser gegeben.[58]

Following this report, Dr Walbaum was immediately dismissed. It is not quite clear whether his dismissal was caused by his report, but one can suppose that this happened through the influence of the Pacific Phosphate Company. His successor, Dr Adolf Müller, did not dare to criticize the company again, and made only statistical reports. The last of these was published in 1911.[59]

CONCLUSION

It is difficult to draw general conclusions about Germany's medical service in the Pacific between 1885 and 1914 from the examples presented in this paper. Nevertheless, they shed light on some special problems Germany had in her distant Pacific *Schutzgebiete*.

Compared with Africa, very few physicians were sent to the Pacific. Such a small number could not hope to provide all islands with medical care, and were completely overwhelmed by work in areas they could visit frequently. The establishment of health services on Germany's Pacific islands was a function of committed *Regierungsärzte*. But adequate medical care could be supplied only with the help of native assistants, trained in medical education projects. Such attempts were made in Germany's *Schutzgebiete* in Africa, especially in Togo, the Cameroons, and in German East Africa. But more doctors and more money would have been needed to realize such projects in the Pacific, and these were not forthcoming. This unsatisfactory situation was mainly caused by Germany's lack of interest in her Pacific islands. This neglect derived from Bismarck's disregard for Pacific colonies; and the attitude did not change very much until 1914. Instead of building up a sufficient colonial infrastructure, including an adequate system of public health, Germany more or less relinquished her Pacific territories to chartered companies, especially to the Jaluit-Gesellschaft.

Although confronted by their capitalistic greed, the colonial government in Berlin was inactive. The companies' ruthless actions in Africa and in the Pacific were known and disliked. But the companies were needed for the exploitation of mineral resources and natural products because the *Kaiserreich* was not interested in financing such enterprises at her own expense. (During the first decade of the twentieth century Germany was much more interested in armaments, especially in making herself a respectable naval power.) In addition, the companies acted on their own initiative. Large areas and even whole groups of islands were owned by them. Judicially, these islands were part of the *Schutzgebiete*; in practice they were 'ruled' by the companies. They only looked to the 'use value' of their low-paid indigenous and Chinese labourers, and had no other interest in the islanders.

Nevertheless, the German *Regierungsärzte* tried to do what they could in providing the native population with medical care and protecting the company's workers against ruthless exploitation, but they were hopelessly outclassed by the unfamiliar conditions, traditional practices, and corporate profiteering. Unlike the companies, they took the islanders and their customs seriously but they had no preparation for such a difficult task, and no ethnological education in Berlin or Hamburg before being sent to the Pacific. At least Dr Born tried to compensate for this lack of experience through regular contacts with his British colleague on the Gilberts. But this was not a frequent phenomenon. Certainly, the *Reichskolonialamt* (colonial government) did not prevent such contacts if they seemed to be useful, but it disliked too close connections with rival European interests.

With Germany concentrating her energies upon the health situation in Africa (sleeping sickness, malaria) and in her 'malaria colony' of New Guinea, her Pacific islands and their medical problems were neglected completely. The so-called *Bevölkerungsrückgang* (population decline) evident on some of the islands was recognized by the *Regierungsärzte* and must have been by the colonial administration, too. However, Berlin did not send out demographic expeditions before 1913 and did not even organize regular censuses in the region. Thus, reasons for the decline could only be guessed. It is unlikely that the administrative situation would have changed dramatically after the 'Külz Expedition' in 1913, even if Germany had not lost her colonies.

As to the question of 'colonial guilt': at no time during Germany's colonial presence in the Carolines, the Marianas, or in the Marshalls was there an adequate system of public health. With an unsatisfactory state of health on most of the islands, with a dramatic decline in population which affected the whole region, and with the companies showing no respect for the dignity of man, the *Kaiserreich* gave up its good chance of establishing an adequate system of medical care. With reference to the Caroline, the Mariana, and the Marshall Islands under the *Kaiserreich*'s colonial administration, Germany's defence against the *Koloniale Schuldlüge* ('colonial guilt lie') turns out to be hollow revisionism.

At the outbreak of the First World War, contacts between the *Reichskolonialamt* and Germany's possessions in the Pacific were disrupted immediately. In most cases it is not known whether or how the colonial physicians left the area. Some colonial civil servants pretended to be Dutch and travelled back to Germany. Ludwig Külz, for instance, used this trick to get back to his mother country in 1915, where he was immediately sent to the Persian front with the German-Turkish 'Persian Mission' led by General Goltz-Pascha. He survived the war. Others may have also been lucky enough to get home from the Pacific, but probably only to die on the European battlefields of the First World War.

NOTES

This article would never have appeared without the great help and support of Professor Roy MacLeod. He kindly reviewed the manuscript several times, corrected many incorrect English expressions and straightened out some of my thinking. He translated the longer German quotations into contemporary English. I also have to thank the staff of the *Zentrales Staatsarchiv der Deutschen Demokratischen Republik* in Potstdam (GDR) which supplied me with manuscripts of German colonial physicians in the Pacific.

1. The best printed sources covering tropical matters in the German *Schutzgebiete* are the *Medizinal-Berichte über die Deutschen Schutzgebiete Deutsch-Ostafrika, Kamerun, Togo, Deutsch-Südwestafrika, -Neuguinea, Karolinen, Marshall-Inseln u. Samoa, 1903/04–1911/12* (Berlin: Mittler & Sohn, 1905–15) and the *Archiv für Schiffs- und Tropenhygiene*, published from 1897. The journal was financed by the *Deutsche Kolonial-Gesellschaft* (German Colonial Society) and an organ of the *Institut für Schiffs- und Tropenhrankheiten* in Hamburg. Although the *Deutsche Medizinische Wochenschrift* normally covered things other than tropical medicine, it also published important articles on this subject from time to time. Especially for the African situation it is also very useful to take note of German political colonial journals before 1914, as for instance the *Deutsche Kolonialzeitung* and the *Deutsches Kolonialblatt*.

2. Hanno Beck, *Germania in Pacifico, Der deutsche Anteil an der Erschließung des Pazifischen Beckens* (Mainz: Akademie der Wissenschaften und der Literatur, Steiner Verlag, 1970); Ernest S. Dodge, *Islands and Empires. Western Impact on the Pacific and East Asia* (London: University of Minnesota Press and Oxford University Press, 1976); Steward G. Firth, *New Guinea under the Germans* (Melbourne: University of Melbourne Press, 1982); Horst Gründer, *Geschichte der deutschen Kolonien* (Paderborn, Munich, Vienna, Zürich: Schöningh, 1985), 169–88; Peter J. Hempenstall, *Pacific Islanders under German Rule: A Study of the Meaning of Colonial Resistance* (Canberra: Australian National University Press, 1978); G. Kurt Johannsen and H.H. Kraft, *Germany's Colonial Problem* (London: Thornton Butterworth, 1937), 18–30; John A. Moses and Paul M. Kennedy (eds), *Germany in the Pacific and Far East, 1870–1914* (St Lucia: University of Queensland Press, 1977); Heinrich Schnee, *German Colonization -Past and Future: The Truth about the German Colonies* (London: Allen & Unwin, 1926); Philip Snow and Stefanie Waine, *The People from the Horizon. An Illustrated History of the Europeans among the South Sea Islanders* (Oxford: Phaidon, 1979).

3. Robert Koch and Paul Kohlstock, 'Gutachten über die Notwendigkeit eines Instituts für Tropenhygiene', *Münchener Medicinische Wochenschrift, 46* (1899), 501–2; Bernhard Nocht, 'Die Umgestaltung des Hamburger Seemanns-Krankenhauses zu einem Institut für Schiffs- und Tropenhygiene', *Deutsche Medizinische Wochenschrift, 26* (1900), 203–4; M. Otto, 'Das Seemanns-Krankenhaus und Institut für Schiffs- und Tropenkrankheiten zu Hamburg', *Archiv für Schiffs- und Tropenhygiene, 5* (1901), 239–44; Bernhard Nocht, 'Das neue Institut für Schiffs- und Tropenkrankheiten', *Beihefte zum Archiv für Schiffs- und Tropenhygiene, 18* (5), (1914) 10–25; Peter Mühlens, 'Forschungsarbeiten des Hamburger Tropeninstituts und ihre Bedeutung für die Medizin und Hygiene der warmen Länder', *Die Medizinische Welt, 8* (1934), 1384–7.

4. See Paul Kohlstock, 'Ueber die Dienstverhältnisse der in den deutschen Schutzgebieten beamteten Aerzte', *Deutsche Medizinische Wochenschrift, 25* (1899), 33–5; Hans Ziemann, 'Über die Errichtung von Tropeninstituten und die Gestaltung des ärztlichen Dienstes in den deutschen Schutzgebieten', *Beihefte zum Archiv für Schiffs- und Tropenhygiene, 13* (6) (1909), 46–54; Claus Schilling, 'Über den ärztlichen Dienst in den deutschen Schutzgebieten', ibid., 33–45; Emil Steudel, 'Der ärztliche Dienst in den deutschen Schutzgebieten', ibid., 17–31; Heinrich Werner, 'Die Organisation des Sanitätsdienstes in den ehemaligen deutschen Schutzgebieten vor und nach dem Weltkriege', *Deutsche Medizinische Wochenschrift, 64* (1938), 268–71, 309–13.

5. Otto Finsch, *Carolinen und Marianen* (Sammlung gemeinverständlicher wissenschaftlicher Vorträge, vol. 60) (Hamburg: Hamburgische Verlagsanstalt u. Druckerei, 1900); M. Friederichsen, *Die Karolinen* (Hamburg: L. Friederichsen, 1902); Hans-Ulrich Wehler, *Bismarck und der Imperialismus* (Cologne and Berlin: Kiepenheuer & Witsch, 1969), 400–7.

6. Johannsen and Kraft, op. cit., n. 2 above, 18.

7. 'Medizinal-Berichte' (über die deutschen Schutzgebiete) 1901/2 (=Anlage H zur

Denkschrift über die Entwicklung der Deutschen Schutzgebiete 1901/2), *Stenographische Berichte über die Verhandlungen des Reichstags*, vol. 196 (Berlin: J. Sittenfeld, 1903), 5503–37; 'Medizinal-Berichte' (über die deutschen Schutzgebiete) 1902/3 (=Anlage H zur Denkschrift über die Enwicklung der Deutschen Schutzgebiete 1902/3, ibid., vol. 205 (Berlin: J. Sittenfeld, 1904), 385–404; *Medizinal-Berichte über die Deutschen Schutzgebiete*, 1903/4–1911/12 (Berlin: Mittler & Sohn, 1905–15).

8. Buse, in *Medizinal-Berichte über die Deutschen Schutzgebiete* (Berlin: Mittler Sohn, 1910), 422.

9. *Zentrales Staatarchiv der Deutschen Demokratischen Republik Potsdam* (hereafter *ZStA* Potsdam), R. Kol. Amt 10.01, no. 5775; Girschner to *Kolonialabteilung des Auswärtigen Amtes*, Ponape, 1 January 1900; Buse, in *Medizinal-Berichte über die Deutschen Schutzgebiete 1909/10* (Berlin: Mittler & Sohn, 1911), 526.

10. See *Deutscher Kolonialatlas mit Jahrbuch* (Berlin: D. Reimer, 1906), 21; 'Denkschrift(en) über die Entwicklung der Deutschen Schutzgebiete', *Stenographische Berichte über die Verhandlungen des Reichstages 1905/6* and *1906/7*, vols 239 and 245 (Berlin: J. Sittenfeld, 1907 and 1908), 81–2 and 4117–19.

11. See Girschner, in *Medizinal-Berichte über die Deutschen Schutzgebiete 1906/7* Berlin: Mittler & Sohn, 1908), 251, and 'Denkschrift über die Entwicklung der Deutschen-Schutzgebiete 1908/9', *Stenographische Berichte über die Verhandlungen des Reichstages*, vol. 271 (Berlin: J. Sittenfeld, 1911), 927.

12. Ludwig Külz, 'Über das Aussterben der Naturvölker. I. Ursachen und Verlaufsformen unter besonderer Berücksichtigung der Eingeborenen in der deutschen Kolonien', *Archiv für Frauenkunde und Eugenetik, 5* (1919), 113–44; Ludwig Külz, 'Über das Aussterben der Naturvölker. II. Der Aussterbe- Mechanismus bei den Karolinern der Insel Jap', ibid., *6* (1920), 44–85; Ludwig Külz, 'Zur Biologie und Pathologie des Nachwuchses bei den Naturvölkern der deutschen Schutzgebiete', *Beihefte zum Archiv für Schiffs- und Tropenhygiene, 23* (3) (1919), 5–182, esp. 112–21.

13. Sunder had been asked by *Bezirksamtmann* Senfft to report about the state of health of the people on Yap because Senfft had noticed a strong decline of the population. *ZStA Potsdam*, R. Kol, Amt 10.01, no. 5732, Senfft to *Kolonialabteilung des Auswärtigen Amtes*, Yap, 2 June 1901. See also 'Denkschrift über die Entwicklung der Deutschen Schutzgebiete 1900/1', *Stenographische Berichte über die Verhandlungen des Reichstags*, vol. 193, (Berlin: J. Sittenfeld, 1902), 2949.

14. *ZStA Potsdam*, R. Kol. Amt 10.01, no. 5775, Sunder to Senfft, Yap. 12 April 1901: 'The population is in a state of constant decline according to the records of the Spanish missionaries and this is confirmed by the presence of numerous abandoned houses and the low number of children. Tuberculosis, syphilis, gonorrhoea, supported by customs and social circumstances, are bringing about the end of the brown population of Yap. It would be a pity if this nice, kind, and culturally advanced people who are also known for their willingness to work were before long to belong only to the past.'

15. For obituaries and more detailed biographies see: *Deutsches Kolonialblatt* (1914), 217; *Vossische Zeitung*, 1909, no. 17, II, Mittagsausgabe; *Geographen-Kalender*, (1910), 247; *Deutsche Rundschau für Geographie und Statistik, 31* (1910), 328; *Globus, 95* (1910), 161; Walther Hubatsch, *Die Schutzgebiete des Deutschen Reiches 1884–1920*, Excerpt from *Grundzug zur deutschen Verwaltungsgeschichte 1815–1945, 22* (Marburg/Lahn: J.G. Herder-Institut, 1984), 506–7, 535. Senfft must have been very successful in his posts before entering Germany's colonial service because he was highly bemedalled: among other things, he was bearer of the Großherzogtum Sächsischer Hausorden der Wachsamkeit, the Württembergischer Friedrichsorden, the Preussischer roter Adlerorden, 4 Klasse, and, interestingly enough, also bearer of the [Spanish] Amerikanischer Orden Isabellas der Katholischen. Senfft's most important articles on 'Germany in the Pacific' were: 'Die Marshall-Insulaner', in S.R. Steinmetz, *Rechtsverhältnisse von eingeborenen Völkern in*

Afrika und Ozeanien (Berlin: Mittler & Sohn, 1903), 425–55; 'Ethnographische Beiträge über die Karolineninsel Yap', *Petermanns Mitteilungen, 49* (1903), 49–60, 83–7, and 'Die Karolineninseln Oleai und Lamutrik', *Petermanns Mitteilungen, 51* (1905), 53- 7.

16. Senfft to *Kolonialabteilung des Auswärtigen Amtes*, op. cit., n. 13 above.

17. Born, in *Medizinal-Bericht, 1901/2*, n. 7 above, 5519–34.

18. ibid., 5520: 'Nachdem ich den Boden so vorbereitet hatte, begann ich die Insel zu bereisen.'

19. ibid.

20. Born, op. cit., n. 17 above, 5533–4.

21. ibid., 5533.

22. Külz, 'Aussterben II.', n. 12 above, 59.

23. ibid., 76.

24. This was combined with a deterioration in nutrition. The Spanish had paid for copra with brandy; this led to single-crop farming and thereby to one-sided nutrition. Stock-farming was unknown, and fishing was not practised; ibid., 80–3.

25. Born, Op. cit., n. 17 above, 5534; 'It was not unusual . . . to see entire villages drunk, men, women, [and] children. Murder, theft, [and] arson [committed] in a drunken state were the order of the day. The mothers fed their children with schnaps; alcohol ruled the entire island and the population declined rapidly.'

26. Born, in *Medizinal-Berichte über die Deutschen Schutzgebiete 1906/7* (Berlin: Mittler & Sohn, 1908), 239.

27. Buse, in *Medizinal-Berichte über die Deutschen Schutzgebiete 1908/9* (Berlin: Mittler & Sohn, 1910), 424: 'Amongst the people of Yap the transmission of tuberculosis from parents to children, the spreading through infection in the home, has always been evident. It seems to me that the question of the great decline in the Yap population must be answered to the effect that a great part of the responsibility for the problem falls upon the tuberculosis bacillus.'

28. *ZStA Potsdam*, R. Kol. Amt 10.01, no. 6047, Ärztliche Expedition der Professoren Dr. Leber und Dr. Külz nach Neu-Guinea (report to Kolonialabteilung des Auswärtigen Amtes, dated May 1914). See also Hans Fischer, *Die Hamburger Südsee-Expedition, über Ethnographie und Kolonialismus* (Frankfurt am Main: Syndikat, 1981).

29. Külz, 'Aussterben II.', n. 12 above, 44–85.

30. Külz, 'Biologie und Pathologie', n. 12 above, 119: 'The Japanese have come into our inheritance, and it is hardly possible to harbour the faint hope that in the [area of the] arduous welfare work the new masters will walk in the old paths [laid down by] the Germans'.

31. Hubatsch, *Die Schutzgebiete des Deutschen Reiches 1884–1920*, n. 15 above, 531–6.

32. 'Denkschrift über die Entwicklung der Deutschen Schutzgebiete 1899/1900', *Stenographische Berichte über die Verhandlungen des Reichstages*, vol. 189 (Berlin: J. Sittenfeld 1901), 1004: 'Der Gesundheitszustand in Rota (südliche Marianen) ist ein sehr schlechter, von 116 zur Arbeit verpflichteten Männern sind 22, d.h. 19 Prozent in Folge von Krankheit arbeitsunfähig. Auch auf Saypan und Tinian (nörlich von Rota) ist . . . der Gesundheitszustand ein wenig erfreulicher. Daher wurde die Hierherkunft des Kaiserlichen Regierungsarztes . . . beantragt.'

33. Girschner, 'Ärztlicher Bericht des auf den Ost-Karolinen stationierten Regierungsarztes über eine nach Saipan (Marianen) vom 26. Oktober 1903 bis 29. Februar 1904 ausgeführte Dienstreise', *Medizinal-Berichte über die Deutschen Schutzgebiete 1903/4* (Berlin: Mittler & Sohn 1905), 277–84, 277.

34. ibid., 277–9.

35. ibid., 279.

36. *Medizinal-Berichte über die Deutschen Schutzgebiete 1909/10* (Berlin: Mittler & Sohn, 1911), 557–9.

37. 'Denkschrift über die Entwicklung der Deutschen Schutzgebiete 1905/6,' *Stenographische Besichte über die Verhandlungen des Reichstages*, Vol. 239 (Berlin: J. Sittenfeld, 1907), 86.

38. *Medizinal-Berichte über die Deutschen Schutzgebiete* (Berlin: Mittler & Sohn, 1911), 558.

39. ibid., 560: 'The Chamorros [major population on the Marianas] are obviously a degenerating race. Probably as a result of inbreeding the children are becoming smaller in such a way that even the natives are already noticing it. As well the children are also poorly developed, especially the boys. Those of the Carolinians [there was always a small group of workers from the Carolines on the Marianas] appear stronger and develop a powerful build during puberty. . . As gratifying as it is in itself that many children are born here. I can ultimately only perceive an unhealthy overproduction in it, which is again detrimental to the race because of the exhaustion of the mothers. Unfortunately the intellectually advanced Chamorros absolutely scorn contact with the strong Carolinians.'

40. ibid., 569.

41. Hans-Ulrich Wehler, op. cit., n. 5 above, 407; Steward G. Firth, 'Die Bostoner Mission in den deutschen Marshall-Inseln', in Klaus J. Bade (ed.), *Imperialismus und Kolonialmission. Kaiserliches Deutschland und koloniales Imperium* (Wiesbaden: Steiner, 1982), 257–68; Jeschke (Captain of the *Kaiserliche Marine*), 'Bericht über die Marshall-Inseln', *Petermanns Mitteilungen, 52* (1906), 270–7; Wilhelm Treue, *Die Jaluit Gesellschaft auf den Marshall-Inseln 1887–1914. Ein Beitrag zur Kolonial- und Verwaltungsgeschichte in der Epoche des deutschen Kaiserreichs* (Berlin: Duncker & Humblot, 1976).

42. 'Denkschrift 1906/7,' n. 10 above, 4125.

43. Walbaum, in *Medizinal-Berichte über die Deutschen Schutzgebiete* 1908/9 (Berlin: Mittler & Sohn, 1910), 452 and *Medizinal-Berichte 1909/10*, (Berlin: Mittler & Sohn, 1911), 546.

44. *ZStA Potsdam*, R. Kol, Amt 10.01, no. 5738, Staatssekretär Dernburg to Kaiserliches Bezirksamt Jaluit, Berlin, 22 November 1908: 'Eine Bezahlung für ärztliche Behandlung durch die Eingeborenen selbst, welche . . . hierzu finanziell gar nicht in der Lage sind und auch früher hierfür eine Entschädigung nicht gezahlt haben, wird auch für die Folge wohl nicht in Frage kommen. Von einer solchen Bezahlung wird aber auch schon um deswillen abzusehen sein, weil andernfalls nach den bisher gemachten Erfahrungen die Eingeborenen sich abhalten lassen würden, den Arzt überhaupt in Anspruch zu nehmen.'

45. Walbaum, in *Medizinal-Berichte über die Deutschen Schutzgebiete 1906/7* (Berlin: Mittler & Sohn, 1908), 256; *ZStA Potsdam*, R. Kol. Amt 10.01, no. 5738, *Jaluit-Gesellschaft* to Dernburg, Nauru, 9 February 1910; Government Herbertshöhe [New Guinea] to *Kaiserliches Bezirksamt* Ponape, Herbertshöhe, April 1912.

46. Born, in *Medizinal-Berichte über die Deutschen Schutzgebiete 1910/11* (Berlin: Mittler & Sohn, 1913), 705, 715. More detailed information about Robertson's work can be found in his report on the health situation on the Gilbert and Ellice Islands in *The Journal of Tropical Medicine and Hygiene, 11* (2) (1908), (15 January 1908); this report was reviewed by B. Scheube, *Janus, 13* (1908), 309. For the health situation on the Gilbert and Ellice Islands see also *Gilbert and Ellice Island's Colony, Medical Officer, Medical and Sanitary Reports* (Suva, Fiji Islands, 1913/14).

47. Born, op. cit., n. 46 above, 703; see also Braunert, in *Medizinal-Berichte über die Deutschen Schutzgebeite* (Berlin: Mittler & Sohn, 1915), 597.

48. Firth, op. cit., n. 41 above, 265, Channon to Boston Mission, 2 June and 27 September, 1902.

49. This led to uprisings on Namorik and Mejit, ibid., 263–6.

50. *ZStA Postdam*, R. Kol. Amt 10.01, no. 5784, Schwabe to *Kolonialabteilung des Auswärtigen Amtes*, Jaluit, 31 December 1894; Bartels, 'Die Lepra auf den Marschall-Inseln' (letter published in the *Deutsche Medizinische Wochenschrift*, Jaluit, 25 June 1898),

Deutsche Medizinische Wochenschrift, 36 (1899), 12–15. On Lai, Arno, and Aur, six cases of leprosy were registered.

51. Bartels, ibid., 13.

52. *ZStA Potsdam*, R. Kol. Amt 10.01, no. 5784, Jaluit-Gesellschaft to *Kolonialabteilung des Auswärtigen Amtes*, Hamburg, 3 November 1898.

53. ibid.

54. ibid.: 'The ordinance which is to be passed to implement this rule should in our opinion be preceded by an introduction which stresses on the one hand the necessity of the isolation and the other the humane welfare work of the government, so that thereby existing prejudices are weakened and the aversion of the natives is overcome if possible.'

55. Marginal note of the *Kolonialabteilung* on the letter from the Jaluit-Gesellschaft (n. 52 above): 'Es scheint, als ob die J. Ges. die für sie nahezu wertlose [!] Insel Killi dem Reich aufhalsen [saddle with] will: "Times Danaos et dona ferentes".' (= 'Quidquid id est, timeo Danaos et dona ferentes', Vergil, *Aeneid*, II. 49).

56. *ZStA Potsdam*, R. Kol. Amt 10.01, no. 5784, Bartels to the *Landeshauptmann* of Jaluit, Jaluit, 1 May 1899: 'But who shall feed them? They themselves are not able to fetch the coconuts down from the trees, remove the shells and scrape out the pulp, to catch fish etc., and much less so are their fellow sufferers who are gravely ill. Shall a number of healthy Kanaks be isolated with them for this purpose [so that they may] become leprous, too? Or shall the orderly climb the coconut palms? That would be fairly much his only occupation which could save him from drink or insanity, because he is in part dispensable and in part unable to do anything to care [for the patients].'

57. ibid.

58. *ZStA Potsdam*, R. Kol. Amt 10.01, no. 5787, Walbaum to *Kolonialabteilung des Auswärtigen Amtes*, Nauru, 6 June 1907: 'The circumstances relating to the health of the workers of the Pacific Phosphate Company need particular discussion. That they were from the outset since the arrival of the [Chinese] coolies very unfavourable has already been mentioned in the last report. The external circumstances are at least in part responsible for that. . . . After a portion of the distributed food was held back from distribution following police intervention in May because it was disgusting and unhealthy, it has perhaps become a little better as far as provisions are concerned. For washing and drinking purposes only the poor quality, brackish water from some waterholes is available to the majority of the workers, and only for cooking are they given rainwater or condensed water.'

59. Müller, in *Medizinal-Berichte über die Deutschen Schutzgebiete 1909/11* (Berlin: Mittler & Sohn, 1911), 546–8.

5

French colonial medicine and colonial rule: Algeria and Indochina

Anne Marcovich

INTRODUCTION

Colonial history usually draws upon documents and reports written by those who witnessed the unfolding of events from the point of view of the dominant culture.[1] Such documents generally celebrate the victories of 'civilization over barbarism'[2] and in this respect the history of French colonization and of the development of colonial medicine is no exception. Triumphant rhetoric to the tune of 'To colonize is to civilize' could still find its way into print as late as 1955.[3]

In medical policy, France, more than any other nation, tended to legislate in the abstract. Programmes were created in terms of a preconceived order, and took little account (if any) of local cultural and political realities.[4] An example of this can be found in the centralizing tendency of the French administration which, faithful to what may be called a pure Jacobin tradition, insisted on the law being the same for all.[5]

Health care played a large role in the implementation of the French ideal of civilization. To partake of the bounty of civilization, the benefits of medical knowledge were often no more than a form of 'seduction' through 'medical diplomacy' declared Henri Salvandy, when, as Minister of Education, he discussed French policy in Algeria at a medical congress in 1845.[6] Conquering peoples by the spirit of justice and humanitarian intentions presupposed a considerable faith in the omnipotence of medicine.[7] As Frantz Fanon argues, in the colonies the doctor is an integral part of colonization, of domination, of exploitation.[8]

However, more prosaic motives may be discerned behind these high-sounding ideals. Many Europeans hoped, in fact, to protect themselves against epidemics by undertaking to heal diseased natives. Even though the 'contagionist' school of thought carried diminishing weight in French medical circles, it none the less maintained a dominant position in French medical practice. Furthermore, as any contact with illness was considered potentially dangerous, treating and protecting native populations was given priority also in order to guarantee and maintain a healthy and efficient workforce.

The history of French colonial medicine can be divided roughly into two periods: a pre-Pasteur and a post-Pasteur era. Medical and sanitary thinking was radically transformed by the Pasteur Institutes, which began in France and spread to the colonies, where they acted as centres for developing public health programmes and for fighting contagious diseases. The first colonial Pasteur Institute was opened in Saigon in 1891, and was soon followed by institutes in Constantinople (1892), Tunis (1893), Algiers (1894), Nha Trang (1895), Tangiers (1914), Hanoi (1922), and Tananarive in Senegal (1927). None of these superseded medical organizations already in place. These pre-existing organizations maintained their importance and even became responsible for a new medical thrust in the colonies in the 1880s,[9] heralding the upheavals caused by Pasteur's discoveries.

In the course of this article I will examine the spread of western medicine in Algeria, a country which was colonized between 1830 and 1848, and in Indochina, which was occupied in 1887.[10] The Algerian case permits a study of French colonial medicine over a relatively long span of time. As a consequence it becomes possible to see the long-term outcomes of decisions taken. It must be remembered that French Algeria was governed under an atypical administrative structure and that the French adopted a much more pronounced assimilationist policy in this colony. Despite these differences, however, solutions applied in Algeria may be considered faithfully to reflect events and policy in other colonies at the same time. The French government always ensured that a direct and centralized administration became operative in each colony and territory under a protectorate status. No matter how diverse the problems encountered in the different dominions of the French empire, they were all dealt with from the same point of view. Even in Indochina, French policy remained highly centralized and thus highly dependent on Paris. In the domain of public health, this policy was noticeably furthered by the founding of Pasteur Institutes. The Saigon Institute, followed by Nha Trang, and Hanoi, were responsible for the establishment of a powerful sanitary organization endowed with far-reaching medical research capabilities. In fact, no other colony could boast such an efficient network.

THE PRE-PASTEUR ERA: ALGERIA, 1830–1880

From the 1830s, medical intervention programmes in Algeria participated in the impetus of colonization, opening the door to the all-powerful civilizing influence of rational and scientific medicine.[11] Indeed, medical staff did not limit themselves to treating the sick or to preventive measures. Medicine was perceived as being the vector of a new civilization, able to transform mentalities and traditions by importing a new way of life.

Such a dream was probably the result of a deeply rooted hope that scientific development would some day solve the remaining problems of medical knowledge. The nineteenth century witnessed a massive development of medical research in France, particularly in theoretical fields. Anatomo-clinical work, pharmacology, physiology and especially neurophysiology developed new insights. Increasingly precise instruments were made to auscultate and examine patients.[12] Progress, however, remained elusive, where practical applications of new discoveries were limited.

What were the actual sanitary problems encountered by French doctors in Algeria? The medical reports which began to pour in after 1851 included fevers, smallpox, cholera or typhus, syphilis, ophthalmic and gall disorders.[13] Fevers (predominantly malaria) afflicted specific regions where they were both generalized and constant. Ophthalmic disorders and syphilis were even more widespread. Cholera killed thousands of people during epidemic outbreaks in 1849, 1850, and 1851. The virulence of cholera did not stop other epidemics, particularly smallpox, which seem to have been ever-present. It is, in fact, quite possible that smallpox did more damage than cholera. Furthermore, poverty, probably aggravated by the arrival of the 'Europeans', certainly weakened the population and exposed it to the spread of disease.

At the outset of the Algerian invasion, the French army availed itself of a large medical service.[14] The surgeons and doctors employed were far more numerous than those needed to take care of sick and wounded soldiers. Excessive personnel, and the medical infrastructure subsequently created by the army, clearly testifies to the larger intention of occupying conquered areas. Hardly had the army moved into an area than colonizers began to settle, with both hospitals and schools being planned. By 1832, a civil hospital was functioning in Algiers; there were two others in Oran, and one in Bône. In 1843 General Thomas Bugeaud, responsible for the French victory in Algeria, drew attention to the need for a regular medical service. Thanks to his lobbying, a medical service was attached to the administrative organization of the Algerian territory. In 1845 a decree called for the creation of colonial doctors whose task would be to take care of the Europeans, and in 1847 a public health service attached to the Arab Bureau was launched for the benefit of the natives.[15]

The military and civilian hospitals, originally intended for the European colonizers, were also open to the local population, but they were soon submerged by the requirements of the military and of European civilians. Furthermore, these institutions could only be viewed with mistrust by the local population, for whom both the European organization and the way of life was so foreign. It soon became obvious that the colonizing and civilizing mission of medicine would not be fulfilled by these hospitals.

In 1835, an itinerant medical service of French doctors was created to look after the Arab population. At the beginning, this service was not restricted to areas controlled by the army. The objective was, quite simply, 'to let them (the infirmaries) precede the army so that the population be controlled not only by military force but also be tied to the benefits of civilization'.[16] Such faith in the power of medicine was sustained by two certitudes: first, that European medicine rested on an irrefutable science; and second, that the Arab population had only to see this medicine at work to be converted. 'It is only . . . by practicing medicine and surgery . . . in the presence of these people, that the Arabs will gain confidence in consultations and remedies.'[17] With the exception of certain specific cases,[18] however, these certitudes were often contradicted. European medicine was often unconvincing, especially when it presented an image of poverty and decrepitude. Moreover, European medicine, which presented itself as scientific and rational, led to a deep misunderstanding which sometimes resulted in total rejection. For the native population, nothing could be more alien: the doctors' way of acting and of thinking, the hospitals, the curative techniques (surgery in particular), and also the cultural models used by the French doctors in dealing with the body, sickness and death. French doctors tried to diagnose the symptoms and precisely define the illness before prescribing treatments. For their Arab patients, sickness was associated with a series of extra-medical causes, and in particular, with the will of God. A medicine was a single entity to be used without distinction. Often Arab patients could not understand why the doctor did not prescribe enough medicine to cure all the family's ills. Sickness was not understood as a sequence of events whose evolution could help the doctor's diagnosis.[19] Often native patients saw the doctor only after the local doctor (*thébib*)[20] had failed, and thus sometimes too late for European therapeutics to work.

Such attitudes and behaviour produced two reactions amongst the French doctors in Algeria: a conciliatory approach and a radical one. The first was often associated with exemplary, isolated individuals who believed that medical help had to be 'created' by means of slowly teaching the native population to see their sicknesses and their bodies in unaccustomed ways. Dr E.L. Bertherand of the *Bureau Arabe* of Algiers (1848–55) thought, for example, that the Arabs had to learn a new way of being sick, and that doctors had to carry out what he called a 'moral graft'. Many doctors realised that any patient-oriented educational enterprise would take a long time to bear fruit, and that the only way was to let the native population decide of its own accord to seek out medical attention which, it must be pointed out, was offered free of charge. Generally speaking, it is in this category of doctors that one finds those most willing to collaborate with the *thébibs*, and to recognize that some remedies of traditional practitioners could be more efficacious than the sulphur, antimony, henna, and honey used by European doctors. Amongst these European doctors, some went so far as to incorporate a magical approach if a specific situation warranted it.

The 'radical' response was nothing less than the expression of colonial domination, and as such was a collective phenomenon. This reaction was at the root of procedures which tended to put European ideas and cultural/political institutions into practice, mostly without adaptation. For a long time it was not deemed necessary to introduce structures to reduce the 'culture shock' created in Algeria. Voices calling for the training of Arab doctors were not raised until 1855, and even then such advice was mainly adopted to help out the European doctors whose numbers were insufficient to meet the needs of the colony. In any case, a school for training Arab doctors was not opened until 1875.

While most visible in the domain of therapeutic practice, the implementation and imposition of the European medical order left a far deeper mark upon the domain of preventive medicine. It is well known that the hygienist school held an important position in French medical thought, and it was through this lens that the European doctors assessed the situation in Algeria. This theoretical framework was also used to try to understand, as well as to prevent, the many sicknesses afflicting the European community in Algeria — sicknesses which posed much less of a problem in Europe. Thus, European doctors searched for the causes of illnesses in mephitic miasma, the winds, the humidity — generally speaking, in the environment. Countermeasures were adopted in order to purify the air and clean up inhabited areas so as to curtail agents responsible for fevers and epidemics.[21] Garbage dumps were removed, cesspools were dried up and trees were planted to protect the European quarters from the dangerous winds which allegedly carried illness.

Such activities partially screened the popular notion that Arabs were better suited to live in given places than Europeans. Natives seemed to be genetically adapted. Racial ideas current in Europe found 'scientific' confirmation in the observations made by colonial Europeans.[22] Moreover, by manipulating the environment, European colonizers began to impose a new way of living — 'hygienic measures' became instruments for the imposition of a European cultural order on the native population. Whether they were considered to be directly or indirectly responsible, the Arab way of life, their habits and even their very culture were accused of causing epidemics. Cleaning and purifying the air and environment created 'healthy' areas for Europeans — and also paved the way for uprooting local culture and for imposing new rules of social interaction.[23]

The Arab population sometimes accepted a few curative health techniques but rejected attempts at prevention. Such refusal was particularly apparent in the smallpox vaccination campaign.[24] Protective techniques had not as yet become a socially accepted procedure even in France,[25] but smallpox was endemic in Algeria, and vaccination was a necessity for the survival of the Europeans.[26] Although vaccination was a personal measure, it was also a protective measure for the population as a whole. As I have argued elsewhere,[27] the success of the smallpox vaccination campaigns rested upon the fact that although they were not compulsory, they were nevertheless well organized by the centralized bureaucracy. In fulfilling these primary conditions in Algeria, however, the programme became a threat to the cultural integrity of the native population, especially as the price paid was a form of coercive assimilation by a foreign cultural element.

In a sense, the Arab population understood what was at stake. Rumours orchestrated by the political and religious authorities warned against vaccination, which would mix the blood of the occupied and the occupiers. As a result, it was thought that all kinds of hybrids could be produced and all kinds of contaminations would be brought about. In some cases it was rumoured that the real intention was not to vaccinate but rather to kidnap children, and submit the boys to a second circumcision.[28]

In all cases, it became apparent that what was at stake was cultural, religious or even 'racial' alienation. In fact, Arab refusal was not strictly a medical issue but rather a form of resistance aimed at the French, since it was felt that each occasion for submission constituted a danger to the integrity of the Muslim nation. In trying to prevent a collective invasion, the 'body' under treatment became Arab society as a whole. The smallpox vaccinations in Algeria were far more than a preventive technique; rather it was more a collective operation which grouped Europeans and Arabs together under the same law.

As time passed, the issue became less sensitive. Often the French did not insist on imposing vaccination procedures, in part because the vaccines were not always of the best quality. In all probability this attitude helped to stop the alarmist rumours which had circulated initially. To a certain extent, the Arab population also grew familiar with the idea. By 1863 the principle of vaccination had become accepted, and this coincided with the emergence of the first Arab doctors who began to administer smallpox vaccine themselves.

By the 1870s the colonization of Algeria had moved into a new phase in which both the French army and the Algerian resistance were less prone to military operations.[29] Within the next two decades (when the borders of French Algeria became fixed), it was obvious that medical and sanitary organization was necessary. This required funds, materials, and personnel. Compared to the beginning of French involvement in Algeria, this second period saw the abandonment of some early goals. The ideal of meeting the medical needs of the entire Arab population and even the tribal minorities, free of charge, implied vast financial and material resources. It soon became evident that this policy was too ambitious. The physical distances involved were enormous and doctors had neither the money nor the horses to undertake long journeys. The medical staff suffered a chronic lack of basic necessities, including surgical instruments and medicines. Years went by before the smallpox vaccine arrived. In 1866 the medical staff in Algeria received instructions to stop the distribution of free medicines as no money was available for replenishing stocks. Still worse was the shortage of doctors. Many of the French doctors in Algeria were, in fact, nothing more than sanitary officers, trained only for three years; and many were military men, or civilians unable to find jobs in France.[30] Generally speaking, French doctors working in France were unwilling to become expatriates, and as a consequence, the medical staff in Algeria was not easily renewed.

In 1845, it was decided that French doctors should also serve the Arab population. However, by 1850 it was apparent that they could not even handle the Europeans living in Algeria. The health service to the non-Europeans suffered accordingly. 'The Arab population is being deprived of medical attention' was a recurrent comment in contemporary reports. The outlying districts were the first to be abandoned. A report written in 1863 stated that 'the medical service is not being organized by the *Bureau arabe* since it cannot be said that there is a regular service when a doctor shows up from time to time at the burial of a cadaver'.[31]

European doctors wished to be both systematic and complete in their approach to illness. In the period preceding the Pasteur revolution, however, they had limited therapeutic and preventive means at their disposal, which could not be applied in an organized and continuous fashion on a large scale. Individual care could not be generalized, against a persisting lack of financial, human, and material means which could not be found locally and had to be imported from France.

The ambitious outlook of French colonial medicine in Algeria can be said to have produced nothing more than a mediocre result. The means at hand in no way measured up to the goals that had been set. Only the medical revolution brought about by the discoveries of Pasteur could fill the gap revealed by the 'Algerian experience'.

PASTEUR AND THE TURNING POINT: INDOCHINA, 1891–1930

Pasteur's work infused colonial medicine with a new dynamism. The medical and sanitary ideas produced by this breakthrough, along with its political and ideological implications, brought about an important break with the past.[32] The bacteriological discoveries of Koch, Yersin, Kitasato, and Ehrlich, and the use of vaccines and serum, put powerful tools into the hands of doctors, tools which gave them an unlimited confidence in their art, a phenomenon not unlike that observed amongst the revolutionary doctors of the eighteenth century. New insights gained in the field of infectious diseases complemented the physiological discoveries made in the course of the nineteenth century. The human body came to be seen as being governed by independent mechanisms which could be considered in isolation. The contagionist theory, which antedated Pasteur, saw the causes of disease and epidemics as being varied and undefined, involving alimentary and hygienic habits, as well as social and natural factors that could not be defined. Pasteur's discoveries brought about an almost total abandonment of 'cultural culprits'. As a consequence, the culture of colonized peoples was no longer seen as a danger and, to a certain extent, was even discounted as an interesting entity. Man could only be seen as a biological factor. A basic idea began to develop: that once nature had been mastered on a global level, western scientific culture would inevitably be adopted everywhere and by all. The struggle to dominate nature was therefore transformed into an instrument of colonization, of economic growth and of new possibilities for settlement. The power able to stop a sickness from spreading or which could resolve a sanitary problem would be able to impose its domination all the more easily and would therefore be able to exploit the wealth of occupied territories.[33]

It is probably due to these economic and political issues that scientific competition developed between different countries to the extent of becoming a motor for political rivalry.[34]

Research was highly diversified. It focused on diseases such as bubonic plague, typhus, typhoid fever, and also on non-contagious diseases such as cancer and beriberi as well as various types of snake venoms.[35] But the main research programmes were those which worked on rabies, malaria, smallpox, cholera, endemic and epidemic intestinal sicknesses, and amoebic and bacterial dysentery. The incidence of these sicknesses was high for both European and native populations. Their medical solution was an absolute necessity for the stability of French control in the colonies.[36]

The approach adopted by the Pasteurians was always the same. The first step consisted in carrying out field observations of a disease, observing its progress, differentiating it from other diseases that might be similar, isolating the agent, and determining the type of transmission and the sequence. At this point work began on a serum, and then on the vaccine. Such research showed a continuous pendulum movement between laboratory and field observation which narrowed the gap between the exterior (natural) environment and the interior (artificial) environment of the laboratory.[37] Fundamental new ideas were born in the process. Beyond the search for a given bacillus or virus developed a new conception which saw these agents as living organisms requiring specific conditions in order to live and reproduce.[38] Once this was understood, the next step was to undertake controlled laboratory reproduction. It is this sequence of events, as well as the search for a micro-organism as the cause of illness, that constituted the basis of Pasteur's contribution to medicine.

The discovery of the bacillus responsible for the bubonic plague illustrates how such research was done, and at the same time shows how international scientific competition, prompted by the colonial powers, left its mark upon the vast new field of epidemic diseases. The nineteenth century witnessed a progressive spread of bubonic plague from the southern provinces of China towards Canton. Hong Kong and Amoy were hit in 1894, and the progression of the disease soon threatened Indochina as well. The French government in the Metropole requested the Indochinese colonial government to send a medical and scientific team to study the plague. Alexandre E.J.Yersin (1863–1943), a student of Pasteur and collatorator of Emile P.P. Roux(1855–1933), had been in Indochina only one year when he was sent to Hong Kong, where the sickness seemed to be particularly virulent.

Arriving in June 1894, Yersin found that his was not the only team studying the phenomenon. A Japanese group led by Professor Shiba Saburo Kitasato (1852–1932) had already started work in the British colony. Between these two teams a strong rivalry developed, encouraged by the British government, which seems to have favoured Professor Kitasato's group.[39] In fact, the later benefited from free access to the main hospital of Hong Kong (Kennedy Town Hospital) and was permitted to use hospital facilities in order to watch the evolution of the sickness and to carry out the necessary autopsies. All cadavers were reserved for the Japanese team. Yersin, on the other hand, had to bribe sailors charged with burying the dead in order to obtain bodies. None the less, he soon formulated a hypothesis that the germ would be found in the bubon produced by the disease. This hypothesis united the Pasteur tradition of enquiry with the anatomo-clinical school of Xavier M.F. Bichat (1775–1802), whose contribution to medicine was to link a sickness to the lesions it produced. Yersin found what he called a '*purée*' of bacillus in the bubon which, he reported, 'I am cultivating on agar before using such cultures on mice and other guinea pigs . . . there are good chances that this bacillus is the one responsible for the plague'.[40] The animals inoculated with the pus from the bubons all died and, after autopsy, were all shown to carry the same bacillus. A complete description of this bacillus was published in September 1894 in the *Annales* of the Pasteur Institute. This discovery nevertheless remained controversial for a long time, being attributed to Kitasato rather than to Yersin, and the debate about who was the first in discovering the bacillus was not resolved until 1975.[41]

Once the bacillus had been isolated, it was hypothesized that mice and rats, who were known to be subject to the disease, might be the carriers. It was not yet known how men picked up the disease, and how it returned to the rats.[42] A serum[43] was developed in 1895 which cured many patients afflicted with the disease. That same year a vaccine was also developed by the French and was sent by the Pasteur Institute in Paris for use in British India where a very murderous plague had broken out in 1895, threatening other countries.

In 1898, the work of Paul Louis Simond (1858–1947) finally unveiled the transmission mechanism. Like Yersin, Simond was an exponent of Pasteur's ideas and at the same time an exponent of the anatomo-clinical tradition of Bichat. He discovered that the disease seemed to occur without direct contact with a plague-carrying rat, and that the bodies of the sick often showed minuscule skin lesions that looked like flea bites. These lesions were usually found in the more delicate areas of the body and were noticeable during the first few hours of the sickness. This led him to look more closely at the role of the flea in bubonic plague. A year later he was able to publish his conclusions, but these were not immediately accepted. It seemed impossible that an insect could play such an important role in the spread of epidemics. Curiously, this refusal had little basis, especially since discoveries made shortly thereafter showed that other insects could be the bearers of sickness. In fact, in 1897 the Englishman, Sir Ronald Ross (1857–1932), demonstrated that mosquitoes were connected with malaria,[44] and in 1898 Giovani Battista Grassi (1854–1925) proved that the mosquito in question was the *anopheles*.[45] The discovery of the bacillus, the site of its reproduction, and the carriers it used, brought about new ways of fighting disease. The first step, however, was to show that the diseases found in field work were actually the same as those isolated and studied in laboratory conditions. Such a link had, in fact, far-reaching economic potential, as we will soon see.

The conquest of sickness was a basic condition for colonial expansion and development. Conquering the Indochinese forests, for example, raised the problem of coping with malaria. The construction of new railway lines, roads, and canals, not to speak of the development of agriculture in regions that had never been exploited, could only be carried out by using 'native' labourers who were exposed to the risks of malaria.

Above and beyond any humanitarian considerations, the *Archives des Instituts*

Pasteur d'Indochine pointed out that only a proper draining and sanitation programme would permit a labour force to remain economically viable. Up until 1917, these programmes remained empirical and often unsuccessful. Nevertheless, they were continued by the Saigon branch of the Pasteur Institute at the specific request of plantation owners. According to Dr N. Bernard (Director of the Saigon Institute in 1925) who was entrusted with research in this field, the first step was to prove that the sudden fevers so often observed were actually a form of malaria. Blood tests carried out on patients showed that they all had massive quantities of the protozon identified by Laveran.[46] Once this was established, steps could be taken to stop the spread of the disease.

In order to destroy the larvae of the *anopheles*, rivers had to be dug out and deepened and their banks had to be turned into pasture land. Such measures were expensive. It was, however, not yet universally accepted that the *anopheles* mosquito was the major malaria-causing factor; therefore a major experiment using human beings was begun. Two camps were set up for the labour force and their families. One, where simple bamboo beds were provided, was set far away from any infected areas, while the other camp, much more comfortably equipped, was pitched next to a stream known to contain large quantities of *anopheles* larvae.

> A few weeks later two-thirds of the coolies of the latter camp had to be taken to the infirmary of the plantation or to a hospital to be treated for malaria . . . The children born in the healthy camp developed normally in the course of the three years during which the experiment continued.[47]

The object of this experiment was to study the preventive measures needed better to exploit those areas infested by malaria. In such a case, 'scientific' investigation was put ahead of any humanitarian consideration. Such experiments show us the very real limits of what it meant to bring 'rational science and Pasteur's medicine' to bear on 'humanitarian' endeavour. The native populations were used explicitly, in this case both as cheap labour and as subjects for medical research.[48]

As the colonial economy expanded, a new epidemiological situation arose, and other diseases became significant. The rapid growth of urban centres, especially in the delta region, and European methods of building, often carried out hastily and without consideration, brought about serious sanitary problems. In particular, a series of diseases linked to water supply, and tuberculosis, became increasingly frequent.[49] After close observation of the schools in Cholon,[50] tubercolosis was fought by frequent check-ups to isolate the afflicted. To prevent diseases associated with the water supply, new sterilization systems were required. The chemical sterilization methods used in Europe often failed to ensure desired results. Out of such needs grew the Saigon Cholon Water Surveillance Service, an organization which was eventually extended to all of Indochina and which became one of the most important departments of the Pasteur Institute in Saigon.[51]

Colonial economics, as well as humanitarian concerns, structured the growth of Pasteur Institutes. In fact, although the research on infectious diseases carried out by the various institutes aimed at helping as many people as possible, this goal was inextricably linked to colonial enterprise. These factors eventually gave rise to the development of nothing less than an industrial production system. This was the case with vaccines,[52] for example, which were produced in large quantities, especially during epidemics. During the 1927–8 anti-cholera campaign, no less than twelve million units of vaccines were used in a period of seven months; this was roughly 100 times more than the productive capacity of the local laboratory. Once such a programme had been carried out, what remained was an industrial plant that had little use. In other cases, however, things worked out differently. In Nha Trang, for example, where serum for the bubonic plague was prepared, the presence of large laboratory animals required suitable stables as well as grazing land. These installations, and the number of animals used, increased when the bovine plague was under study. The installations remained useful, because the animals were needed for further research as well as for producing vaccines and serums.

Each successful discovery bore the germ of further expansion. Such was the case with the quinine venture.[53] In 1917, in order to start plantations, Yersin undertook the adaptation of the quinine tree to local conditions. The project was started to offset supply problems caused by the First World War,[54] but the ultimate aim was to make France self-sufficient in this drug.[55] The cultivation of the tree could only take place after clearing suitable land, and planting and managing new plantations.

Programmes entailing research into a disease, making vaccines, sterilizing water supplies, examining the diet of workers in developing areas,[56] and cultivating of trees for the production of quinine, all reveal the mechanisms of economic and geographical expansion at work. Each discovery and each new undertaking fed the increasingly powerful Pasteur Institutes of Indochina. Although the original objectives were primarily medical and sanitary, they were soon swept up in the politics of colonial expansion. The institutes thus played a key role in the occupation of foreign soil and facilitated the exploitation of the colonies. Microbiological discoveries and solutions to sanitary problems automatically became instrumental in fostering geographical and economic occupation. The revolution brought about by Pasteur in the field of medicine was the starting-point for institutes that saw their work in terms of biological research and yet still became the tools of a highly successful cultural colonization.

CONCLUSION

E. Friedson has pointed out that hospitals have replaced parliament and the church as the most representative institutions in western culture.[57] French colonial history would seem to show that medicine as a whole was also eligible for such a role. Curiously, it became successful precisely at the moment when it least sought to play this part. Before Pasteur, it was thought that the world could be conquered with medical knowledge, yet the method and knowledge available produced limited practical results and could only be applied in limited fields and in geographically circumscribed areas. As a result, conflict arose between co-existing cultures in which colonized peoples still had the means to resist a medical institution which was not altogether convinced as to the practical value of what it was offering.

The post-Pasteur era brought about radical changes in modern scientific medicine. If, in the past, hygienic and moral measures were deployed — village by village and community by community — in order to prevent the spread of contagious diseases, the only factor which concerned medical authorities 'after Pasteur' was the existence (or absence) of the micro-organisms which cause diseases and the implementation of the means (preventive vaccinations and curative serums) to cope with them. The ultimate goal of post-Pasteur medicine was to protect society as a whole from 'invisible actors', to use the term coined by B. Latour.[58] Only specialists, however, had the knowledge and techniques to cope with this new development — a new state of affairs which also entailed a redefinition of professional linkages in society. Micro-organisms thus took on the role of social actors, able to 'disorganize' society, and post-Pasteur medicine ended up fighting a series of isolated phenomena rather than cultures which housed the micro-organic foe. Ultimately, however, this indifference turned out to be a powerful tool in the transformation of colonial societies.

As we have seen, the logic governing the direction which research took, and the use made of the results so obtained, caused the Pasteur Institutes to investigate increasingly diversified fields and to concern themselves with geographically diverse areas of the world.[59] Originally concerned with isolating a specific bacteria or protozon, the Pasteur Institute 'network' ended up influencing French society as a whole and eventually contributed to the changing of the world economic order. Paradoxical as it may seem, European culture was never exported as successfully as when its sole aim was to export its medicine.

NOTES

This paper was translated by A.J. Grieco and S.F. Matthews Grieco.

1. See M. Ferro, *L'Histoire sous surveillance: science et conscience de l'histoire* (Paris: Calman Levy, 1985).
2. In another area, see C. Herzlich and J. Pierret, *Malades d'hier et d'aujourd'hui* (Paris: Payot, 1984) in which the authors try to describe medical history as viewed by patients. The book is a pioneer effort in trying to 'see things from the other side of the bed'.
3. E. Sergent, 'La Médecine française en Algérie', *Archives de l'Institut Pasteur d'Algérie, XXXIII* (1955), 281–5.
4. G. Hardy, *La Politique coloniale et le partage de la terre aux XIXè et XXè siècles* (Paris: Albin Michel, 1937), 348.
5. P. Guillaume, *Le Monde colonial XIXè siècle–XXè siècle* (Paris: Armond Colin, 1974), 133.

6. Y. Turin, *Affrontements culturels dans l'Algérie coloniale* (Paris: Maspero, 1971), 19.

7. J.P. Peter, 'Le Grand Rève de l'ordre médical en 1770 et aujourd'hui', *Autrement*, no. 4 (1975–6), 183–93.

8. F. Fanon, 'Medicine and colonialism', in J. Ehrenreich (ed.), *The Cultural Crisis of Modern Medicine* (New York: Monthly Review Press, 1978), 229–51, argues that western medicine became part of the oppressive process of colonization and, as such, was considered by the natives as an enemy, foreign to the native culture of the colonized countries; and shows how, as natives became trained and involved in the liberation of their country, they became part of the social body.

9. A. Bordier, *La Colonisation scientifique et les colonies françaises* (Paris: Reinwald, 1884); Paul Brau, *Trois siècles de médecine coloniale française* (Paris: Vigot Frères, 1931); P. Nosny, 'Propos sur l'histoire de la médecine coloniale française', *Médecine Tropicale, 24* (4) (1964), 375–82; *Le Domaine colonial française* (Paris: Editions du Cygne, 1930), vol. 4, ch. IX, 'La Médecine et l'assistance médicale aux colonies', 338–400; J. Loubert,'Oeuvre civilisatrice du Corps Médical Français en pays d'outre mer', *Progrès médical, 84* (1956), 397–98; R.Frey, 'Colonisation et médicine', *Presse médecine, 63* (1955), 1245.

10. X. Yacono, *Histoire de la colonisation française* (Paris: PUF, 1969); Nguyen Khac Vien, *Histoire du Vietnam* (Paris: Editions Sociales, 1974).

11. See for example Dr Serge Agnely, 'Influence politique de la médecine — influence morale du médecin comme instrument de conquête et de civilisation en Algérie', Rapport pour l'année 1847, quoted by Turin, op. cit., n. 6 above, 307.

12. J. Leonard, *La Médecine entre les pouvoirs et les savoirs* (Paris: Aubier, 1981), 153–4.

13. Turin, op. cit., n. 6 above, 313.

14. W.B. Cohen, *Rulers of Empire: In the French Service of Africa* (Stanford: Hoover Institution Press, 1971).

15. Dr Pouzin quoted by Turin, op. cit., n. 6 above, 282.

16. Dr Agnely quoted by Turin, op. cit., n. 6 above, 148.

17. Quoted by Turin, op. cit., n. 6 above, 307.

18. Although western medicine had slender therapeutic means at this time, some of its remedies were efficacious. Quinine and its derivates were known from the eighteenth century. A.J Pelletier (1788–1842) isolated the alkaloid of this plant in 1820. Quinine was much used against periodically recurrent fevers and quite successfully against malaria. Its high degree of success and the rapidity of the cure soon overcame the reticence of the Arab population. Furthermore, quinine was much used by the occupying army which distributed it to the local population. Syphilis was treated with mercury and, after 1855, with potassium iodate. Western medicine also disposed of fairly efficacious eye-drops. On the other hand, epidemic conditions were often beyond the control of western medicine.

19. See F. Fanon's description of the gap existing between the behaviour of the physicians and of the arab population, and the deep misunderstanding resulting from this. Fanon, op. cit., n. 8 above.

20. The magical and religious role of the *thébib* went beyond the domain of the western doctor. *Thébibs* were consulted for medical reasons but also for personal (and collective) spiritual problems. In larger towns they were often full-time. Village *thébibs* often healed their patients in exchange for services and, at times, for free.

21. 'We must increase the number of water holes and the light masonry works. This will be a powerful means to keep the tents away from rivers and streams and thus in healthier places.' (Dr Bertherand, 1849) quoted by Turin, op.cit., n. 6 above, 328.

22. Such notions are even more apparent when examining tropical colonies. See, for example, M. Worboys, 'The emergence of tropical medicine: a study in the establishment

of a scientific specialty', in G. Lemaine *et al.* (eds), *Perspectives on the Emergence of Scientific Disciplines* (The Hague: Mouton, 1976), 75–95. The author of this article shows to what extent emergent tropical medicine seemed to confirm racist theories as to a differential resistance to parasitic sicknesses between European and native subjects. For French nineteenth-century racial theories, see Leonard, op. cit., n. 12 above, 168.

23. I have shown elsewhere ('Contagion et santé publique: une représentation du lien social au XVIIIème siècle', *Sciences sociales et santé, 11* (2) (1984), 45–70) that rules of hygiene were used against the poor in order to impose a specific moral code. Medical ideas concerning contagion can reveal both political ideologies and the way in which societies perceive individual and collective interaction. For the economic aspect of this question, see James A. Paul, 'Medicine and imperialism', in J. Ehrenreich (ed.), op. cit., n. 8 above, 221–86.

24. In 1798 Edward Jenner discovered the principle of inoculating cow pox as a preventive measure against smallpox. His technique replaced an earlier procedure which consisted in inoculating smallpox itself.

25. Claudine Marenco and S. Govedarica, *La Vaccination des enfants en France, 1880–1980* (Paris: CNRS, DGRST, University of Paris IX Dauphine, 1980).

26. A.M. Moulin, 'La Vaccination anti-variolilque — approche historique de l'évolution des idées sur les maladies transmissible et leur prophylaxie' (Unpublished PhD thesis, University of Pierre and Marie Curie, Paris, 1979). Concerning the medical institution's propensity for circulating knowledge and discoveries, see J.Clavreul, *L'Ordre Médical* (Paris: Seuil, 1978), 34.

27. A. Marcovich, 'L'Introduction de la vaccination Jennerienne — un révélateur des idéologies et des politiques de santé', *L'Année sociologique, 36* (1986), 57–73.

28. Turin, op. cit., n. 6 above, 358.

29. The last resistance in Southern Algeria and in the Kabil region capitulated in 1871. Despite revolts at the end of the Second Empire (1864), the French occupation of Algeria continued until the 1950s.

30. There were great differences in teaching quality depending on the faculty attended in France. See Leonard, op. cit., n. 12 above, 49–89.

31. Quoted by Turin, op. cit., n. 6 above, 326.

32. J.P. Bozon, 'Quand les Pastoriens traquaient la maladie du sommeil', *Sciences sociales et santé* (special issue on Anthropology, Society and Health), *III* (34) (1985), 27–56.

33. It must be pointed out that when it came to practical applications the attitudes could be different. Thus Sir P. Manson (1844–1922) and Sir R.Ross (1857–1932), two leading doctors in the field of tropical medicine, saw things differently. Manson considered field sanitation measures to be quite unimportant as compared to the 'greater knowledge of the pathology and etiology of tropical disease [which] would facilitate better control measures and increased the chance of effective protection, mainly for Europeans'. Ross saw 'general living conditions, diet and sanitations as the main determinants of health. His approach to tropical medicine was therefore holistic, practical and preventive', Worboys, op.cit., n. 22 above, 90.

34. The French Pasteur Institutes were not, however, the only ones of their kind. The British Empire had an equivalent in its Lister Institute, Germany had the Koch Institutes, and the USA had Rockefeller Institutes. The Pasteur Institutes were nevertheless, more evenly distributed throughout the French colonies than were the institutes of the other colonial powers.

35. H.G.S. Morin, H. Jacotot, and J. Genevray, 'Les Instituts Pasteur d'Indochine en 1934', *Archives des Instituts Pasteur d'Indochine, 20* (December 1934), 442.

36. L.A. Bordès, 'Les Premières Recherches sur le paludisme en Indochine', *Archives des Instituts Pasteur d'Indochine, 12* (October 1930), 11.

37. See B. Latour, 'Give me a laboratory and I will raise the world', in K. Knorr

and M. Mulkay (eds), *Science Observed: New Perspectives in the Sociology of Science* (London: Sage Publications, 1982).

38. B. Latour, *Les Microbes: guerre et paix* (Paris: Metaillé, 1984), 38.

39. S. Kitasato (1852–1931) was a student of R. Koch (1843–1910) and might have shared the same feelings, for Koch did not think very highly of Pasteur and his students.

40. H.H. Mollaret and J. Brossolet, *Alexandre Yersin ou le Vainqueur de la Peste* (Paris: Fayard, 1985), 137.

41. See N. Howard Jones, 'Kitasato, Yersin and plague bacillus', in *Clio Médica* (1975), 10, quoted by Mollaret and Brossolet, op. cit., n. 40 above. Concerning this dispute see also H. Harold Scott, *A History of Tropical Medicine*, 2 vols (London: Edward Arnold, 1939–1942), vol. 2, 729–39 and 765.

42. These problems were discussed during the Tenth International Sanitary Conference held in 1897. See Mollaret and Brossolet, op. cit., n. 40 above, 163.

43. Progressively improved (particularly by Yersin), it managed to improve the chances of surviving this sickness.

44. A. Laveran (1845–1922) had discovered in 1880 in Constantine that malaria was caused by a protozon living in human blood.

45. One can also mention M. Nicole (1862–1932) who proved in 1909 (Tunis) that lice are the vector for typhus. The virus of the sickness was not discovered until 1916 by H. La Rocher (1879–1956) in Lima.

46. See n. 44 above.

47. Bordès, op. cit., n. 36 above, 14.

48. Medical experimentation on native populations seem to have been frequently perpetrated by the colonizers — see F.Fanon, op. cit., n. 8 above.

49. ibid., 15.

50. F.H. Guérin, P. Lalung Bonnaire and M. Adrien, 'Premiers Résultats de l'enqête sociale sur la tuberculose dans les écoles de Cholon', *Archives des Instituts Pasteur d'Indochine, 1* (1924), 189–207.

51. R. Pons and J. Guillerm, 'L'Approvisionnement en eau des villes de Saigon et Cholon', *Archives des Instituts Pasteur d'Indochine, 5–6* (1927), 250.

52. Mollaret and Brossolet, op. cit., n. 40 above, 24.

53. ibid., 212.

54. Holland and its colonies were the world's greatest quinine producers. With reference to quinine as an instrument for colonization see D.R. Headrick, *The Tools for Empire: Technology and European Imperialism in the Nineteenth Century* (New York: Oxford University Press, 1981).

55. Mollaret and Brossolet, op. cit., n. 40 above, 212.

56. J. Guillerm and H.G.S. Morin, 'Determination statistique de la ration alimentaire du travailleur indigène en Cochinchine', *Bulletin Société Pathologie Exotique, XIX* (2–3) (1926), 905.

57. E. Friedson, *Profession of Medicine: a Study of the Sociology of Applied Knowledge* (New York: Dodd, Mead, 1970).

58. Latour, op. cit., n. 38 above.

59. Bozon, op. cit., n. 32 above.

Part II

European Medicine and Colonial Practice

6

Temperate medicine and settler capitalism: on the reception of western medical ideas

Donald Denoon

The great advances in European medical knowledge, from the 1860s onwards, made it technically possible for the whole world's population to enjoy better and more diffuse well-being.[1] As western medicine began to become scientific, it spawned further disciplines such as 'tropical medicine', which even promised to transform the evil reputation of most tropical environments.[2] It happened that well-being was conferred very selectively, and it is the purpose of this paper to enquire how medical possibilities were subordinated to political purposes. The approach is comparative, surveying the experience of a mix of 'temperate' and 'tropical' communities in Australasia and southern Africa, seeking out the particular social and political conditions which most favoured the acceptance and application of the most beneficial pieces of medical knowledge, during that most decisive of generations, from the late nineteenth century to the Great War.

I

The regions under review were either British colonies (such as New Zealand, the Australian colonies, British New Guinea, the Cape and Natal) or else subject to some degree of British imperial oversight (the Afrikaner republics which became British colonies during the Boer War). These British societies drew their medical knowledge and personnel mainly from Scotland or England or (in the case of the Cape Dutch) the Netherlands. Late in the nineteenth century, medical graduates began to enjoy greater public esteem in western Europe.[3]

The careers of two prominent colonial doctors exemplify many features of their profession. Sir William MacGregor, son of a Scots farm labourer (a disproportionate number of British doctors were Irish or Scots), graduated from Edinburgh and was attracted to the guaranteed income of the colonial service. He then graduated from colonial medicine (in the Seychelles and Fiji) to colonial administration (in Fiji, British New Guinea, and Lagos).[4] His near-contemporary Sir Leander Starr Jameson graduated from London, and achieved notoriety by inventing a disease in Kimberley, bearing all the symptoms of smallpox but requiring no quarantine. That mis-diagnosis may have been a medical crime, but it was a political triumph, since diamond mining could continue despite the demise of much of the labour force.[5] Jameson graduated from medicine to politics, bringing both his practitioner's charm and his questionable judgement to his new profession. MacGregor and Jameson were both involved in persistent public acrimony with their professional colleagues, and that was only to be expected in an era when scientific criteria were only beginning to be used in arbitrating conflicts between raving egotists.

During the last quarter of the nineteenth century 'germ theory' was giving a scientific basis to medical practice, and widening the distinction between university-trained doctors and self-educated 'quacks'.[6] At the same time, the rise of professional associations created a forum where rival opinions could be discussed and a professional judgement reached, behind closed doors. These institutional changes transformed the public reputation of the medical profession, in the colonies as in Britian — and Jameson and MacGregor were among the last of the great public brawlers in their profession.

The rise of the medical practitioners, and the evolution of ideas within their profession, combined to play upon the sensibilities of politicians and bureaucrats in the colonies. And one of the most significant developments in medical research towards the end of the nineteenth century was the separation of 'tropical medicine' from the rest of medical thinking.[7] The careful research of Ross (who established the role of the anopheles mosquito in the malaria cycle) and of Manson (who incriminated mosquitoes in elephantiasis) provided the scientific impetus, although neither disease was necessarily tropical in its provenance. The sharp-eyed Joseph Chamberlain seized upon this research, in pursuit of ways of keeping administrators and other Europeans alive in the new, undeveloped estates of the British tropical empire. The discipline was more secure financially than scientifically. Ross himself believed that the proper approach to tropical well-being was to extend to the dependencies those public health measures which had already transformed the quality of life in western Europe — clean drinking water, clean food, and careful sanitation. Such measures were likely to have a generally benign influence on whole populations. Ross was several generations ahead of his times. Under Manson's direction, the new discipline veered towards laboratory work and curative measures. When he opened the London School of Tropical Medicine in 1899, and struggled to define the discipline which should animate this institution, he fell back on a dubious distinction: tropical diseases were commonly parasitic in origin, whereas other diseases were more commonly bacterial.[8] This distinction was not taken up by researchers. As research began to flow into the journals, it mainly contrasted the human biology of European and non-European patients, stressing race to the virtual exclusion of social and environmental circumstances.

Now racial comparisons can and do yield useful scientific insights: as one among several perspectives, it would be unobjectionable. And even with its racial enthusiasm, the new discipline did not entirely stultify research. The Institute of Medical Research in Kuala Lumpur added to the body of Dutch and American data (from Java and the Philippines) confirming the dietary basis of beriberi, and generated the modern study of vitamins.[9] The social assumptions and political pressures which shaped the infant discipline did not prevent it from being useful; but they did influence its general strategy and its particular methods.

II

If doctors were to impose their ideas upon colonial society and to protect their public image and incomes from unseemly brawling, they had first to form professional associations (as they were doing so successfully in Britain). From about 1875 onwards, colonial Australian doctors formed a plethora of such associations, independent of each other and often in competition. At the turn of the century most of these associations became branches of the British Medical Association.[10] In the several colonies they pressed upon governments the need for registration procedures which separated the university-trained sheep from the self-taught goats; and the professional associations then enjoyed the right to advise colonial governments on matters of health policy. The evolution of medical associations in New Zealand was essentially similar.[11] In southern Africa, the convergence of local medical associations was delayed by the balkanization of the region, and by the divisive issue of imperial intervention during the 1890s and the Boer War. None the less South African doctors achieved the substance of the dominance enjoyed by their Australian counterparts, by about the turn of the century.[12] These professional bodies, stating their points of view as scientific truths, were influential upon politicians and bureaucrats who shared their respect for seemingly scientific, rational and efficient procedures. It is during the same era that the colonial states accepted a general responsibility for the condition of livestock:[13] much the same kind of thinking sustained the entry of the colonial governments into responsibility for the health of their human subjects.

The consequences are most clearly seen in the microcosm of New Zealand. When Frederick Truby King returned from medical studies in Edinburgh, he involved himself in public affairs, devising a system of maternal and child care to arrest the moral and physical degeneration of the white race, prescribing to mothers precisely how they must nurture their infants.[14] Before 1910, New Zealand was losing between 60 and 90 of every thousand white infants before their first birthdays. By 1915 the mortality rate had fallen to 50, and continued to decline, until New Zealand became one of the healthiest countries in the world.[15] These were ideas whose time had come. The Plunket Society, formed to popularize Truby King's ideas, represented the most respected and influential elements of colonial society. Newly enfranchised women, the target of the campaign, now had their behaviour regulated by seemingly God-given rules of conduct. Costly immigrants could be supplemented by uterine immigration. Whole generations of disciplined, unspoilt babies would grow to healthy and self-disciplined adulthood. Whether or not the Plunket Society was entitled to the credit for declining mortality rates, it was a powerful coalition of state and scientific authority.

Public health legislation and institutions were often triggered by epidemics.[16] Perhaps the most serious was influenza, which arrived at the end of the Great War, carrying off more than 6,000 people from a population of about a million. The public response revealed the values and techniques available to the society. One Member of Parliament calculated that 'within the last three weeks New Zealand has lost £20,000,000 worth of humanity', and a Royal Commission was empanelled to determine how public health measures could be improved.[17] The Minister of Health now regretted that Public Health budgets had been outstripped by veterinary expenditure. In expiation, the government gave renewed attention to slum clearance and to sanitation. It re-emphasized hygienic training for women and involved them more directly in health administration — and wondered how to raise Maori standards of living.

Concern for the perceived deterioration of the white race might lead us to expect that Maori well-being would be neglected. Certainly, Maori mortality and morbidity rates were worse than those for the Dominion as a whole: but Maoris were too well entrenched in the wider society to be neglected entirely. Dr Maui Pomare and his colleagues devoted themselves to the survival of the race. Combining up-to-date western medical knowledge with an intimate understanding of the dynamics of rural life, they mobilized the enthusiasm of their own people and directed government resources towards improved housing, clean water, and effective sewage.[18] The demographic decline was first arrested and then reversed. In its role as Good Shepherd, the New Zealand state cared for its brown sheep as well as its white flock. If doctors themselves were the main beneficiaries of New Zealand health policy, it must be conceded that well-being was fairly evenly distributed during that heroic era from the depressed 1890s to the tranquil 1920s. There was a very narrow gap between what was technically possible and what was actually accomplished.

II

If we divide Australian health services into three geographical zones, some interesting contrasts emerge. In the temperate southern half of the continent, where almost all white Australians lived, advances in western medicine — and in the organisation of the caring professions — were very swiftly adopted. When Victoria introduced a four-year medical degree programme, as against the three-year programme of British universities, Australia was assured a flow of well-trained practitioners. Australian doctors were also quick to assault all other health personnel, restricting their practices or subordinating them to the control of registered doctors.[19] When private capital and state support established a medical research centre in 1915, the Walter and Eliza Hall Institute began a research programme similar in general purpose to those of Europe, and of comparable quality.[20] As in New Zealand, so in Australia, the reproductive behaviour of women (or rather the lack of it) was a matter of government anxiety.[21] And as in the other colonies, exogenous epidemics often triggered legislation and public health reorganization.[22]

Whereas Queensland health services were not merely provoked by epidemics: they focused persistently upon quarantine. That colony had a border within bow-shot of a genuinely tropical country; until the turn of the century its sugar industry relied upon Pacific islanders; and its pastoral industry employed significant numbers of Aboriginals. As we have seen, the discipline of tropical medicine was implicitly racist: in Queensland that implicit tendency became explicit. The Australian Institute of Tropical Medicine in Townsville — the first medical research institute on the continent, in 1910 — had a clear brief to promote the health of whites in tropical areas. Much of its work was to train quarantine officers (though there was also room for veterinary research).[23] Its scientists debated the possibility of a white population, permanent and healthy, in a tropical climate: Queensland was the critical test of the debate, being the only tropical community in which whites were numerically dominant.[24] When the colonists resolved the issue on their own, Sir Raphael Cilento put forward his explanation for their triumph:

> the absence of any teeming native coloured population, riddled by endemic disease [combined with effective quarantine measures, improved standards of living, and an increase in the Queensland-born population] . . . it was with the arrival of swarms of coloured labourers that the situation became critical.[25]

That perception forged an important link between tropical *disease* and tropical *people*. The former could be prevented if the latter were excluded. During the 1920s the Institute trained most of the doctors who proceeded to the Australian tropics. The Institute's purpose was stated in these terms:

> From the earliest days of colonisation European diseases were introduced in quantity among the early settlers; various tropical diseases were introduced by the Kanakas from the islands of the Pacific; and by the hordes of Chinese and other Asiatics that poured in before the days of Federation . . . . Three sets of disease conditions consequently present themselves for control:
> (1) those introduced from European countries;
> (2) those introduced from neighbouring tropical lands;
> (3) those indigenous to the country.[26]

The Institute concentrated on diseases in the second and third categories.

That medical strategy was well attuned to the time and place. It was the medical dimension of 'fortress Australia', from which Pacific Islanders were being deported, and to which only white immigrants would be admitted. Queensland quarantine officers formed the backbone of the new federal Quarantine Service, which became increasingly salient as swift sea-passage brought exotic infections (and exotic people) ever closer.[27] Whenever it was absolutely necessary for islanders to enter Australia, stringent measures applied. The parties of Papuan medical students who attended courses at Sydney University in the 1930s, for instance, were domiciled (symbolically enough) in the old Quarantine station across the harbour for the duration of their courses.[28]

III

If tropical, continental Australia enjoyed a blend of temperate medicine and quarantine measures, the third tier of Australia's medical responsibilities — New Guinea and Papua — were exclusively the stage of tropical medicine. It is in this Melanesian environment that we may most vividly perceive the blinkering effect of the new discipline.

Colonialism arrived very late in western Melanesia, partly because health conditions were daunting. The first European resident — the Russian scientist and Tolstoyan, Nikolai Miklouho-Maclay — was lucky to survive a few months' residence on the north coast in 1873. He came to the conclusion that

> it is not the Papuans or the tropical heat or the impassable forests that guard the coasts of New Guinea. Their mightly ally protecting them from foreign invaders is the pale, first shivering and then burning fever.[29]

Nevertheless Bismarck consented to the annexation of New Guinea in 1884, provoking the Australian colonies to demand British protection over Papua (British New Guinea) in the same year. Medical difficulties continued to constrict colonialism for almost another generation. Missionaries, gold-miners, administrators, and their Papuan and Polynesian co-workers died in appalling numbers in British New Guinea.[30] German planters survived in the Bismarck Archipelago, but they and their labourers and their plantations collapsed on the New Guinea mainland, where some settlements had to be abandoned in the face of malaria and dysentery.[31]

One of very few doctors to survive for any length of time in early colonial Papua was Dr William MacGregor, Administrator from 1888 to 1898. Trained before the invention of tropical medicine, he struggled to impose upon Papua (and then upon Lagos, to which he was promoted) those measures of clean water supplies, good sanitation, and dry accommodation which had transformed the health of temperate western Europeans. Denied the resources of money and personnel he required, he was mainly restricted to a series of precise and incisive observations reflecting his pre-tropical training. Many of the maladies common to Europe were absent from British New Guinea: some he considered might be the products of civilization, such as cancer and diphtheria; others were absent through the good fortune of isolation. Though malaria was clearly the most dangerous infection for Europeans (before the development of prophylactic regimes of quinine), he thought it less destructive in the native population. For them, the most serious infection was dysentery — 'the chief agent in the rapid depopulation of the Pacific'. Unknown before the advent of Europeans, and so diverse that each epidemic required a new treatment, it posed a sharp problem to medical authorities. Whoever developed an effective regime of prevention or treatment might claim to be 'the saviour of the Pacific Islander'.[32]

As these observations suggest, MacGregor was acutely aware of social and political circumstances which promoted infection. Had he remained in Papua, and assembled the resources for a strong Department of Public Health, these perceptions would probably have led him to extend to Melanesia many of the measures which had succeeded in Europe and in temperate Australia. He was a friend of Robert Ross, and kept abreast of the burgeoning literature in tropical medicine, but he remained fundamentally a 'pre-tropical-medicine' doctor. Addressing the cadets of the new Institute of Tropical Medicine, he argued that the circumstances of a tropical colony made quarantine a better strategy than it was in Britain. But he went on to impress upon tropical doctors

> the extreme desirableness of becoming experts in the examination of water. The quality of the water used by a community may have as much, or almost as much, influence on them as has the quality of the food they eat or of the air they breathe.[33]

MacGregor (and Robert Koch, who brought the good news of anopheles and quinine to the German tropical empire shortly afterwards)[34] were surveyors rather than institution-builders. By the time that public health was institutionalized in Papua (shortly before the Great War) the notions of tropical medicine had thoroughly permeated the officers in charge. In practice, the main strategies were international quarantine and internal racial segregation (Dr Strong in Papua published the advice that European settlers should live at least a quarter of a mile away from Papuans).[35] There were small hospitals, racially segregated and very unpopular. In Table 6.1 the *Papuan Annual Report* for 1918/19 reveals how people found their way into the Port Moresby Native Hospital. Most Papuans attended because their employers sent them.

Papuans encountered western medicine in the form of extension patrols, and the activities of the patrols are indicated by the statistical summaries of treatments provided. The *Papuan Annual Report* for 1925/6, for instance, gives us the breakdown in Table 6.2.

The popularity of hookworm treatment owes much to the Rockefeller campaign against hookworm throughout northern Australia and the Pacific islands. Led by the redoubtable Dr Sam Lambert, the campaign captured the imagination of plantation managers and government officials who imagined that pit latrines and oil of chemopodium injections would yield a healthy, vigorous labour line and

Table 6.1: Admissions to Port Moresby Native Hospital, 1918/19[36]

Indentured labourers	524	
Time-expired indentured labourers	36	= 71%
Rejected recruits	57	
Prisoners	44	
Government employees	162	= 20%
'Non-Papuan coloured'	10	
'Villagers'	38	= 5%
Total patients	871	

Table 6.2: Treatments given by health extension officers in Papua, 1925/6

Hookworm treatments	49,518
Yaws	12,643
Venereal diseases	186
All others	51
Total	62,398

multiply production. Lambert himself recognized that the campaign was inconsequential, and in the 1930s he transferred himself to the Central Medical School in Fiji.[37] By then the damage was done: a general concern for environmental conditions had yielded to enthusiasm for the treatment of specific maladies, including hookworm but also yaws, which responded very dramatically to a single novarsenobillon injection.

Not only did this redirection of energy and attention divert medical personnel from improving the health of the population at large: it did not serve the long-term interests of the plantation economy itself.[38] In the virtual absence of maternal and child health services, population did not increase and may indeed have declined. Intrusive tuberculosis, malaria, dysentery and pneumonia were unrestrained. On the plantations themselves, where a strict enforcement of hygienic standards might have helped, they were not enforced. Even the dietary standards necessary to sustain a healthy labour force were not policed. Cilento reveals much in this chilling account:

> in 1925, when several hundred [people] suffering from venereal disease were placed in concentration camps at Rabaul and Kavieng for treatment, an unexpected failure in the supplies of fresh food producd an almost immediate outbreak of beri-beri . . . . At that particular time the diet that was official for natives was absolutely lacking in vitamins of any kind whatever.[39]

The cumulative effect of this evidence is very clear. The social and political perceptions of medical personnel, and especially their increasingly powerful belief that 'tropical medicine' was quite different from ordinary (or 'temperate') medicine, led them astray. The measures which were technically possible were not implemented: what was implemented was a series of attacks upon specific diseases which were medically fashionable but socially of little consequence. At a time when New Zealanders and temperate Australians were increasing their health standards and their life expectancy, the well-being of Pacific islanders either remained static, or else declined.

IV

The dislocation of the Boer War revealed how fragile was the well-being that South African settlers enjoyed. Half a million British soldiers were passed fit to fight the Boers. One in ten came down with enteric fever alone, and 8,225 died of it (battle casualties were fewer, at 7,582).[40] Warfare was more dangerous to civilians than to soldiers. In the Boer concentration camps, the mortality rate peaked at 334 per thousand per annum before British public opinion recoiled from these 'methods of barbarism' and forced an improvement in medical and hygiene services. Death mirrored life in its unequal opportunities: the peak mortality rate in African concentration camps reached 380.[41] War was the pursuit of mortality by other means: many black men were no more at risk in warfare than they had been in the Kimberley mining compounds before the outbreak of fighting.[42]

War brought other intimations of mortality, when plague reached all ports (from Buenos Aires through the Cape to Sydney and Auckland) linked by the movement of troops and horses and provisions.[43] The panicky response of settlers — to blame the poor, and especially the coloured poor — was neither strange nor in itself significant. (During the influenza epidemic in Auckland, twenty years later, some commentators blamed the 'dagoes', while a newspaper remarked that 'the Hindoo hawkers . . . live in pestilence, filth, and under conditions shocking in the extreme. These people are licensed by the City Council to sell fruit, and therefore to disseminate disease.'[44] What did prove significant was the collusion between the last of the Cape Liberals and the loudest of the Cape doctors, to introduce urban segregation allegedly as a public health measure.[45]

The engine of economic and social change in southern Africa, however, was not white sentiment at the Cape but the gold-mining industry in the Transvaal. As war petered out in 1902, High Commissioner Sir Alfred Milner transferred his headquarters from Cape Town to Johannesburg and set about the construction of a modern bureaucracy,[46] the better to harness the mining industry to his imperial purposes. He expected that scientific principles would infuse the Crown Colony bureaucracy, instead of the superstition and special pleading which had characterized the Kruger Republic. Accordingly the British non-elected administration established an elaborate and up-to-date Department of Agriculture, to demonstrate its superiority to the old regime of landowners. What the new administration crucially failed to do was to lavish as much attention on human health as it did on veterinary research.[47]

Milner poached many of his officers from the Cape, including Dr George Turner as his Medical Officer of Health. Born in England in 1848, Turner trained in medicine during the 1870s and 1880s. He was involved in public health in Britain before he came to the Cape in 1895.[48] In the Transvaal his public image was tarnished by parliamentary speeches in which he endorsed the claim of certain respectable blacks to travel in second-class railway compartments instead of the customary third-class accommodation. His credibility as a champion of science probably suffered in consequence.[49] He was also unhelpful in framing medical arguments to justify municipal segregation. In 1906 he applied to withdraw into two years of leprosy research before retiring from the public service. His boss Lionel Curtis was quick to grant the request. He was impressed by Turner's rinderpest research but glad to see the back of him as a medical administrator:

> his faults are due in great measure to the fact that as an administrator he is a round man in a square hole . . . . Remember we have been unable as yet to produce a Public Health Act and the real reason has been that Dr Turner could devise nothing that would fit in with the system of local government in this country.[50]

The nub of the problem in framing a public health act was urban segregation. Milner himself wished to create separate townships for Indians and Africans at the end of the war, to forestall white agitation. Chamberlain (and the India Office) argued that separate locations could only be justified on the grounds of hygiene rather than race.[51] What was required of Turner was a quasi-medical vindication of urban segregation, on the lines which every other public health officer in southern Africa had been able to invent.[52] This was his square hole.

Curtis was less squeamish. Reflecting on his work in the Transvaal, he described it thus:

> the duty of excluding British subjects with a certain number of favoured exceptions, from a British country, is the most odious which a British Government could legitimately undertake . . . . [The real justification for doing so] is that if the doors were thrown open to Asiatics . . . the white population would begin to assume to the coloured population . . . the same proportions which are to be found in India . . . . The real object we have in front of us is not to exclude dirty Asiatics and to admit clean ones . . . but it is to shut the gate against the influx of an Asiatic population altogether.[53]

He was not oversimplifying. After the war, Indians returned to the Transvaal only under permit. Once it became clear that returning Indians would be entitled legally to compete against white traders, the permit system was applied stringently. The following letter was sent to the relevant official in Durban, the main port of entry:

> seeing that [Indians] have now a perfect right to take out trading licences, it is important to fence with them in the matter of [residence] permits as long as possible. The plague has formed a very good reason for keeping them out for the past five months and now there is an outbreak of smallpox in Natal which we are also making the most of.[54]

What was being created was politically expedient disease.

Surrounded by such cavalier views of disease and well-being, Turner was often baffled. The most urgent public health issue of the day was the appallingly high mortality rate among mining workers. The government appointed a medical commission to investigate living conditions in the compounds; Turner quoted the best up-to-date advice, which laid down a minimum of 300 cubic feet of space for each miner; the other doctors considered this recommendation too expensive; and in the event the government advised (but did not enforce) a minimum of 200 cubic feet.[55] After a series of such decisions, it is not surprising that the Transvaal was no healthier after five years of Crown Colony administration than it had been before. Ironically, a more thorough application of public health perceptions to the industrial scene might have averted the acute labour shortage which drove the Government to import Chinese labour, an experiment which hastened the demise of the Crown Colony regime.

Kimberley diamond-mining compounds were held to be models of hygienic working conditions in the first years of this century. They had only recently achieved that reputation, more as a consequence of managerial calculation than of government regulation.[56] Much the same process may be observed in the Witwatersrand mining compounds from the end of the Boer War until the outbreak of the Great War. Managers made their own assessments, and devised remedies suitable to them, at their own unhurried pace. In the aftermath of war, rinderpest and concentration camps, the health of the rural population was miserable. Combined with wretched working and living conditions at the work site, this gave rise to a mortality rate which peaked at 112 per thousand per annum *in the compounds* in mid-winter 1903. The rate fluctuated between 30 and 60 plus during the next two years.[57] The obvious device for increasing the migrant labour force was to recruit in the tropical hinterland: but tropical recruits died more swiftly than the others.[58]

One definable problem afflicting black and white workers alike was silicosis, which further predisposed its victims towards pulmonary tuberculosis. Morbidity and mortality among white miners was highly visible — through Cornish as well as South African statistics — and became a public issue after the Boer War. That issue was nevertheless neglected until 1907, when a Responsible Government was elected in the Transvaal and Labour Party supporters of the Afrikaner cabinet insisted upon an enquiry. By about the time of the Great War some preventive measures had been adopted in the mines, and a system of workers' compensation was adopted.[59] While black miners may have benefited from the preventive measures, they were excluded from the compensation schedule. From the Great

War onwards, mine managers certainly improved the health services for all their employees; but tuberculosis could rarely be arrested during the few months of a labour contract, and labour migration disseminated the disease throughout the rural hinterland.[60]

The more immediate cause of death and disability, with the greatest incidence, and killing black miners especially, was pneumonia. Managements tackled it first by making perfunctory efforts at warm, dry, ventilated accommodation. When this strategy proved expensive, the Transvaal Medical Society (which included all the doctors who worked part-time in the compounds) directed experiments with an 'Anti-Pneumococci Serum' developed by the government bacteriologist. When that failed, Sir Julius Wernher recruited Sir Almroth Wright and a team of technicians to develop a vaccine. Only when all these laboratory-based strategies failed did attention return to working conditions.[61]

Samuel Evans, the brains of Wernher & Beit and of the Chamber of Mines, read press references to the health hazards of the Panama Canal project. A visit to Panama in 1912 impressed upon him the efficacy of the programme devised by the Chief Sanitary Officer, Colonel Gorgas, which had reduced the annual mortality rate among workers from 39 per thousand in 1906 to 6 in 1912. At Evans's insistence, Gorgas was brought to the Witwatersrand the following year, and reported on compound conditions in 1914. His report criticized the scattered hosptial facilities, the part-time and untrained medical staff, the barracks-style accommodation, the crowding and filth and poor sanitation of the compounds, and the carbohydrate-rich diet. Few of his recommendations were accepted, but his assistant Dr Orenstein was recruited as Superintendent of Sanitation, to co-ordinate medical services for the mining companies. Under his supervision, health services were centralized and became more professional, with full-time doctors instead of part-time consultants; sanitary conditions were improved in the compounds; and in 1917 he initiated the training of black and white nurses to replace the untrained ex-servicemen who functioned as medical orderlies. By that year, in any case, the annual mortality rate in the compounds had been brought down to 8.45 per thousand from disease, and to 2.94 from accidents.[62]

It is often argued that the function of the state in a capitalist society is to cater to the long-term needs of capital. The southern African medical evidence sits uncomfortably with that theory. Confronted by epidemic and exotic diseases, the holders of state power opted for short-term, politically popular solutions. Facing a dying labour force in the mining compounds, administrators took evasive action: it was left to the managers of capital to find their own solutions. In the circumstances it is hardly surprising that they did not solve the problem but shifted it from the work place to the rural areas, paying careful attention to the labour force at the work site and turning a blind eye to the environmental matrix of industrial disease.[63]

V

We may now broach general questions about the uneven distribution of well-being in the societies under review. And first we should try to elucidate the relationship between the authority of doctors and the power of the state. At first sight we seem to be witnessing the origins of that 'medical dominance' which infuriates democratic socialists in the 1980s. Scrambling out of the skilled working class, doctors entered the comfortable petty bourgeoisie in the late nineteenth century. Their status and incomes were protected by the state, through registration procedures. They could now band together in professional associations and largely determine the conditions of their individual employment. They were represented on commissions and boards which advised governments. Their voices were louder, and better modulated, than ever before: and they spoke the dogmatic language of absolute scientific judgement.

Yet that power was limited and conditional. Erik Olssen ascribes Truby King's influence to his skill in 'articulating and imposing coherence upon a cluster of anxieties' which troubled white New Zealanders.[64] Much the same judgement could be passed upon all the most impressive medical accomplishments of this generation. Drs Maui Pomare, Peter Buck, and Apirana Ngata certainly combined European knowledge of sanitation with revived Maori decline, on the tinder of the Maoris' own anxieties.[65] In temperate Australia, the social anxieties were much the same as in New Zealand — to achieve for the whole population at least the health status of western Europe, and to sustain a high birth-rate. For these purposes, the techniques of medication and of medical organization could most conveniently be adapted from western Europe. Tropical Australians were prey to the additional anxiety about their ability to establish themselves permanently in the tropics. The racially specific quarantine and immigration provisions of Queensland and of the new federal government, so passionately endorsed by the Director of the Institute of Tropical Medicine, may be seen as devices to assuage those fears. Across Torres Strait, in the Melanesian archipelago, colonists were worried primarily about their own survival, secondly about the vigour of the indentured labour force, and only peripherally about the health of the population as a whole. The clamour of the feverish colonists, combined with the vogue for the techniques of tropical medicine, prevented the application of those public health measures which (as MacGregor knew, and his successors forgot) could really save lives and enrich them.

For the southern African situation, Olssen's formula needs elaboration. If doctors had been the socially neutral voice of disinterested science, they would have embarked upon the kinds of public works programmes which MacGregor initiated in Lagos.[66] There was scant scientific evidence to sustain the policy of urban racial segregation which became standard throughout the continent.[67] George Turner, who took his Hippocratic oath seriously, was twice martyred while the trimmers of his profession flourished.[68] The expensive housing measures which did save the lives of miners in the compounds were not adopted until the managers of the mines were convinced that cheaper, laboratory-based measures would fail. Doctors succeeded when (and only when) they worked through the political force field which refracted their opinions. Those who tried to work against the political grain became powerless. The complication in the southern African milieu is that there were two distinct 'clusters of anxiety' which could generate medical policy and practice: the white electorate in general, and the largest lump of coherent capital in the southern hemisphere.

At the turn of the century, the medical profession had the knowledge and skills to transform the lives of the whole human race. Manson claimed for tropical medicine that

> I now firmly believe in the possibility of tropical colonisation by the white race. Heat and moisture are not in themselves the direct cause of any tropical disease. The direct cause of 99% of these diseases are germs . . . . To kill them is simply a matter of knowledge and the application of this knowledge.[69]

Yet these available benefits were very selectively bestowed. Maoris — who were never subjected to 'tropical medicine' — began their demographic revival at the turn of the century. Every other Pacific islander society languished (under tropical medicine) until the 1930s (in Fiji) or the 1950s (everywhere else). In Africa the same lack of benefit is clear: tropical medicine neither opened up large areas to dense white settlement nor improved the well-being of Africans.[70] 'Tropical medicine' may best be seen as a mental framework which reconciled professional health workers to providing a lamentable and inadequate service.

The greatest benefits were enjoyed by Europeans. Hobart Houghton puts it this way:

> The presence of persons of European descent was an important, if not decisive, factor in promoting economic progress . . . for they provided a seed bed where the imported innovations could be cultivated and acclimatised.

What ideas precisely were planted in this seed bed?

> These innovations ranged from the biological theories of Darwin to modern methods of transport, from new educational techniques and the establishment of newspapers to joint-stock banking and the limited liability company, and from the application of power in the manufacturing process to the introduction of new skills and the organisation of labour. Above all it made Africa aware of advances in preventive and curative medicine for man and beast.[71]

This is, of course, exactly the opposite of the truth. What Africans in this generation experienced was Rhodes's organization of their labour, Jameson's mis-diagnoses, urban segregation justified by spurious science, the introduction of tuberculosis and rinderpest, and a pseudo-Darwinian discrimination. From the Africans' point of view, the seed bed was a nursery for triffids.

Yet the settlers were certainly able to acclimatise those technical and organizational innovations which served their immediate purposes. Great Britain generated the ideas and the terms in which medical debate and research were conducted in the antipodes. The colonists did not passively replicate these western European institutions: rather, the introduced ideas and institutions could be ignored, or they could be re-ordered and perhaps re-interpreted (as in the distinct emphasis placed upon tropical medicine in Queensland). In health care, then, the settler capitalist societies were simultaneously dependent and autonomous, derivative and yet creative; and it is this degree of autonomy and innovativeness which distinguishes the settler capitalist societies from their peasant neighbours. In brief, the availability of life-giving and death-dealing ideas and institutions was not random. It depended partly upon the presence or absence of a settler capitalist mode of production; and within each settler society it depended further upon the distribution of political and economic power.

NOTES

1. I follow F.B. Smith, *The People's Health, 1830–1910* (Canberra: Australian National University Press, 1979) in this usage, and in much else. 'Well-being' describes a less precise condition than the mere absence of specific sickness.
2. Michael Worboys, 'The emergence of tropical medicine: a study in the establishment of a scientific specialty', in G. Lemaine *et al.*, *Perspectives on the Emergence of Scientific Disciplines* (The Hague: Mouton, 1976), 75–98.
3. For the evolution of the medical profession in Britain, see Smith, op. cit., n. 1 above; for the Australian colonies see T.S. Pensabene, *The Rise of the Medical Practitioner in Victoria* (Canberra: Australian National University Press, 1980), and Evan Willis, *Medical Dominance: the Division of Labour in Australian Health Care* (Sydney: Allen & Unwin, 1983); for New Zealand, see F.S. MacLean, *Challenge to Health: A History of Health in New Zealand* (Wellington: New Zealand Government Publication, 1964); and for southern Africa, see E.H. Burrows, *A History of Medicine in South Africa up to the End of the Nineteenth Century* (Cape Town: Balkema, 1958), and World Health Organization, *Apartheid and Health* (Geneva: WHO, 1983).
4. Roger Joyce, *Sir William MacGregor* (Melbourne: Oxford University Press, 1971).
5. Burrows, op. cit., n. 3 above, 258–9.
6. Pensabene, op. cit., n. 3 above, 33–56.
7. Worboys, op. cit., n. 2 above, 87–92.
8. ibid., 88.
9. I am grateful to Lenore Manderson for restraining my intemperate attack on tropical medicine. For its value in colonial Malaya, see Anon., *The Institute of Tropical Medicine* (Kuala Lumpur: Institute of Tropical Medicine, 1960).
10. Pensabene, op. cit., n. 3 above; Willis, op. cit., n. 3 above.
11. MacLean, op. cit., n. 3 above.
12. Burrows, op. cit., n. 3 above, and M.W. Swanson, 'The sanitation syndrome: bubonic plague and urban native policy in the Cape Colony, 1900–1909', *Journal of African History*, XVIII (1977), 387–410.

13. Donald Denoon, *A Grand Illusion* (London: Longman, 1973); A.G.L. Shaw, *The Economic Development of Australia* (Melbourne: Longman, 6th edn, 1973).

14. Erik Olssen, 'Truby King and the Plunket Society. An analysis of a prescriptive ideology', *New Zealand Journal of History*, *XV* (1981), 3-23.

15. MacLean, op. cit., n. 3 above.

16. For example, the smallpox epidemic at the Cape in 1882 (discussed later in the chapter), and in New South Wales in the same year; and plague in New Zealand and in South Africa during the Boer War. See C.J. Cummins *A History of Medical Administration in New South Wales, 1788-1973* (Sydney: Health Commission of New South Wales, 1979); Burrows, op. cit., n. 3 above; and MacLean, op. cit., n. 3 above.

17. Geoffrey Rice, 'Christchurch in the 1918 influenza epidemic. A preliminary study', *New Zealand Journal of History*, *XIII* (1979), 109–37.

18. John A. Williams, *Politics of the New Zealand Maori: Protest and Cooperation, 1891–1909* (Auckland: Auckland University Press, 1977), ch. 8.

19. Pensabene, op. cit., n. 3 above.

20. F. Macfarlane Burnet, *The Walter and Eliza Hall Institute, 1915–1965* (Melbourne: Melbourne University Press, 1971).

21. Neville Hicks, *'This Sin and Scandal': Australia's Population Debate, 1891–1911* (Canberra: Australian National University Press, 1978).

22. Cummins, op. cit., n. 16 above; Pensabene, op. cit., n. 3 above.

23. R.A. Douglas, 'Dr Anton Breinl and the Australian Institute of Tropical Medicine', *Medical Journal of Australia*, (7, 14, 21 May 1977) *1* 713–16, 748–51, 784–90.

24. For example, A. Grenfell Price, 'The white man in the tropics', *Medical Journal of Australia*, *1* (1935), 106–10.

25. Sir Raphael Cilento, in R.W. Cilento and C. Lack, *Triumph in the Tropics: An Historical Sketch of Queensland* (Brisbane: Smith and Paterson, 1959), 426. For a scholarly account of north Queensland history, see G.C. Bolton, *A Thousand Miles Away* (Canberra: Australian National University Press, 1963).

26. Australian Archives (Sydney), School of Public Health and Tropical Medicine, Series, SP 1061/1, General Correspondence 1908–55, file 65, AITM circular letter, signed by Cilento, 30 November 1922.

27. Cilento, in Cilento and Lack, op. cit., n. 25 above.

28. Hank Nelson, 'Brown doctors: white prejudice', *New Guinea*, *V* (1970), 2.

29. N. Miklouho-Maclay, *Travels to New Guinea: Diaries, Letters, Documents*, compiled and introduced by D. Tumarkin (Moscow: Progress Publishers, 1982).

30. S. Latukefu, 'Oral history and Pacific island missionaries', in D. Denoon and R. Lacey (eds), *Oral Tradition in Melanesia* (Port Moresby: Institute of Papua New Guinea Studies, 1981), 175–87.

31. W.H. Ewers, 'Malaria in the early years of German New Guinea', *Journal of the Papua New Guinea Society*, *VI* (1973), 3–30. See also R. Fleming Jones, 'Tropical diseases in British New Guinea', *Transactions of the Royal Society for Tropical Medicine and Hygiene*, *V* (1910–11), 93–105.

32. Sir W. MacGregor, 'Some problems of tropical medicine', address at London School of Tropical Medicine, 3 October 1900, *Lancet* (13 October 1900), 1055–1061.

33. ibid.

34. S.G. Firth, *New Guinea Under the Germans* (Melbourne: Melbourne University Press, 1983).

35. Walter Mersh Strong, in Staniforth Smith (ed.), *Handbook of the Territory of Papua* (Melbourne: Australian Government Printers, 3rd edn, 1912).

36. I. Maddocks, 'Medicine and colonialism', *Australian and New Zealand Journal of Sociology*, *XI* (1975), 27–33.

37. S.M. Lambert, *A Doctor in Paradise* (London: J.M. Dent, 1942).

38. This issue is taken further in Donald Denoon's *Doctors' Dilemmas* (in preparation).

39. R.W. Cilento, *The White Man in the Tropics: With Especial Reference to Australia and its Dependencies*, Commonwealth of Australia, Department of Health, Service Publication (Tropical Division) no. 7 (Melbourne: Government Printer, 1925); and his 'Nutrition and numbers', the Livingstone Lectures 1936.

40. William Osler, *The Principles and Practice of Medicine* (London: Appletons, 8th edn, 1918).

41. Peter Warwick, 'The African refugee problem in the Transvaal and Orange River Colony, 1900–1902', *University of York, Centre for Southern African Studies, Collected Papers*, vol. 2 (1977). For a participant's account, see Emily Hobhouse, *The Brunt of the War and Where It Fell* (London: Methuen, 1902).

42. Rob Turrell, 'Kimberley's model compounds', *Journal of African History, XXV* (1984), 59–75.

43. Swanson, op. cit., n. 12 above.

44. Quoted in L. Bryder, ' "Lessons" of the 1918 flu epidemic in Auckland', *New Zealand Journal of History, XVI* (1982), 97–121, at 106.

45. Swanson, op. cit., n. 12 above.

46. Shula Marks and Stanley Trapido, 'Lord Milner and the South African State', *History Workshop, VIII* (1979), 50–80.

47. Cf. Denoon, op. cit., n. 13 above.

48. Burrows, op. cit., n. 3 above.

49. Transvaal Legislative Council Debates, second session, 21 December 1903, for a characteristic Turner intervention; and Transvaal *Leader*, 23 December 1903, for a characteristic response. Attenborough's film, *Gandhi*, opens with the hero's experience on a Transvaal train.

50. Sir Patrick Duncan Papers (unsorted in 1965, in the University of Cape Town), Curtis to Duncan, 31 May 1906.

51. Public Record Office, C.O. 291/39, Milner to Chamberlain, 21 June 1902; and C.O. 291/46, India Office to Colonial Office, 29 July 1902, leading to Chamberlain to Milner, 6 August 1902.

52. Swanson, op. cit., n. 12 above.

53. Transvaal Archives, Pretoria, Lieutenant-Governor series, LtG. 94. 97/3. Confidential memo by Curtis, 1 May 1906.

54. ibid., Governor series, P.S. 56, vol. 156 (1904), unsigned copy of letter to 'Noel', 20 August 1904.

55. Transvaal Government, Report of Compound Air Space Commission; and Chamber of Mines Archives, Confidential Circulars, copy of Dr Porter to Secretary, Chamber of Mines, 7 July 1905. The Report is also mentioned in A.P. Cartwright, *Doctors of the Mines: A History of the Mine Medical Officers' Association of South Africa* (Cape Town: Balkema Press, 1971). Some of Turner's further difficulties are mentioned in Denoon, op. cit., n. 13 above.

56. Turrell, op. cit., n. 42 above.

57. *British Parliamentary Papers*, Cd. 1904 (lxi) 1895, enclosure in 101; report of Government Mining Engineer, 1 September 1903; and Cd. 1905 (lv) 2401, enclosure in 10; report of Secretary for Native Affairs.

58. The evidence is presented in D. Denoon, 'The Transvaal labour crisis', *Journal of African History, VII* (1967), 481–94.

59. G. Burke and P. Richardson, 'The profits of death: a comparative study of miners' phthisis in Cornwall and the Transvaal, 1876–1918', *Journal of Southern African Studies, IV* (1978), 2.

60. ibid.; and World Health Organization, op. cit., n. 3 above.

61. Cartwright, op. cit., n. 55 above.

62. ibid.
63. World Health Organization, op. cit., n. 3 above.
64. Olssen, op. cit., n. 14 above.
65. Williams, op. cit., n. 18 above.
66. Joyce, op. cit., n. 4 above.
67. P.D. Curtin, 'Medical knowledge and urban planning in tropical Africa', *American Historical Review*, *90* (3) (1985), 594–613.
68. Many people could claim to have been martyred by Curtis. In Turner's case, Curtis not only confounded his professional career but, by permitting him to move into leprosy research, signed his death warrant. Turner died of leprosy in 1915.
69. Worboys, op. cit., n. 2 above.
70. Curtin, op. cit., n. 67 above.
71. D. Hobart Houghton, 'Economic development, 1865–1965', in M. Wilson and L.M. Thompson (eds) *The Oxford History of South Africa*, (Oxford: Oxford University Press, 1971), vol. 2, 6.

7

Medical professionalism in colonial Carolina

Diane Sydenham

INTRODUCTION

Throughout the eighteenth century, the journals and correspondence of South Carolinians sounded one pervasive theme — the profound precariousness of life in the colony. This precariousness in turn produced an abiding preoccupation with personal health. Rarely did the colonists neglect an opportunity to comment on the present state of health of either themselves or their family and friends. Sometimes, as in the correspondence of merchant Robert Pringle, this concern appeared in polite salutations prefacing or closing otherwise formal business communications.[1] At the other extreme were those colonists like Mrs Ann Manigault whose whole world seemed to focus on the health of family and acquaintances.[2] Illness, disease and death — these seem clearly to have been the chief protagonists of South Carolinians in their struggle to wrest a comfortable living from the New World.

This essay focuses upon the relationship between white South Carolinians and their medical practitioners. It argues that, despite the intense interest in health maintenance in the colony, medical practice offered little in the way of personal satisfaction to the ambitious professional medical practitioner. Consequently many looked beyond medicine and, especially, beyond South Carolina's borders for challenge and stimulation. South Carolinians, for their part, withheld respect and full social acceptance from all but a few practitioners who did achieve international reputations. Except for a brief period at the end of the eighteenth century the majority of citizens clung to their belief in self-treatment as the cheapest and most reliable form of medical attention.

In this essay the words 'doctor' or 'practitioner' are used interchangeably. Both were used with no discernible distinction in eighteenth-century South Carolina. The terms, as they are applied here, refer to those individuals identified as professionals and distinct from smaller groups of handymen, dilettantes, and planter/practitioners.[3] Seventy-five per cent of the 170 doctors practising in South Carolina in the eighteenth century constitute this professional category. They offered South Carolinians sincere and dedicated attention and, while a few complained of difficulties in maintaining a viable practice, these professional practitioners continued to offer medical attention to colonists throughout most of their working lives. Their education and training were diverse and did not always include formal medical training, although such training became more common in the last third of the century when it was no longer necessary to leave America to study. All had made some educational commitment to a career in medicine and, depending upon their circumstances, their preparation was as thorough as possible and often included a lengthy apprenticeship.[4]

A PECULIAR DISEASE ENVIRONMENT

Since the very beginnings of settlement, when ill health forced the early settlers to move in 1680, South Carolina's inhabitants had engaged in a continual battle against diseases that attacked the colony.[5] For many of them, the battles merged into an almost constant war which structured their daily existence and further accentuated the seasonal rhythms of Carolina's climate. Decade after decade, the colony was beleaguered by yellow fever, smallpox, and what are now understood to be malaria and dysentery.[6]

South Carolina's particular combination of unhealthy climate and numerous wealthy inhabitants preoccupied with personal health proved attractive to a wide variety of medical practitioners. The very learned, the very desperate, and every shade in between aspired to the title of doctor and were sought after by South Carolinians. In a few parts of the province, colonists were able to choose between a variety of quacks and Edinburgh graduates and, even in remote areas of the backcountry, Carolinians could frequently elect self-treatment or call in outside assistance.

The peculiar disease environment of South Carolina, a combination of natural conditions and individual psycho-social adjustment to that environment, produced not only a particularly unhealthy population but a population vitally concerned about its health. Eighteenth-century South Carolinians seemed to have understood the concept of health in its very fullest extent, defining it not just in terms of 'the absence of disease or infirmity' but also, as twentieth-century health workers have defined it, 'complete physical, mental and social well being'.[7] Health was thus far more than the absence of obvious painful or uncomfortable symptoms: it was manifest as well in more spiritual and psychological ways. The state of a patient's 'spirits' could be just as important as his physical condition.[8] Emotional manifestations of health, the colonists recognized, 'ever . . . effect[ed] the spirits'.[9] South Carolinians' emphasis on 'seasoning', the process by which new arrivals gradually adjusted physically and mentally to their new environment, highlights Carolinian acceptance of this twentieth-century concept of true health as embodying 'total adaptation to an environment and a balanced relationship of . . . body and mind'.[10]

At the end of the eighteenth century South Carolina had still not accepted legislation establishing criteria for the legitimate practice of medicine. The sole exception, unique in colonial medical history, was the banning of negroes from the practice of medicine under pain of death. Nor were slaves able 'to attend in the Business of any Doctor of Physic' out of a fear that they might gain 'knowledge in the use of medicines'.[11] With regard to whites, however, the colony remained wide open, and receptive, to anyone who fancied himself a healer and could convince others that he possessed these skills. Many practitioners, along the spectrum of those offering their services to South Carolinians, took advantage of the absence of institutional controls upon medical practice to embroider sketchy knowledge and experience to the point where they might acquire the appellation 'Doctor'.

The old medical categorizations of Britain and Europe characterized by 'exclusiveness, selfishness and slothfulness' had not survived transplantation to the American colonies. Stringent dividing lines between professional groups on the eastern side of the Atlantic had produced 'rigid corporations and petrified bodies of learning', resulting in continual bickering over precedence and status among physicians, surgeons, and apothecaries that was rarely evident in the colonies.[12] While a colonial doctor might style himself 'surgeon', 'physician', or more formally, 'Practitioner of Physic', these labels meant little in terms of limitations upon the way he practised medicine and even less to most of his patients who were primarily interested in his success with their particular ailment.

Since their earliest settlement the colonies had been marked by the absence of defined occupational structures. These were only just beginning to appear towards the end of the eighteenth century, although medical practitioners in one or two colonies had been attempting to introduce some systematic organization for several decades. The Virginia Anatomical Club had tried to introduce British medical divisions in that colony in 1761 in the hope that 'every member of the Club shall make it his endeavour, if possible, for the honour of his profession not to degrade it hereafter mingling the trade of an apothecary or surgeon with it'.[13] Later in the century, the controversial Philadelphia physician John Morgan argued for the introduction of European divisions. Morgan contended that each field was master of its respective sphere of competence and, while he did not envisage the divisions being introduced in the hierarchical European manner, Morgan certainly felt that internal medicine (as opposed to surgery) should command greater respect, while pharmacy was a separate and lower calling altogether.[14] But this 'attic full of institutions' and artificial categorization of skills and treatments was impossible to maintain even outside London, let alone in the colonies.[15]

In South Carolina, where competition for patients in the towns or scarcity of patients in the backcountry encouraged and perhaps forced doctors to utilize their talents with as much versatility as possible, division and specialization were totally impractical. Occasionally a Carolinian confessed his confusion at the blurring of distinctions known to exist in Europe.'I won't pretend to say', wrote one, 'whether an Apothecary or Chirugeon can be calculated a *graduate* Physician, or a graduate Physician is of course an Apothecary and Chirugeon'.[16] In general, the South Carolina practitioner performed as physician, pharmacist, and surgeon, thereby enhancing his reputation with each patient and able to charge more for his tripartite attention. Doctors' social aspirations might have argued for their eschewing drug selling and apothecary duties, but economic considerations usually overwhelmed these pretensions. Apprentices in many practices did most of the pharmacy work, enabling the fastidious practitioner to avoid the more mundane aspects of his occupation. It seems clear that the prevailing system worked to the advantage of both the patient, who found it more convenient to receive complete service from the one doctor, and the practitioner, who could earn more by preparing and supplying a drug, or carrying out a surgical procedure he recommended.

Without legislative action, pressure groups, or professional organizations such as the Royal College of Surgeons to set and enforce agreed standards of training and practice, create boundaries on specialists, or determine who could practise, where and when — who or what constituted a doctor in South Carolina in the eighteenth century is difficult to discern. Those who did practise did not attempt to establish any kind of self-regulating body among themselves, except for the purposes of fee setting, until almost the last decade of the century. The South Carolina Medical Society was formed in 1789, partly in response to doctors' perception of their increasing power, sophistication, and importance, but its emphasis was less on overt professional limitations than on educational exchange, community service, and financial return.

While the absence of strict controls may have encouraged some would-be doctors, the range of seemingly endless, vaguely definable illnesses from which inhabitants were rarely free was probably the main factor that attracted medical practitioners to the colony. Although there were seasons and areas in which the disease environment was less prejudicial to health, South Carolina's reputation for ill health was well earned. Even medical practitioners found themselves unable to maintain their health during the sickly season. Alexander Garden, who was kept busy by a large and successful practice in Charleston, concluded that he was 'generally sick every year' during the summer.[17] William Fyffe found that his 'usual Sickness in the Fall' undermined the income from his practice.[18] The death and drama of major epidemics of smallpox, yellow fever, influenza, dysentery and malaria more profoundly affected the demography and perhaps the reputation of the colony. Certainly such outbreaks were not kind to a doctor's sense of professional expertise and to his income. So often there was little that could be done; frequently, what could be tried was at the risk of personal exposure. In the worst epidemics the decimation of whole families and the scramble to escape proximity to the disease reduced the patient pool and made collection of doctors' accounts extremely difficult. Nevertheless, although other colonies certainly experienced epidemic disease, it was South Carolina's notorious reputation for unhealthiness, the unending stream of minor complaints, the numerous plantations with large slave populations that had to be kept healthy, and an economic boom unparalleled in the eighteenth century, which proved a magnetic combination for medical practitioners of every kind.

PROFESSIONAL CIRCLES

Despite the demands upon his knowledge and time, the practitioner who became wealthy from a practice in South Carolina was the exception rather than the rule.[19] The rewards of medicine, especially for ambitious Charleston practitioners, often lay not in the amassing of an estate but rather in the accumulation of intellectual capital. Medicine, they found could provide a respectable base from which to launch a satisfying and stimulating career in the world of science and letters.

Colonial life and private practice were insufficiently challenging for medical men whose background, education, and hopes prepared them for something quite different. These practitioners sought to relieve their disappointment in part by promoting arts, letters, and culture on the local scene, making a contribution in this area far beyond what might have been expected in terms of their numbers in the population. Extensive correspondence with colleagues, family, and public figures both in the colonies and abroad also generated some of the mental stimulation that the everyday practice of medicine in South Carolina could rarely produce.

As South Carolina had made little attempt to control medical practice or support an appropriate code of ethical conduct for medical practitioners, the colony lagged behind other colonies such as Pennsylvania and New York in encouraging medical excellence and the emergence of a well-trained, responsible medical community.[20] Unprotected from pretenders or avaricious quacks, a practice in South Carolina could be a source of frustration for the dedicated and formally trained. Career satisfaction had to be sought elsewhere and many found it in their scientific and literary pursuits. Several doctors wrote and published extensively. Much of their work was scientific, but it ranged across a broad spectrum in both content and purpose. In publishing, practitioners achieved the renown that could never otherwise have come to them in status-conscious South Carolina.

Until the close of the eighteenth century, there were no medical journals within the colony to serve as a specific outlet for their work, so South Carolina practitioners looked elsewhere. Local printers trailed behind those of Philadelphia, New York, and Boston (all of which supported comparable medical communities) in publishing the works of local physicians. Medical historian John Blake has argued that throughout the eighteenth century 'the potential audience on this side of the Atlantic was not large enough to justify ordinarily the expense of publishing works of this limited appeal in America'.[21] Moreover, while American editions were usually less expensive than the imported European equivalent, the quality of the product was rarely so good, and to Carolinians, never as significant. For South Carolinians continually measuring themselves against overseas standards, publication in Europe carried far greater prestige. In their revolutionary fervour after 1780, some South Carolina practitioners patronized American printers. For the most part, however, they continued to send their manuscripts to Europe, often through influential friends.[22]

Occasionally, a local issue provided an opportunity to promote a practitioner's ideas and reputation. For example, the appearance in several colonies of a smallpox epidemic in 1738 occasioned a public debate among practitioners over the efficacy of inoculation, and provided a forum for two South Carolina practitioners — Dr Thomas Dale and Dr James Killpatrick — to air their views and display their scientific, intellectual, and literary skills. Inspired by the success of inoculists in Boston, Killpatrick and several other practitioners decided to try inoculation on a larger scale in Charleston. Probably as many as one thousand South Carolinians were treated and Killpatrick reported an extremely low mortality rate thereafter. But Dale disagreed with Killpatrick and entered into a lengthy debate over the efficacy of inoculations.[23] The *South Carolina Gazette* reported the controversy in several editions, and ultimately issued both arguments in separate pamphlets. Printer Lewis Timothy concluded that 'the generality of my customers shew a Dislike to have anymore inoculation in the Gazette'.[24]

Pamphlets such as those by Dale and Killpatrick were a common mode of communication in the eighteenth century, and Killpatrick's *Full and Clear Reply* typifies their polemic style and documentation bolstered with quotations from prominent medical practitioners. Its tone vacillates from laboured argument to amusing and bitter denunciation.[25] Dale's contributions were similar.

Thomas Dale was one of the most intellectual members of the medical community. The son of an English apothecary and a graduate of Leyden, Dale had already ventured into print with several translations of Latin works, all published in London. Prominent in social and literary circles in Charleston, Dale also wrote for the Dock Street theatre. (His humorous epilogue to a production of *The Recruiting Officer* appeared in the popular *Gentlemen's Magazine*.)[26] Dale maintained an extensive medical practice throughout his life, his varied interests typifying him as the eighteenth-century ideal of a well-rounded gentlemen.[27]

Shortly after this controversy, and perhaps because of it, Killpatrick departed for England, where, as Dr James Kirkpatrick, he 'became fashionable and famous as an inoculator'.[28] Kirkpatrick continued his writing and published *An Essay on Inoculation* in 1743, and *An Analysis of the Inoculation Comprising the History, Theory and Practice of It* in 1754. His continued contact with South Carolinians in England, and his correspondence with both prominent South Carolina families and members of the Charleston medical community, are indicative of the esteem in which Kirkpatrick was held. Eliza Pinckney was much 'obliged to him' for his care of her sons who were still at school in England.[29] Kirkpatrick corresponded with the prominent Charleston practitioner Lionel Chalmers, who 'promised to send him a letter' describing a further outbreak of smallpox in the colony in 1760.[30] Local practitioners were proud of his achievements in England and continued to view him as a valuable member of their circle.

Few ambitious practitioners, however, were content with the rarely expressed approval of South Carolinians, and, like so many colonials before and since, often found that even this came only after they had established a reputation elsewhere. They sought to expand their reputation and their knowledge through numerous contacts with friends and colleagues in other colonies and, particularly, with the world beyond the Atlantic. South Carolina practitioners took advantage of the general and widespread interest in North American and initiated correspondence with prominent scientists, naturalists, medical practitioners, and intellectuals. A few correspondents were perhaps more interested in what they could obtain from eager South Carolinians, but most were flatteringly enthusiastic in their pursuit of an exchange of letters, ideas, information, and local flora and fauna.

Dr John Fothergill, a well-known Quaker physician who often extended London hospitality to young practitioners, students, and travellers from America, requested botanical samples on numerous occasions from his many colonial correspondents. Fothergill, whose father had spent several years in South Carolina for the Society of Friends, corresponded with Lionel Chalmers. Occasionally Fothergill offered advice on specific medical problems but more often he requested help in enlarging his botanic collections. Chalmers also acted as Fothergill's fiscal agent to William Bartram, whom Fothergill had engaged to supply drawings of South Carolina plants and animals. Pleased to be the recipient of letters from a member of European scientific circles and thus indirectly a part of that circle, Chalmers appeared unoffended by Fothergill's frequent requests and sometimes arrogant manner. Rather, to Chalmers, Fothergill's wide-ranging interest in America was personally rewarding and even flattering. In one letter Fothergill expressed a wish

> that some person can be found in America capable of describing the present time with the state of agriculture, commerce, and the dawn of the arts; and that every twenty years a fresh account of the present state of the colony should be authenticated by their respective assemblies.[31]

In another letter he detailed the best method of sending plants and seeds, requesting particularly 'the useful, the beautiful, the singular or the fragrant'.[32]

Although such correspondence enhanced their sense of being part of significant international scientific, intellectual, and cultural exchanges, South Carolina practitioners continued to feel isolated from the 'real' scientific and intellectual world they believed only existed overseas. Knowledge of their distance from the centre of activity heightened their frustration with practice in America at least until the Revolution caused them to rethink their relationship with America.

Alexander Garden frequently lamented his isolation and was never particularly content in South Carolina because of it. Garden hoped to establish his reputation in European scientific circles, but complained that his medical practice never allowed him time to pursue his real interests in botany, 'our people preferring a slavish attendance to any other qualification'.[33] Garden's earliest local publications reflect both his botanical interests and his medical training.[34]

Bemoaning his isolation in the belief that 'what has been passing in the literary world is entirely unknown to us', Garden relied on correspondents to keep him informed of the latest findings in medicine, natural history, and botany.[35] He was delighted with the appearance in the *Philosophical Transactions* of one of his letters to John Ellis concerning the electric eel, and another to Dr Hope on the use of tobacco ashes as a cure for dropsy.[36] These publications encouraged Garden's hope that his physical isolation did not also mean that his work was out of touch with the interests of researchers overseas. Such recognition and appreciation were more significant to Garden than his warm reception and busy practice in Charleston and its environs.[37] Writing to Linnaeus in 1763 he announced his intention to 'withdraw myself from [medicine] in two or three years at most, I shall then wholly devote my time and thoughts to the cultivation of the delightful and engaging study of Nature'.[38]

Born and educated in Scotland, Garden had been drawn to South Carolina because, ironically, its climate appeared to suit his health, and because its wealthy, unhealthy citizenry promised a good financial return. A scholar, explorer and linguist, Garden's attempts to develop his interests among his Carolina colleagues met with little success. Even his hope of establishing a local college came to nothing. Ultimately his loyalty to the Crown had him banished from South Carolina, and he returned to London where he was received as 'a most welcome addition to the scientific circles'.[39] In contrast, though South Carolinians were in some measure pleased by Garden's international reputation, what really counted was his doctoring — the time and attention he gave to his patients' ills. 'Slavish attendance', as Garden called it, was what mattered in this most plagued of colonies. It is clear however, that Garden was welcome in homes where the ordinary practitioner was not.

Correspondence with the luminaries of their era assuaged some of the doubts and disappointments of local practice. David Ramsay, who corresponded with among others, John Adams, Noah Webster, and Benjamin Franklin, was 'much honored' by letters from Thomas Jefferson, then resident in Paris.[40] Jefferson assisted Ramsay in arranging for the French edition of his first book. In exchanging ideas, books and pamphlets with such men and with his mentor Benjamin Rush, Ramsay found some of the excitement and satisfaction absent from medical practice. This was particularly true at the turn of the century, as Ramsay's political influence waned. Publishing his research and his memories of South Carolina's history offered Ramsay the hope of improving his precarious finances. He believed such publications provided a clear demonstration of his intellectual capabilities. In spite of the fact that his practice was busy and successful, both his income and his abilities were hampered by the fact that medical practice was rarely effective and early death was a constant reminder of medicine's deficiencies. Nor did it open the door to Charleston society and upward mobility.

With few exceptions, Ramsay directed his considerable literary output away from medicine. His writing was historical and political rather than scientific. History, he believed, gave him an appropriate medium through which he could express his 'opinions on a variety of subjects'.[41] Ramsay's *History of the Revolution of South Carolina from a British Province to an Independent State* was in many senses a labour of love, but it was a financial disaster.[42] The venture left Ramsay severely out of pocket; undeterred, he launched into *The History of the American Revolution*.[43] His correspondence provides evidence of the enormous vitality and enthusiasm with which he tackled these projects. Contemporary reviews were, on the whole, favourable when *The History of the American Revolution* appeared, but it is doubtful that it was a financial success.[44]

Aside from these substantial studies Ramsay produced numerous shorter pieces, the first of which appeared anonymously as the humorous *Sermon on Tea*, and his 4 July orations were regularly published.[45] Two of Ramsay's best-known publications began as addresses before the South Carolina Medical Society and were printed at the behest of the Society, and the later *Review of the Improvements, Progress and State of Medicine in the Eighteenth Century* originated from a proposal to the Society.[46] Ramsay's medical practice certainly flourished, but a great deal of his time was spent writing and ensuring the circulation of what he had written. He believed his writing was significant and sought recognition of it from others. Benjamin Rush, impressed by the persuasive 'spirit of freedom' disliked Ramsay's ornamental style, preferring 'simplicity to everything in composition'.[47]

Although Ramsay lamented the absence of good, modern medical texts relevant to American conditions, he declared proudly in his study of medical progress that there were 'more medical writings ushered into public view, by the physicians of Charleston, than any other part of the American continent'.[48] Although this appears to have been correct, Ramsay failed to take the *quality* of these writings into consideration. Little of the scientific or medical work produced by South Carolinian practitioners was pathbreaking in design or conception. Most of it conformed to established eighteenth-century tradition and style — describing, measuring, capitalizing on the novelty of South Carolina and sustained interest in America.[49] These practitioners were observers and recorders and they wrote of the climate rather than technical advances in surgery or the definitive identification of a disease.

One of the most prolific practitioners in the field of medical or scientific publication was John Lining, best known for his *Description of the American Yellow Fever*, published in Charleston in 1735 and believed to be the first description of the disease's symptoms to come from America.[50] Like so many other practitioners, Lining found it easier and more stimulating to achieve status outside medicine. He established his international reputation with the publication of his letters in prestigious English and Scottish journals. For the most part these were descriptions of his observation and measurement of South Carolina climate.[51] By 1754 Lining had practically abandoned his medical practice for the greater rewards and satisfaction he found in science.[52] He experimented with electricity and with raising indigo, and so won the recognition and respect of the international scientific community.[53]

Lionel Chalmers, contemporary and sometime partner of Lining, was also gratified to find himself included in these circles. Initial contacts were made through Fothergill. Chalmers, who possessed no formal degree in medicine, published a letter discussing tetanus and sent through Fothergill in *Medical Observations and Inquiries* in 1757.[54] Chalmers lobbied influential friends to ensure that his work was published. Chalmers' material also appeared in his *Account of Weather*.[55] His *Essay of Fevers* was published in several countries[56] and was serialized in *The American Magazine* and *The Pennsylvania Chronicle*.

David Ramsay pronounced Chalmers 'the best medical character here', and he was certainly patronized by many prominent Charleston families.[57] Nevertheless Chalmers was continually frustrated by delinquent accounts and looked beyond medicine for a satisfying life.[58] He was a Justice of the Peace, an active member of the Library Society and maintained a voluminous correspondence. The day-to-day practice of medicine in the eighteenth century could not contain his energies. Chalmers searched for these qualities elsewhere, and found them in a local, national and international circle of colleagues.

TOWARDS A PROFESSION

Historians of medicine and science have made much of the botanical expertise, eye for detail and sound observation preserved in the publications of South Carolina practitioners such as Chalmers, Garden and Lining. However it is difficult to determine precisely what affect this may have had upon South Carolina's inhabitants or upon the relationship between doctors and their patients. It would take more than an international reputation to alter the deep-seated belief in the community at large that medical practitioners were too expensive, indecisive, unsympathetic and unable to cure even the most common complaints. To many South Carolinians medical practice was not the best way to get ahead in the world.[59] Scientific publication enhanced their reputation, if not as colonial doctors, then certainly as members of the metropolitan culture. Such a reputation, advanced by publication, made palatable an occupation otherwise frustrated by South Carolina's inadequate prospects, a reluctant patient pool sustained by a philosophical ideal of 'every man his own doctor' and the insufficient and inadequate knowledge available from a relatively undeveloped discipline.

Significantly, but less tangibly, the development of this metropolitan outlook and commitment among men of medicine helped to promote the first brief period of professionalized medicine in South Carolina.[60] From the limited evidence available, Charleston practitioners who established themselves internationally had the busiest practices and were welcomed socially in the homes of the town's influential citizens. Ironically, in reaching beyond routine practice, practitioners helped to allay for a time the doubts of laymen over the utility of restricting medical practice to those practitioners who could demonstrate formal training and/or extensive experience. The slow relinquishing of those misgivings is partially evident in the establishment of the South Carolina Medical Society in 1789.

The years of war marked a transition from a time when any educated layman could read the few available texts and perform as adequately as the practitioner with years of training and experience. The complex health problems occasioned by the war brought about some loss of faith in self-treatment.[61] The growing acceptance of inoculation was just one element of health care which could not be dealt with alone or with the assistance of family or friends. Many South Carolinians prided themselves on their independence and this loss of control was distressing.[62] But medicine held out the promise of great things. The gradual improvement and acceptance of less expensive American medical school training especially after the Revolution helped to widen the gap between self-treatment and the now more numerous professional practitioner.[63] South Carolinians slowly recognized the futility of trying to maintain the traditional image of the gentleman practitioner who came when you needed him, offered his undivided attention, and reluctantly accepted your offer of payment in gratitude for his successful services. Growing admiration for the experience and skill of doctors, and awareness of their overseas reputation, helped to develop a shortlived confidence in local medicine and in community practitioners. This tentative receptiveness injected new life into the practitioners' spasmodic attempts at organization which had been rejected so vigorously in 1755. (In that year a group of doctors agreed to discontinue treating patients unless they received immediate payment. This blunt attempt to determine fees through organization elicited only public derision.)[64]

Once established the Medical Society was cognizant of its responsibility to the public to record its findings, medical or climatological. Thus the Minutes of the Society note that members were encouraged to relay information on 'weather & diseases' which the Secretary would record. Details of 'remarkable cases' were also requested.[65] At the monthly meetings members took turns presenting papers for discussion, enlightenment and entertainment. Eventually the Society collected and published these. The papers offered at these gatherings reflected the practitioners' eclectic interests and were by no means confined to medical topics. They ranged from Dr John Budd's humorous 'Dissertation on Porter' to a joint report of an investigation into Charleston's water supply.[66] Interest was also generated by papers pertinent to South Carolina's health problems such as a Philadelphia College of Physicians study of epidemic fever.[67]

The Society was enthusiastically received by members who were reminded of 'the importance of the study of Natural Knowledge, particularly an acquaintance with the principles & effects of Mechanic Powers as connected with the Science of Medicine'. The Society provided a focus for medical practitioners, and individuals and organizations outside South Carolina — such as the American Philosophical Society — looked to it for specific information and advice.[68] Attendance at meetings, though, was frequently poor and more than one meeting was cancelled. Disillusionment set in quickly and the hopeful aspirations of ambitious practitioners for the Society remained largely unfulfilled.

Nevertheless, the Society did achieve some of its aims. A second fee bill was established in 1792. In comparison with the failed attempt of 1755, practitioners were far more sure of their professional status and the public appeared more ready to accept their articulation of that status. Other states had by this time established the precedent of regulating doctors' charges. Virginia had established a medical fee bill in 1763, and one of the first actions of the embryonic New Jersey Medical Society was the preparation of 'A Table of Fees and Rates' in 1766. The fees contained in the South Carolina bill of 1792 appear to have been accepted with little public reaction by either patients or practitioners.[69] In addition, a library was begun, a water safety programme for the Charleston foreshore, where several drownings had occurred, was established, and a dispensary set up.

By 1822 however, a prominent citizen, Edward Ravenel, could find little in the doctors' actions 'to sanction their opinion of their own charity and dignity . . . . Various attempts have been made to stimulate them to some literary exertion and all have failed.'[70] The Society struggled on through the disputes surrounding the establishment of a local medical school, but was unable to defeat the legislative decision to rescind licensure requirements in 1838. Medicine had not lived up to its enlightenment promises and there was once again strong reaction against any attempt to enhance the status of the practitioners by establishing rules for admission to practise.

In the short term then, the Charleston practitioners of the eighteenth and early nineteenth centuries improved the situation for their generation and established the rudiments of professionalism. Spurred by the establishment of medical societies, South Carolinian practitioners became more interested in local outlets for publication of their research. Occasionally journals such as *American Museum* published medical articles, but the increasing volume of such materials and the apparent growth in audience highlighted the demand for specific medical journals. The South Carolina Medical Society quickly saw the utility of New York's *Medical Repository* which began publication in 1797.[71] The *Charleston Medical Register* thus began to appear in 1803 under the editorship of David Ramsay. This newly developing genre of American medical journalism also gave practitioners a fresh medium through which to bring their work to a larger local audience. The journals also encouraged the growing sense of professional identity embodied in the infant medical societies. By 1810 four other American journals competed with the *Medical Repository* and the *Charleston Medical Register*.[72] Clearly the local and national intellectual community had sufficiently expanded to support such publications.

Charleston's practitioners' search for challenge and stimulation, their research and their publications had inspired, encouraged and improved intellectual exchange within North America. Most significantly for their own careers, their efforts to involve themselves in the metropolitan intellectual community had, in some measure, paved the way for the first acceptance of professional medical practice in South Carolina. This opened fresh avenues of exchange, thereby increasing the potential for improved and enlightened medical practice. Out of frustration had come satisfaction, pleasure, social status, and recognition of their role as men of science and letters.

These advantages did not extend to their role as practical healers. In the long term, South Carolinians demanded more than the approbation of European intellectuals to persuade them of the necessity for regulated medical practice. Until medical practitioners could demonstrate their value to society in practical terms — in lives saved, in pain relieved — South Carolinians, in common with many others around the world, withheld their complete acceptance and support. Practitioners were welcome at the social festivities, trusted in legal matters, and worthy members of numerous organizations but, when it came to questions of health, an international reputation and a list of publications only advanced the professional practitioner up the long line of those consulted. These assets placed him before other practitioners but, with the resurgence of interest in self-help, behind relatives, friends, and local authorities.

NOTES

1. See, for example, Walter B. Edgar, *The Letterbook of Robert Pringle*, 2 vols (Columbia: University of South Carolina Press, 1972), vol. I, 62, Robert Pringle to Humphrey Hill, 22 January 1738/9.

2. Mabel L. Webber (ed.), 'Extracts from the journal of Mrs Ann Manigault, 1754–1781', *South Carolina Historical and Genealogical Magazine* (hereafter *SCHGM*), *21* (1920), 10–23.

3. Two hundred and twenty individuals have been found who practised medicine in some form in South Carolina in the eighteenth century. Sufficient information was available to permit classification of 170 — almost 78 per cent — of these. The remaining 23 per cent could not be traced beyond a bare skeleton of their lives and so had to be eliminated from a typology based primarily upon teasing out an individual's perspective of his occupation. The categorization used here was constructed upon four criteria: the range and diversity of a doctor's practice, the character of his reception by both the public and other doctors, his ultimate career choice and, especially, his self-perception — his view of himself, his occupation, and his expectations. Thus it distinguishes among four groups of practitioners: handymen or jack-of-all-trades, dilettantes, planter/practitioners and professionals.

4. Medical apprenticeships could be as long as seven years and were often stringent, binding agreements, demanding high standards. In New Jersey, for example, a student could not even be accepted as an apprentice unless he was competent in Greek. For useful discussion of colonial apprenticeships in medicine see Genevieve Miller, 'Medical apprenticeships in the American colonies', *Ciba Symposia*, *8* (1946), 502–10, and Henry Viets, 'The medical education of James Lloyd in Colonial America', *Yale Journal of Biology and Medicine*, *31* (1958), 1–13.

5. St Julien Ravenel Childs, 'Health and disease in the early history of South Carolina (Unpublished MA thesis, George Washington University, 1931), chs 3–8.

6. John Duffy, *Epidemics in Colonial America* (Baton Rouge: Louisiana State University Press, 1953); St Julien Ravenel Childs, *Malaria and Colonization in the Carolina Low Country, 1526–1696* (Baltimore: Johns Hopkins University Press, 1940).

7. Defined in the Constitution of the World Health Organization, *Basic Documents* (Geneva: WHO, 1970).

8. A recovering patient might thus be described as 'eat[ing] well, and . . . in high spirits', Elise Pickney (ed.), 'Letters of Eliza Lucas Pickney, 1768–1782', *South Carolina Historical Magazine* (hereafter *SCHM*), *76* (1975), 145, Eliza Pickney to Mrs Daniel Horry (undated).

9. Read Family Papers, South Caroliniana Library, University of South Carolina, Columbia, South Carolina, Box 1, Folder 7, Cornelia Read to sister Betsey, 16 September (1790?).

10. G. Melvyn Howe, *Man, Environment and Disease in Britain* (Harmondsworth: Penguin, 1972), 19. For a useful summary of the problems of defining health, see Douglas Gordon, *Health, Sickness and Society: Theoretical Concepts in Social and Preventive Medicine* (St Lucia: University of Queensland Press, 1976), ch. 4.

11. The Negro Act of 1740 with additional clauses included later in the year, contained in Thomas Cooper and David J. McCord (eds), *The Statutes at Large of South Carolina* (Columbia: A.S. Johnston, 1836–41), 7, 402, 422–3.

12. Daniel Boorstin, *The Americans: The Colonial Experience* (New York: Random House, 1958), 227–30. See also Richard S. Shryock, 'Public relations of the medical profession in Great Britain and the United States, 1600–1870: a chapter in the social history of medicine', *Annals of Medical History* n.s., *2* (1930), 310.

13. Quoted in Judith Ward Steinman Karst, 'Newspaper medicine: a cultural study of the colonial south, 1730–1770' (Unpublished PhD thesis, Tulane University, 1971), 75.

14. John Morgan, *A discourse upon the institution of medical schools in America delivered at a public anniversary commencement, held in the College of Philadelphia, May 30 and 31, 1765. With a preface containing, amongst other things, the author's apology for attempting to introduce the regular mode of practising physic in Philadelphia* (Philadelphia: W. Bradford, 1765).

15. R.S. Roberts, 'The personnel and practice of medicine in Tudor and Stuart England, Pt. 1, The Provinces', *Medical History, 6* (1962), 217–34.

16. *South Carolina Gazette*, 12 June 1755.

17. James Edward Smith, *A Selection of the Correspondence of Linnaeus and other Naturalists from the Original Manuscripts* (London: Longman, 1821), *1*, 59, Alexander Garden to John Ellis, 17 February 1759.

18. Fyffe Letters, William Clements Library, University of Michigan, Ann Arbor, Michigan, William Fyffe to Elizabeth Fyffe, 15 November 1771.

19. Diane Sydenham, 'Practitioner and patient: the practice of medicine in eighteenth-century South Carolina' (Unpublished PhD thesis, Johns Hopkins University, 1979), ch. 4.

20. John Spears and Diane Sydenham, 'The evolution of medical practice in two marginal areas of the western world, 1750–1830', *Historical Reflections* (Spring/Summer, 1982), 195–212.

21. J. Blake, 'Early American medical literature', *Journal of the American Medical Association, 236* (1976), 44.

22. See for example, the letters of David Ramsay published in the *Transactions of the American Philosophical Society, 55* (4) (1965) as 'David Ramsay 1749–1815: selections from his writings', edited by Robert R. Brunhouse.

23. Official action consisted primarily of quarantine measures embodied in 'An Act for better preventing the spreading of the infection of Smallpox in Charles Town', passed 18 September 1738 by the General Assembly.

24. *South Carolina Gazette*, 1, 8, 15 June; 17, 24, 31 August, 1738. The debates appeared in pamphlet form as *The Case of Miss Mary Roche who was Inoculated June 28, 1738, fairly related and etc. with some occasional remarks on the smallpox and a few seasonable observations on the practice of inoculation*, by James Killpatrick, 1738; *The Case of Miss Mary Roche, more fairly related and etc.*, by Thomas Dale, 1738; *A Full and Clear Reply to Doctor Thomas Dale . . .*, by James Killpatrick, 1739; *The Puff: or a proper reply to Skimmington's last crudities . . .*, by Thomas Dale, 1739; *South Carolina Gazette*, 7 September 1738.

25. Joseph I. Waring, 'James Killpatrick and smallpox Inoculation in Charlestown', *Annals of Medical History*, n.s., *10* (1938), 301–8. Waring maintains that the copy of this

pamphlet in the British Library is the earliest extant medical publication from the colony.

26. See Robert A. Law, 'A diversion for colonial gentleman', *Texas Review, 2* (1916), 79–88 for a brief discussion of this epilogue.

27. Dale's estate inventory and his will revealed a library of nearly two thousand books and an extensive collection of dried plants and botanical specimens, *South Carolina Inventories, 9* (1753–6), 369ff; *South Carolina Wills, 6* (1747–52), 403. Both *Inventories* and *Wills* are held at the South Carolina Department of Archives and History, Columbia, South Carolina.

28. Waring, op. cit., n. 25 above, 304.

29. Elise Pinckney (ed.), *The Letterbook of Eliza Lucas Pinckney, 1749–1762* (Chapel Hill: University of North Carolina Press, 1972), 109, 105, Eliza Pinckney to George Morly, February 1759; Eliza Pinckney to (Mrs Euancel?).

30. ibid., 161, Eliza Pinckney to George Morly, 8 February 1761.

31. Betsy C. Corner and Christopher C. Booth, *Chain of Friendship: Selected Letters of John Fothergill of London, 1735–1780* (Cambridge, Mass.: Belknap Press, 1971), 266, John Fothergill to Lionel Chalmers, 10 September 1766.

32. ibid., 393, John Fothergill to William Bartram, 22 October 1772.

33. Smith, op. cit., n. 17 above, 364, Alexander Garden to John Ellis, 13 January 1756.

34. *An Account of the Medical Properties of the Virginia Pink Root* (Charleston, 1764), no extant copy.

35. Smith, op. cit., n. 17 above, 288, Alexander Garden to Linnaeus, 15 March 1755. For a brief discussion of Garden's correspondence, see Andrew Kerr, Jr, 'Doctors afield: Alexander Garden (1728–1793), colonial botanist', *New England Journal of Medicine, 253* (1955), 610.

36. 'An account of the Gynmatus Electricus or electrical eels, in a letter from Alexander Garden M.D. F.R.S. to John Ellis Esq., F.R.S', *Philosophical Transactions, 65* (1775), 102–10; 'An account of the use of ashes in tobacco in the cure of dropsy . . . in a letter to Dr. Hope', *Medical and Philosophical Commentaries by the Society of Physicians in Edinburgh*, 1775–6.

37. For example, Martha Logan wrote to John Bartram, 'Dr Garden has so much business he has not time to think of me', Mary B. Prior (ed.), 'Letters of Martha Logan to John Bartram, 1760–1763', *SCHM, 49* (1958), 40.

38. Smith, op. cit., n. 17 above, 310. Garden to Linnaeus, 2 June 1763.

39. Edmund Berkeley and Dorothy Smith Berkeley, *Dr. Alexander Garden of Charles Town* (Chapel Hill: University of North Carolina Press, 1969); Smith, op. cit., n. 17 above, 283.

40. Brunhouse, op. cit., n. 22 above, 110, David Ramsay to Thomas Jefferson, 7 April 1787.

41. ibid., 163, David ramsay to Jonathon Lettsom, 1808.

42. 2 vols (Trenton: Isaac Collins), 1785.

43. 2 vols (Philadelphia: R. Aitken & Sons), 1789.

44. Opinions of the study have differed. For a summary of the controversy see Brunhouse, op. cit., n. 22 above, 224. Also useful is Elmer Douglas Johnson, 'David Ramsay: historian or plagiarist', *SCHM, 57* (1956), 189–98 and, especially, Arthur H. Shaffer, *The Politics of History* (Chicago: Precedent Publishers, 1975).

45. Brunhouse, op. cit., n. 22 above, 179–82; (Francis Barley: Pennsylvania, 1774).

46. *A Dissertation on the Means of Preserving Health in Charleston, & the Adjacent Low Country, read before the Medical Society of South Carolina, the 29th May, 1790* (Charleston: Markland & M'Iver, 1790); *A Sketch of the Soil, Climate, Weather, and Diseases of South Carolina, read before the Medical Society of that state, by David Ramsay, M.D., Vice-President of that Society* (Charleston: W.P. Young, 1796); *A Review of the Improvements, Progress and State of Medicine in the XVIIIth Century* (Charleston: W.P. Young, 1801).

47. L.H. Butterfield (ed.) Letters of Benjamin Rush, 2 vols (Princeton: Princeton University Press, 1951), vol. I, 218–19, Benjamin Rush to David Ramsay, 5 November 1778.

48. Brunhouse, op. cit., n. 22 above, 213.

49. Other South Carolinian practitioners were also adding to the corpus of American scientific literature. One student of Ramsay's, John Lewis Edward Whitridge Shecut, who later studied with Benjamin Rush, was particularly interested in botany. His publications in this field attracted some attention in the early nineteenth century and the first volume of a projected two-volume *Flora Carolinaenis* was highly praised.

50. The recurring, seasonal fevers which afflicted most South Carolinians and which, for those who could afford it, motivated an annual migration to cooler, healthier climates, gave rise to numerous publications. Even as doctors were debating the arguments of John Lining and Lionel Chalmers, Dr George Carter produced another essay on fevers, followed by a study of yellow fever: *An Essay on Fevers: particularly on the Fever lately so rife in Charleston S.C. together with some Useful Remarks on the Symptoms thereon, and a Mode laid down towards the Curative Part* (Charleston: W.P. Harrison, 1796); *A Physiological Essay on Yellow Fever, with some Critical Notes and Careful Observations* (Charleston: J.J. Negrin, 1806).

51. See, for example, 'Extract of two letters from Dr. John Lining, physician at Charles-Town in South Carolina to James Jurin M.D., F.R.S. giving an account of statical experiments made several times in a day upon himself for one whole year, accompanied with meteorological observations; to which are subjoined six general tables, deduced from the whole years course', Royal Society of London, *Philosophical Transactions, 42* (1743), 491–509; 'A letter from John Lining, M.D. of Charles-Town, South Carolina, to the Rev. Tho. Birch, D.D. Secr. R.S. concerning the quantity of rain fallen there from January 1738 to December, 1752', Royal Society of London, *Philosophical Transactions, 48* (1753), 284–5.

52. See, for example, Court of Common Pleas, South Carolina Department of Archives and History, Judgement Rolls 046A 0138A, 1758.

53. 'Extract of a letter from John Lining M.D. of Charles Town in South Carolina, to Charles Pinckney, Esq; in London: with his answer to several queries sent to him concerning his experiment of electricity with a kite', Royal Society of London, *Philosophical Transactions, 48* (1754), 757–64, replicated Benjamin Franklin's experiments which had earlier been described in the same journal.

54. *Medical Observations and Inquiries, 1* (1757).

55. London: E.& C. Dilly, 1776.

56. Charles Town (1767); London (1768); Riga (1773).

57. Brunhouse, op. cit., n. 22 above, 52, David Ramsay to Benjamin Rush, 29 July 1774.

58. See for example, Court of Common Pleas, Judgement Rolls 074A 0602A, 1767; 088A 0174A, 1770.

59. Henry Laurens, for example, would have preferred his son, John, to follow him 'into Merchandize' or even the clergy but was relieved when John set aside his 'favourite Physick' and decided to study law. See Philip Hamer *et al.* (eds), *The Papers of Henry Laurens* 10 vols. (Columbia: University of South Carolina Press, 1968–85), vol. *7*, 327; vol. *8*, 447–8, Henry Laurens to Richard Clark, 25 August 1770; Henry Laurens to Richard Clark, 25 August 1770.

60. 'Professional' is used very cautiously, given the extensive debate this topic has generated. While I am not persuaded by any particular definition, I find R.H. Tawney's simple description useful: 'a body of men who carry on their work in accordance with rules designed to enforce certain standards for the better protection of its members and for the better services of the public', *The Acquisitive Society* (New York: Harcourt, Brace & Howe, 1920), 92–3.

61. For discussion of the variety of medical problems faced by practitioners during the war see Philip Cash, 'The Canadian military campaign of 1775–1776: medical problems and effects of disease', *Journal of the American Medical Association, 236* (1976), 52–6.

62. Daniel H. Calhoun, *Professional Lives in America: Structure and Aspiration, 1750–1850* (Cambridge, Mass.: Harvard University Press, 1965); ch. 2 is suggestive on this point.

63. On the significance of the Revolution in persuading intending practitioners of the value of local training, see Benjamin Waterhouse, *The Rise, Progress and Present State of Medicine: A Discourse Delivered at Concord, July 6, 1791 before the Middlesex Medical Association* (Boston: T.J. Fleet, 1792), 26.

64. Almost nothing is known about this association apart from a newspaper announcement of the doctors' agreement, *South Carolina Gazette*, 5 June 1755.

65. Minutes of the South Carolina Medical Society, 28 August 1790, held at the South Caroliniana Library.

66. The former was read before the Medical Society, 28 May 1800, and printed in that year by Markland & M'Iver, Minutes of the South Carolina Medical Society, May 1800.

67. Minutes of the South Carolina Medical Society, March 1799.

68. ibid., 24 December 1790.

69. Bill of Medical Fees, 9 July 1792. Pamphlet in the Francis A. Countway Library of Medicine, Boston.

70. Cited in Joseph I. Waring, *A History of Medicine in South Carolina, 1825–1900* (Columbia: South Carolina Medical Association, 1967), 94.

71. The journals twenty-three volumes attracted an enormous variety of scientific articles, from swallow migration to geology.

72. *Philadelphia Medical Museum* (1804); *Philadelphia Medical and Physical Journal* (1804); *Baltimore Medical and Physical Recorder* (1808); *New York and Philosophical Journal* (1809).

8

Public health and the medical profession in nineteenth-century Canada

Geoffrey Bilson

The year 1815 saw British North America secured against United States' aggression. The war of 1812 was marked by forays into the United States and checks to invasion attempts. It was clear that there was little support in British North America for the ambitions of United States' expansionists and despite continuing American interest in Canada there would continue to be little interest in joining the United States for the rest of the century. An English Canada has been founded largely by people who had fled the United States. The Catholic and francophone population of French Canada had good reasons to fear anglophone and Protestant America. Both preferred to remain within the British Empire. In 1815, that empire offered military support, economic opportunity and, for many English-speaking Canadians, an emotional link and an influential model.

Even in the aftermath of 1815, however, there were ambivalences in the relations both with Britain and the United States. The terms of membership in the Empire were hotly debated in British North America. The forms of government, with an appointed Governor, Executive Council and Legislative Council and an elected Assembly, gave great power to the imperial government within each colony and there was growing criticism of government in the twenty years after the war. Those Canadians who benefited from the system and had access to the patronage it dispensed supported it with vigour and defended it by drawing the contrast between the stability and order of Canada and the turbulence of the United States. Canadians who felt excluded from the system grew increasingly critical of it and urged reforms in government which would increase the role of the voter and bring a greater measure of what came to be called responsible government to the colonies. Many of the reformers looked to the Whigs of England and their triumphs in 1832 as their model but for a few the United States of the years of Jackson offered a more relevant example. In Lower Canada and Upper Canada these more radical politicians led open rebellions against the government in 1837 which were easily crushed. A number of radicals fled to the United States but most found it not to their liking and returned to Canada under amnesty in the years after their retreat.

Political reforms followed the crisis of 1837 and the demands for responsible government were met. In Central Canada, Lower and Upper Canada were united in 1841 but the Union suffered from the fact that anglophone and francophone Canadians could not co-operate easily. The francophones felt threatened by the growing numbers of anglophones and in protecting themselves against cultural assaults they helped to bring about a political deadlock in the United Canadas.

The political deadlock was resolved by creating a new nation, Canada, in 1867 as a federation of Central Canada and some of the maritime colonies which had found life increasingly difficult in these years as the protection of the British Empire declined in the face of free-trade triumphs. The drive toward confederation was intensified, especially in Ontario, by the view westward. The huge area of what is now western Canada was then in the hands of the Hudson's Bay Company. The region was home to Indian and Metis communities who lived by hunting, trapping, and farming. A small settlement of white farmers had existed at Red River for a generation but to Ontarians the west was 'empty' and ripe for settlement by European farmers. A Dominion of Canada could reasonably offer to take over the west from the Bay and secure it from the threat of annexation by the United States. This was done in the years following Confederation, and white settlement of the prairies, sustained by migration from Ontario and immigration from Europe, became a priority of the new nation in the later nineteenth century.

A role within the Empire was the path to independence from the United States in the nineteenth century for all but a few continentalists who advocated annexation in the last decades of the century. Defining the role was a difficult political question — one man's autonomy was another's disloyalty — and always the United States' presence was there. The United States continued to be viewed ambivalently by Canadians attracted by its vigour and rapid growth but fearful of its power on the continent. The new government attempted to protect the industrial base of Canada against United States competition but the United States remained a lure for Canadians. Not until the twentieth century would more people enter Canada in any decade than left it to live in the United States. Canada remained predominantly an agrarian country with over half the jobs provided by agriculture and extractive industry based on the forest, the sea, and the mine. The population was served by small towns and villages with a few major urban centres — Quebec, Montreal, Toronto, Halifax, Winnipeg — dominating their regions and providing the commercial and financial focal points for the nation.

The scattered settlements of the colonies were linked by water in the 1830s. Steamships began to operate on the St Lawrence early in the century. Improvements in transportation focused on canal building in the years after 1815 but the improvements to navigation on the St Lawrence were hampered by political squabbles and by the decision of the imperial government to spend money building a canal between Kingston and Ottawa for defensive military purposes rather than to encourage trade. In the 1840s, attention began to turn to railways and by 1860 about two thousand miles of railway had been laid in Canada to speed the passage of goods and people between the main centres of settlement. But such major centres as Quebec, Montreal, and Ottawa were linked by rail only in 1879 and the problem of overcoming distance continued to plague the country. In 1881 Halifax and Quebec were linked by rail and in that year the Canadian Pacific Railway Company was incorporated to build a line that would cross the continent to British Columbia and open the prairies to settlement by farmers by mid decade.

THE MEDICAL PROFESSION BEFORE CONFEDERATION

The medical profession functioned within the colonies as they developed in the early nineteenth century. Like Canada itself, the profession was shaped by influences from Britain and the United States and by the peculiar political and social circumstances of British North America. At the head of the profession stood the so called 'regular' doctors. These men were trained by apprenticeship or study at medical schools abroad or in Canada after the first schools were established in Lower Canada in the 1820s. The 'regular' doctors were consulted on medical questions by governments and appointed to what offices were available in the public service. They benefited from the assumption of the rulers of the colonies that entry to the medical profession should be regulated and doctors licensed to practise. Medical Boards were established by statute in the colonies, staffed by 'regular' doctors who were given the power to examine candidates and admit them to the practice of medicine. The members of the Medical Boards used their power to lay down the terms for entry to the profession — insisting, for example, that candidates have a good knowledge of Latin and rejecting applicants who failed to meet their arbitrary and unclear standards. The Upper Canada Medical Board between 1819 and 1837 passed 122 of 233 applicants. No doubt many of the candidates deserved to fail, given the state of medical education in these years, but quarrels between members of the profession were often reflected in the decisions of the Boards in Lower and Upper Canada.[1]

The Boards themselves emphasized the colonial nature of British North America. While they were empowered to examine and license applicants for entry to the profession, whole categories of practitioners were exempted from their control. Men with commissions in the military medical services could practise without a license. Graduates of universities in the British Empire were also exempt from examination. The professional bodies in Britain protected the interests of their members who moved to the colonies. In Upper Canada, the 'regulars' persuaded the Assembly to pass legislation in 1839 establishing a College of Physicians and Surgeons of Upper Canada as a step toward self-regulation. The Royal College of Surgeons protested that the legislation infringed their liberties and the Privy Council in London accordingly disallowed the Act and rendered it null and void. As the colonies were granted a greater degree of self-government, these imperial restraints on professional self-government declined.

Despite protests over the operation of the Medical Boards in the early nineteenth century, Canadian politicians never succumbed to the idea of abolishing all restrictions on entry to the profession. They did not wish to follow the American example where state after state in the 1820s and 1830s removed restrictions on entry. There were a few Canadians who supported open entry but they had little influence on legislation. Ideally, at least, the majority of Canadian politicians accepted the argument that medicine should be practised by trained and competent men. The 1820s saw a number of doctors establish medical schools in Lower Canada. François Blanchet and Anthony Von Iffland opened the Quebec Dispensary in 1823 both to serve the poor and to provide a setting in which to teach medicine. Teaching medicine brought doctors some prestige and a little income, and Canadian medical schools were supported by men such as Archdeacon John Strachan of Toronto, a leading conservative in the 1830s, who feared that without schools at home students would go to the United States and return with dangerous 'democratical ideas'.[2]

Doctors who taught medicine in their proprietary schools did so to increase their prestige, to raise the standards of the profession and to make money. Teaching did raise a doctor's prestige. Many of the doctors sufficiently prominent in pre-Confederation Canada to be memoralized in the pages of the *Dictionary of Canadian Biography* are there because teaching made them leaders in the profession. Some could be ruthless in defence of their income. Dr John Rolph is supposed to have used his political influence in the Assembly to close the University of Toronto's Medical School in 1851 to protect his own School of Medicine. The growth of medical schools in Canada, however, differed significantly from the parallel growth in the United States. Training in a medical school was not in itself a path to entry into licensed medical practice. It was followed by examination by the Medical Board unless the school had an affiliation with a degree-granting university. To protect their students from the vagaries of the Boards, most medical schools sought affiliation with a university and entry to the profession was channelled through universities in the 1830s and 1840s. The open market of Jacksonian America never developed in Canada.

This account of the 'regular' doctors suggests a degree of cohesion which requires modification. The history of the profession in pre-Confederation Canada is marked by division and bitterness which mirror the divisions of the colonies. Division, conflict, and factionalism flared frequently in these years. Lower Canada was the site of some of the bitterest factionalism. The profession was dominated by English-speaking doctors who had the ear of the Governor. They were frequently Army or Navy officers who treated civilians, among them influential members of the anglophone community, in their off-duty hours, and who continued to practise in the colony on their retirement from military life. Their dominant position was resented by other 'regulars', among whom could be found English, American and German practitioners. Most resentful of all, however, were the francophone doctors. In Lower Canada, medicine was one of the professions favoured by the sons of francophone farmers as the means of rising socially. The younger sons crowded into the professions in the first decades of the century and came to resent the anglophone dominance. It was in the ranks of the professions that many of the leaders of French Canadian *patriote* opposition to British colonial rule would be found in the 1830s.[3] François Blanchet, educated in the United States and a published writer on medical questions, bitterly-resented being examined by the Medical Board for a licence on his return home. He regarded military medical men, who were rarely university trained, as among the least competent practitioners in the British profession. The division between francophone and anglophone, while never total, did endure into mid century and beyond. In 1847 a College of Physicians and Surgeons of Quebec was established-but drew little support until Confederation. At that time it was strengthened mainly by francophone doctors as a protective agency against anglophone efforts to standardize medical education and licensing.[4]

While the ethnic division was dramatic, there were differences which erupted from time to time to entertain the newspaper-reading public. Doctors were capable of challenging each other's competence to practise and quarrelling over access to hospitals and challenging one another's right to hold a public position. The challenges were sometimes rooted in the political factions of a community but took the form of attacks on the rival's competence. Toronto was entertained in 1844 by an attack on the performance of Dr William Rees as medical superintendent of the Provincial Lunatic Asylum, led by Dr Walter Telfer. Rees was removed and Telfer appointed. Telfer, in his turn, was attacked in 1848 and removed amid a barrage of pamphlets and newspaper articles, to be replaced by Dr George H. Park, a protégé of the politician and doctor, Dr John Rolph.[5]

Divisions between rural and urban practitioners were wide through the first seventy-five years of the century. The drive for reform, improved education and professional organization came from the urban 'regulars', and rural practitioners tended to resent the condescension of their colleagues. Even when the profession was gaining standing and power to govern itself, the gap between rural and urban doctors remained, and rural doctors were noticeably less enthusiastic about professional development than were their city colleagues.[6] 'Regulars' were themselves capable of dividing over the question of professional organization. In the 1830s, for example, some were content with establishing licensing as the means of regulating entry to the profession, and had little interest in developing collegial self-government.

Divisions between 'regulars' entertained the public, which followed the quarrels as they were reported in the newspapers, but they also undermined the 'regulars'' claim to special privilege in the community. The public was not so convinced as spokesmen for the 'regular' professionals that they had a monopoly on medical knowledge. Nor did the rural population have easy access to 'regular' doctors, most of whom preferred to practise in the towns. The small number of doctors licensed by the Medical Boards could not meet the needs of a widely scattered rural population and in the course of the century many patients, if given a choice, turned away from 'regulars' because of the therapies which they employed. These therapies had their own logic and had offered patients some hope in illness in the past.[7] They depended on combinations of bleeding, blistering, purging and dosing with calomel to restore the body's balance and the health of the patient. The traditional therapy faced growing patient resistance and the heroic bloodletting practised in the 1830s was modified by mid century, although 'regulars' continued to rely on large doses of mercury.

Many Canadians turned to the 'irregular' doctors either from choice, preferring the therapies they offered, or because they were the only doctors available in their district. In the scattered communities of British North America it was difficult to police and enforce licensing laws and unlicensed practitioners practised widely. Many of the 'irregular' physicians came into Canada from the United States. They practised a variety of therapies, with Thomsonian medicine being the most popular. This was a system of medicine based on a book of treatments written by Samuel Thomson which came complete with a license to fill in and cut out. It was based on herbal remedies but, like conventional medicine, relied on purging and vomiting for many of its treatments. Thomsonians were joined by others, dismissed by the 'regulars' as Root doctors or Indian doctors. In the towns, 'regulars' faced their biggest challenge from homeopathic practitioners. Many of these men had trained as 'regular' doctors, but their use of minute doses of medicine in place of the heroic remedies of their 'regular' colleagues proved attractive to many patients.[8] When 'irregular' doctors were charged with unlicensed practice, they could often rely on sympathetic juries. The 'regular' doctors faced a serious challenge to their claim to special privilege in pre-Confederation Canada. While they retained the support of governments the public tended to see 'regulars' as one sect among many.

PUBLIC HEALTH AND THE MEDICAL PROFESSION BEFORE CONFEDERATION

Public health offered the 'regulars' an arena in which to consolidate their claim to special skills. Where Thomsonians and homeopaths might treat a disease, the 'regulars' were called upon to prevent it occurring. When governments faced public health problems they turned for advice to 'regular' professionals. Unfortunately for the 'regulars' the skills which they had and the advice they offered were of limited value in the early years and their failures tended to undermine their position rather than to strengthen it.

Public health questions in the early years of the century arose from the problems of the towns. Dirt, inadequate sewage disposal, poor water supplies and overcrowded and often dangerous housing were cited as problems needing action. The problem of cleanliness reflected the functions of the towns with emphasis on the need to regulate slaughter houses and remove accumulated household filth, rather than on the consequences of large-scale industrialization. Little attention was given to the public health aspects of epidemic disease — malaria in Upper Canada, tuberculosis which was especially devastating to the native population, the childhood diseases — or to the dangers of work in the mines and forests or in the fisheries and at sea. The public health aspects of work conditions would begin to be debated only at the end of the century. A few doctors did begin to compile medical statistics early in the period, but the material was unreliable and difficult to collect.[9]

Public health had a low priority among politicians of the early nineteenth century. Few of them were advocates of extensive and expensive programmes of social amelioration. The Lower Canadian *patriote* invoked cultural nationalism, the Upper Canadian reformer invoked Jacksonian democracy, but neither *patriote* nor reformer had much more time for sustained public health efforts than the ruling conservative elites whom they opposed in the 1820s and 1830s. The Reform party used a public health question in Upper Canada in 1832 when it criticized the magistrates of York for their inept handling of the response to the cholera that year. They won control of the newly chartered City of Toronto in 1834 and were in office when the second cholera epidemic struck in 1834. Their response was essentially the same as that of the magistrates of 1832 and public disgust at their handling of the epidemic helped to bring them down in the next elections. In Canada, the complex debate between conservative, liberal and radical approaches to public health questions is not clearly obvious between political parties.

Amid the widespread indifference to public health there was one area of great concern to large numbers of Canadians. Immigration was a highly charged political issue in the early nineteenth century. In Lower Canada, the *patriotes* accused the colonial government of plotting to swamp the French and anglicize the nation by flooding it with British immigrants. The pressure of immigration on a limited land base helped to intensify the political divisions which led to open rebellion in 1837. Upper Canadians tended to welcome British immigrants, but they were made uneasy by the presence of large numbers of poverty-stricken immigrants. Destitute immigrants had to be relieved by public and private agencies in the 1830s. The issue of poor relief entered politics in that era but even more pressing in the opinion of many commentators was the public health danger allegedly posed by immigrants. The one question which was guaranteed to provoke widespread interest in public health was the outbreak of a life-threatening explosive epidemic. Smallpox, typhus and above all cholera caught public attention and brought demands for action. Colonial governments were attacked for allowing cholera to enter the colonies by their ineffectiveness and out of a callous disregard, or worse, for the population. The year 1834 brought charges in Lower Canada that cholera had been imported to destroy the French population.

Immigration and public health were intertwined in the nineteenth century. It was in response to the danger of cholera in 1831 that the government of Lower Canada consulted members of the Quebec Medical Board and established a quarantine station at Grosse Isle which would continue to operate for a century. The stations at Grosse Isle and at Halifax and St John, New Brunswick were among the few permanent public health provisions made before the late 1860s. Other measures against epidemics were short term and made with an eye for the expense involved. Cholera hospitals were set up, often in crude temporary buildings, doctors' services provided to the indigent at public expense and preventive measures taken against the disease. Those colonies, such as Nova Scotia, which had no public health legislation on the statute books passed acts in the aftermath of the cholera epidemic of 1832. Each epidemic was met by the establishment of Boards of Health to deal with the crisis and was followed by the winding up of the Board. The pattern of shortlived responses to immediate dangers persisted into the 1860s. In 1866, the City of Toronto responded to the new danger of cholera by establishing what was intended to be a permanent Board of Health. Economy-minded aldermen abolished it three years later only to be forced to re-establish a Board in 1872, this time in the presence of an outbreak of smallpox.[10] Parsimony was bound to triumph while the need for permanent Boards and public health provisions remained uncertain.

The 'regular' doctors stood to profit when the public became interested in public health. Any government which wanted medical advice turned to the 'regulars' and consulted the existing medical boards. There was personal profit, too, as the posts which were available in cholera hospitals, serving the indigent, manning the quarantine stations and serving on Boards of Health, went to 'regulars'. There was eager competition for all posts which were created and patronage was the key to success. While 'regulars' won immediate rewards from public concern with the epidemics the debate over cholera did little to consolidate the position they claimed in early-nineteenth-century Canada.

Cholera was a mystery and it terrified the men and women of British North America. Laymen wanted to know the nature of the disease, the way in which it was spread and how to help its victims. They turned to their doctors for the information and found no convincing answers but only a debate which emphasized the divisions within the profession and undermined, in laymen's eyes, the 'regulars' claim to special knowledge. From the first debate on cholera in 1831, Canadian doctors disagreed whether cholera was a contagious disease. The debate was central to the questions of the nature of the disease and the best means of defending communities against it. In the first epidemics in 1832 and 1834 the weight of opinion tended to favour the argument that cholera was not contagious. In the later epidemics more Canadian doctors were convinced that the disease was contagious to some extent, but the extent was uncertain and 'regulars' were drawn toward contingent contagionism — that is, that it was possible for the disease to become contagious in certain circumstances. Dr Archibald Hall, one of Canada's most prominent medical journalists, wrote in 1849, 'when we reflect that contagious diseases frequently exhibit themselves in a form apparently epidemic and that epidemics assume many of the features of contagious disease, it becomes a matter of exceeding difficulty to draw the line of demarcation between them'. As late as 1873, a pamphlet on cholera issued by the Canadian government defined it as 'portable', and capable of being carried 'by persons, effects and merchandise and even by the winds of the air and currents and streams'.[11]

This debate was common to the profession in Britain and the United States and most of the ammunition for the battle in Canada was drawn from British sources as medical journals and newspapers reprinted articles from the British press on these questions. Canadian doctors were able to follow the debate in Britain and the work of Snow was reported in the Canadian press.[12] Canadian doctors added their own observations from their practices but no one contributed anything original to the debate which divided the profession, nor was it resolved in a way that comforted laymen.

In the current state of knowledge about the social history of Canadian medicine, it is not possible to say with certainty whether the division between contagionists and anti-contagionists reflected political and social divisions, with contagionists socially conservative and the opponents liberal and radical. Dr Joseph Workman, for example, was well known as a medical reformer. He had arrived in Canada in 1829 from Ireland at the age of 24 and taught school while attending lectures in medicine at the General Hospital and McGill. He wrote a thesis *On Asiatic Cholera* for his degree at McGill in 1835. After a decade in the family business he returned to medicine at the suggestion of his friend, the radical Dr John Rolph, who had participated in the rebellion of 1837, and taught in Rolph's medical school in Toronto while participating in municipal politics where he exercised his interests in reform of education and medical services. Eventually he became medical superintendent of the Toronto Lunatic Asylum. In his thesis, Workman declared himself a contagionist and remained one throughout his career.[13] Dr Wolfred Nelson, on the other hand, was an anglophone *patriote* and more a radical than a reformer. Trained by apprenticeship to an army surgeon, Nelson was a practising doctor when he took part in the rebellion of 1837 and was banished to Bermuda on its failure. He returned to Canada and re-entered municipal politics, and while mayor of Montreal in 1854 published *Practical Views on Cholera*. Nelson was not convinced that cholera was contagious.[14]

There were some doctors who specifically associated medical with social opinions. Dr Anthony Von Iffland argued in 1849 that a belief in contagion was socially dangerous because it produced panic, and also gave the medical profession an unjustified claim to skills which they did not in fact possess.[15] A full study of the profession might reveal clearer patterns but the evidence does not exist to determine the attitudes of the majority of 'regulars' on the question at specific times. The repeated claims of medical journalists that the majority became convinced of the contagiousness of the disease may reflect a profession growing more socially established and conservative; but 'regulars' were far from confidence and security in 1854. Some doctors may have been disposed to one school or the other by social concerns. Perhaps the attraction of the contingent contagion explanation was that it allowed the doctor to reconcile contradictory evidence in the absence of strong social reformist attitudes.

One consequence of the debate on the nature of the disease was to call into question the advice 'regulars' offered for its prevention. The Boards of Health established in the colonies on British models combined laymen and medical men. Public health questions were not regarded as exclusively medical questions in early-nineteenth-century Canada by those who governed the towns and colonies.

They were also matters of policing and government. The medical men were there to deal with the sick and to advise on preventive measures. The usual advice was to clean the streets and inspect the houses to remove the filth which was thought to sustain the disease. The citizens of many towns responded by asking what link really existed between dirt and disease which justified the expense of street-cleaning schemes and the invasion of privacy of house inspection. Why did dirty streets bring cholera in 1832 but not in 1833? And why did clean streets not protect communities in 1834? Where was the proof that quarantine and sanitary laws had any effect, or that anything beyond immediate provision for the victims of an epidemic was needed?[16] Men and women at all social levels resented and resisted public health laws which rested on uncertain justifications.

The opposition to public health laws was strengthened by the widespread conviction in the first half of the century that individual responsibility not social legislation was the key to good health. Sobriety, personal cleanliness and moderation were urged on the people by doctors and politicians in a community threatened by an epidemic. The moral approach to disease retained a strong appeal in the absence of any compelling explanation for preventive measures. Dr Nelson, in his 1854 pamphlet, wrote 'there is a close affinity between moral depravity and physical degradation'. Cholera 'respects cleanliness, sobriety and decent habits. It seldom intrudes where industry and good morals prevail. Hence, in regard to this dreadful pestilence, man is, in no small degree, the arbiter of his own fate.'[17]

By that time, however, the growing cities of Canada were forcing consideration of the need for clean water and safe sewage-disposal. Britain again provided the chief source of support for those who advocated improvements. In St John, New Brunswick, the committee formed in 1854 to consider the city's public health needs following a devastating cholera epidemic quoted extensively from Charles Dickens in support of its recommendations for improvements. British engineering provided examples of what could be done, and even while the health issue remained unresolved the aesthetic argument for clean water was appealing. Fresh mountain and river water should replace the brackish well water and contaminated lake water many Canadians drank. As the towns grew in size, however, one of the most convincing arguments for a good water supply piped to different parts of the town was to protect the citizens from the fires which devastated a number of Canada's predominantly wooden cities. By mid century water supply was becoming a major concern in Canadian towns.

'Regulars', when asked for advice on how a community could protect itself against imported diseases, had shown themselves divided and unsure, and offered advice which was ineffective and unpopular. That did them little good with the public, but if they had been able to offer practical and effective help to patients they would have stood higher in public opinion. The doctor-patient relationship was based on curing rather than preventing disease. The growing number of medical schools in the 1840s and 1850s hoped to increase the scientific knowledge of their students to make them more effective curers. The therapies adopted by Canadian doctors did not cure cholera. They tried every cure reported in the

British press, including transfusions of water and even of milk to relieve its victims, but without success. In therapeutic terms there was no reason to choose a 'regular' over an 'irregular' physician. Many patients preferred the 'irregulars' and a few attributed their recovery to the fact that no 'regular' had his hands on them while they were sick.

THE MEDICAL PROFESSION AND CONFEDERATION

Despite the lack of acceptance of the claims of 'regulars' to special skill and consequently their right to a special position in the community, leaders of the 'regulars' pushed their claims in the years before Confederation. The number of medical schools increased and 'regulars' continued their efforts to become a self-governing profession. The increasing autonomy of British North America reduced the likelihood of interference from London which had destroyed the College of Physicians and Surgeons of Upper Canada in 1839, but 'regulars' still had to convince local politicians that they deserved the special status they sought. The College of Physicians and Surgeons of Quebec was established in 1847 with the support of many 'regulars' who feared that the legislature might extend privileges to the 'irregulars' if action was not taken quickly. After its formation, the College struggled to consolidate the profession by initiatives in education, by organizing practitioners and by pressing for its members to have the exclusive right to practise and calling for stronger laws against the illegal practice of medicine. Its success was limited.

In Nova Scotia, the elite members of the profession centred in Halifax opened what would prove to be a twenty-year campaign in the mid-1850s. They stimulated professional solidarity by organizing medical societies, by participating in the establishment of hospitals and a medical school, by publicizing advances made in 'regular' medicine and by supporting legislation permitting dissection in 1869. The 'regulars' published attacks on 'irregulars' and in 1872 were successful in winning self-regulation for the medical profession.

In Ontario, the 'regulars' were not as successful as their Nova Scotian colleagues. Here, too, the leading doctors of the dominant urban centre — Toronto — led a fight to win privileges for the 'regulars' in the 1850s. A Bill to abolish the Medical Board and do away with all licensing requirements failed by only one vote in the Provincial Assembly in 1851. Stimulated by that threat of open competition, the leading 'regulars' fought for self-regulation of a medical profession by 'regulars'. Their campaign was hampered by division especially between rural and urban practitioners and by successful opposition by the 'irregulars'. The 'irregulars' formed their own medical societies, professional organizations, and educational institutions. They made the case that 'regulars' had no right to exclusive control of the practice of medicine and they won the support of many rural and small town voters who relied on 'irregulars' for care.

The 'regulars' lost the fight for exclusivity in Ontario. 'Irregulars' were allowed to establish boards to examine and license practitioners and the patient was given the choice between examined and licensed 'regular' or 'irregular' practioners. Despite the protests of 'regulars', subsequent legislation confirmed the view that so-called 'irregular' practioners were acceptable to many residents. In 1869, the 'regulars' did succeed in winning legislation to create a College of Physicians and Surgeons of Ontario but were shaken when the Bill was amended to permit 'irregulars' to become members of the College. The legislature preferred one licensing authority to three and allopaths, eclectics and homeopaths were allowed into the College. The forced union lasted into the twentieth century and after bitter opposition the 'regulars' accepted their colleagues. Some hoped that the 'irregulars' would be overwhelmed in the College, others feared that if they did reject the union the legislature would permit open access to the practice of medicine.[18]

Ontario provides a striking example of laymen's reluctance to accept the claims of 'regulars' to a superior position in the profession at mid century. They did, however, accept the argument for the need to have some degree of organization and regulation in medicine as in other aspects of public life. This was the age of organization, the age of the railway company and the corporation, the years in which Samuel Cunard was building his transatlantic empire in the Maritimes, the age of bankers and brewers. South of the border, for many Canadians, was an example of what would happen if things were allowed to fall apart. For a short while, the threat from the United States eased as that nation drifted towards division and civil war. When the war was over, many Canadians again felt vulnerable before the reinvigorated industrial nation whose Secretary of State could suggest that Canada be annexed to the United States in compensation for claims against Great Britain. The response of many of Canada's political elite was to work for the creation of the new nation in 1867 out of the loosely scattered collection of British North American colonies.

July, 1867 saw the birth of Canada and October, 1867 the birth of the Canadian Medical Association (CMA). Dr William Marsden, yet another author of works on cholera and a medical reformer with a long career, suggested the need for a CMA after serving as a delegate from Quebec to the American Medical Association that summer. The time was right and delegates from the new provinces of Canada met in Quebec City and established the CMA. They elected Charles Tupper, a future Prime Minister, as the first president of the CMA, and attracted a considerable number of medical reformers to their ranks. What the reformers wanted was to improve the status of medicine in Canada by increasing professional control over it, and to create a uniform medical profession in Canada by a system of Dominion-wide registration with generally agreed standards of education and competence. Some commentators have pointed out that a major impetus behind the pressure for Dominion registration was to increase the pressure to exclude 'irregulars' from full participation in a reformed profession and to improve the prospects for 'regular' doctors by reducing competition. Similar efforts continued in the provinces.[19]

The formation of the CMA signalled an important shift in the context of medical practice in Canada. The organizers specifically associated themselves with a United States model and the earlier suspicion of the United States which had marked, for example, the opinions of advocates of Canadian medical schools in the 1830s and 1840s, began to evaporate. Britain and Europe remained important sources of ideas and procedures but increasingly Canadian doctors would look South, and those interested in education and organization would be more sympathetic to the United States than were earlier generations. Some of the problems in Canada were different — the American Medical Association was fighting to restore a licensing procedure abandoned in the 1830s, the Canadians never had abandoned licensing — but the objectives were the same and for some Canadian reformers the North American context encouraged an emphasis on similarities over differences.[20]

The CMA did not signal the triumph of a consolidated profession in a newly consolidated country. Canada itself was created with a careful eye on provincial privileges and a division of powers between Dominion and provincial governments. The CMA soon found that its proposals for Dominion-wide registration ran up against provincial governments determined to protect their place in the Confederation against too much central power and against suspicion and opposition from within the medical profession itself. The old division between francophone and anglophone endured. The CMA was dominated by anglophone doctors and that aroused suspicion in Quebec. The members of the Montreal Medical Society led an effort to reinvigorate the College of Physicians and Surgeons of Quebec as an instrument to protect provincial jurisdiction over medical matters. They were especially concerned about medical education, a chief instrument for control of entry to the profession, and were eager to protect medical education from anglophone domination.[21]

The francophone doctors were as interested in reforming medical education as were their anglophone colleagues. Control of medical education, however, did provoke arguments with the universities, who called on academic freedom to protect their right to define curricula and set standards. As provincial medical colleges won the power to examine and license practitioners, the automatic entry to practice guaranteed by a university degree was abandoned. But the professional bodies recognized the value of insisting on formal education. It had the advantage of emphasizing the special status of medicine and of limiting entry to what some contemporaries believed was becoming an overcrowded profession. Compromises were reached between professional bodies and the universities over entry requirements and curricula. In Quebec, for example, the College of Physicians and Surgeons actively supported the requirement that students had to complete a classical education before entering medical school.[22] A profession which, in the 1820s and 1830s, had been one of the avenues to social movement for the sons of francophone farmers now began to restrict access as it consolidated its position in society.

'Regular' doctors had always claimed that their superiority lay in their better education and profounder knowledge. The claim had not been widely accepted outside the profession before Confederation. Now, however, it would be reinforced and more widely accepted by the appeal of scientific medicine in the later nineteenth century. The new scientific medicine, if we date it from Lister, arrived with the new country. Reports of Lister's techniques were published in Canada in 1867, and by early 1868 Canadian surgeons were reporting their own experiments with the system. At least six Canadians studied with Lister and others travelled to Britain to learn his methods.[23]

The new medicine required new curricula and an emphasis on the laboratory. When William Osler came to teach at McGill in the early 1870s he imported microscopes from Germany for his students. McGill became the centre of Canadian scientific medicine in the 1870s but was overtaken by Toronto in the next decade.[24] If the original impetus to the new medicine came from Edinburgh and London the focal point of interest for Canadian doctors increasingly was the United States. A number of Canadian doctors followed Osler's lead in the last decades of the century and took positions in Johns Hopkins and other leading institutions of the new medicine. Links to Britain, of course, remained strong in the last years of the century, but the process of moving from being a projection of Britain to an adjunct of the United States was under way. Perhaps the clearest symbol of that transition at least in medical education can be seen early in the twentieth century. In 1910 Abraham Flexner published *Medical Education in the United States and Canada* which was subtitled *A Report to the Carnegie Foundation for the Advancement of Teaching*. It is now seen as a key document in the drive by the profession in the United States to consolidate its hold on entry to the profession by limiting the numbers of medical schools while raising standards of education to meet the challenge of the new science.

Flexner found a doctor population ratio in Canada of 1:1030, noted that the country was 'thinly settled and doctors much less abundant than in the United States' and proposed 250 new doctors a year as the annual need. This need could be met by four universities. Three of Canada's eight medical schools were described as having 'no present function' and a fourth — Queen's University at Kingston — was seen to have a doubtful future. The reports on individual schools occupied seven pages following the state-by-state reports which make up about one-third of Flexner's book. Western was 'as bad as anything to be found on this side of the line'; Laval and Halifax 'are feeble'; Winnipeg and Kingston 'represent a distinct effort towards higher ideals'; McGill and Toronto 'are excellent'. In three short visits in May, March and October 1909 Flexner examined Canada's medical schools and suggested shutting down half of them. He spent half a day at Queen's and about the same time at Western. The spokesmen for those universities pointed out the fleeting nature of his visits but beyond that there was little protest about Flexner but instead 'reorganization and upgrading of teaching facilities in the province' according to a recent historian of medicine in Ontario.[25] None of the medical schools was shut down but an American report which devoted seven and a half of its 326 pages to Canada was treated with respect by a profession eager to confirm its position by demonstrating its grasp of the new knowledge.

PUBLIC HEALTH AND THE MEDICAL PROFESSION AFTER CONFEDERATION

Public health questions had undermined the claims of 'regulars' to expertise early in the century. The questions were not regarded as exclusively medical ones when Health Boards were set up nor was the conflicting advice offered by medical men reassuring to the public. These attitudes began to change after Confederation as doctors made the case that they did know how to protect the public health and that the means of doing so required the specialized knowledge of medical men. Bacteriology replaced engineering as the key to public health. A Health Board needed men, and by the end of the century women, who knew how to test samples of water or milk. It did not need men who knew how to clean the streets or inspect houses for dirt sharing the seats around the table with medical professionals. The argument was widely accepted by the end of the century.

From the beginning of the period, doctors eager to advance the position of their profession emphasized their public health role. One of the first committees formed by the CMA agitated public health questions and lobbied for the collection of vital statistics as an essential tool of public health. The American Public Health Association was founded in 1872 and a number of Canadians became prominent in its activities, including Dr Frederick Montizambert who would become Canada's first Director General of Public Health in 1899. Dr Edward Playter founded the *Sanitary Journal* in 1874 in Toronto and had sufficiently strong contacts in the Dominion government to receive a subsidy for his work. The next year, in Montreal, George A. Baynes established the *Public Health Magazine and Literary Review*. McGill introduced the first courses on public health in Canada in 1874 and Université Laval soon followed suit. Public health quickly opened up as a field which attracted Canada's doctors and offered careers to nurses in the years after 1880. The Association of Executive Health Officers of Ontario was founded in 1886 to represent the interests of over 300 Medical Health Officers.[26]

Public health in the 1880s gave the medical profession visibility and authority. Gone were most of the divisions and uncertainties of the earlier years. 'The germ theory is a fact', Dr Montizambert announced in 1885. The doctor could now trace a typhoid epidemic to a specific milk supply. Milk and water supplies could be made safe. Diseases could be identified and the sufferers isolated to check an epidemic. The health of children could be improved by work in the schools. Public health had much to offer the doctors and the politician. Dr E.-P. Lachapelle was a leading spokesman for the francophone doctors of Quebec through his positions on the Conseil D'Hygiène and in the College of Physicians and Surgeons. He saw the future of the nation and of the profession tied to the advances made possible by developments in public health. Some have argued that the public health doctors made the impact they did at this time because they offered the leaders of industrializing Canada what they wanted — a healthy workforce living in conditions which would reduce the chance of disruptive social tensions.[27]

Immigration continued to be a concern for Canadians after Confederation and the immigrant continued to be seen as a potential danger to the nation's health. Here, too, the new medicine appeared to offer more security than the old. Public health advocates usually supported the demand for compulsory vaccination of immigrants, especially after a devastating smallpox outbreak in Montreal in 1885. Dr Montizambert, in charge of Canada's Quarantine Service, became internationally recognized for his work. He modified the operations of the quarantine according to developing medical ideas and replaced the old system of landing and examining immigrants with a new one of disinfecting ships and their passengers. In quarantine, the growing pressure of the United States could be felt as the service struggled to refute charges of laxness which allowed diseased immigrants to enter the United States through the St Lawrence. US health standards were tightened in the 1880s and Canada, in turn, stiffened its standards to avoid becoming a 'dumping ground' for immigrants refused admission to the USA. As Canada's need for immigrants was greater than the USA's in the late nineteenth century, when more people continued to leave Canada than entered the country, she never adopted the most stringent standards developed in the USA.

Canada did, however, increase the health barriers to immigrants in the course of the late nineteenth century. The Dominion government shared responsibility for immigration with the provinces and in 1869 the Federal Immigration Branch was established to encourage immigration. It sent medical inspectors to Europe to examine prospective emigrants and spare the families the distress of having some members refused entry at a Canadian port. As the last decades of the century passed, a growing number of doctors argued for the need for a more careful selection of immigrants to protect the nation from physical, moral, and mental degeneration. They came to believe that they had the skills to pick the best stock for the nation and they found an ear in government. From 1882, health standards for immigrants began to exclude whole categories of people. The feeble-minded, morally degenerate and potentially criminal could be recognized by a trained doctor and barred from the nation. Deportation for medical reasons became a part of Canada's immigration policy.[28] The public health nurse moved among the immigrants in Canada's cities and rural villages, teaching them the new rules of hygiene and emphasizing the 'Canadian' way of doing things. Even in the new age of scientific medicine a person was still responsible for protecting his own health.

Not everyone was as inspired by the new public health as the Medical Health Officers. Toronto appointed Dr William Caniff as its first permanent Medical Health Officer in 1883 but he ran into frequent opposition from politicians and the public. There were many who found the public health laws costly and intrusive just as they had in the 1830s. They resented Caniff's suggestion that annual house-to-house surveys should be made in the city. When Ontario attempted to impose compulsory vaccination during the smallpox epidemic of 1885 there was widespread resistance, especially among Toronto's working classes. Prosecutions brought by the Health Officers were often dismissed by the courts. A vigorous anti-vaccination movement was created in 1885 which continued to argue against the need for compulsory vaccination into the twentieth century.[29]

SUMMARY

In the early nineteenth century the medical profession in the colonies of British North America was weakened by internal divisions and factionalism which reflected the divisions of the larger societies. Ethnic and professional division was common. The 'regular' doctors benefited from the assumption of the governors of the colonies that there ought to be regulation, examination, and licensing and thus never faced the open competition characteristic of the unlicensed United States. Some of their efforts to organize, however, were set aside by London when they interfered with the privileges of British professional colleges. When governments sought medical advice and gave out positions they confined themselves to 'regular' doctors. The drive of the 'regulars' to consolidate their position by education was supported by many who feared that without Canadian medical schools, students would go to the United States for training and return with dangerous political ideas. A British university training qualified men to practice without further examination.

The 'regulars' faced constant competition from 'irregulars' who met the needs especially of the rural population. The claim of 'regulars' to be superior in skill and knowledge was not generally accepted by the public. Public health provided one area in which the claims of 'regulars' were tested and found wanting. Nothing that 'regulars' advised protected the colonies from the explosive epidemics, especially of cholera, which terrified nineteenth-century Canadians. The therapies offered by 'regulars' were ineffective and not, for many, demonstrably superior to those of 'irregulars'. Under these circumstances, 'regulars' could not dominate the medical life of British North America.

At mid century, in a time of organizational activity in many spheres and in the years of self-government for the colonies, the medical profession did win a large measure of self-government through bodies sanctioned by colonial legislation. The self-government did not exclude 'irregulars', many of whom were allowed to participate in collegial activity by the legislatures of the colonies which accepted the argument that there was nothing to choose between an educated 'regular' or 'irregular'.

In 1867, Canada was created. The new country created a new setting for medical life but the efforts of the CMA to create a single profession in Canada were thwarted by francophone suspicion and provincial jealousy of Dominion power. The Canadian profession would be organized on a provincial basis for the rest of the century. The founding of the CMA at the moment of Canada's creation signalled a shift from the predominance of British models for Canada to a growing association with the United States, through professional organizations and the increasing attraction of the United States for Canadians as the two nations moved into the industrial era. The price paid was a growing acceptance of United States leadership and authority most dramatically demonstrated in the Flexner report of 1910.

Coinciding with the creation of Canada came the beginnings of the new scientific medicine. The successes of that medicine helped to sustain the claims of 'regulars' to special prominence in medicine. Public health gave the scientific doctor a chance to display his (and, after the 1880s in Canada, her) new skill. Public health offered doctors a career and hundreds entered that branch of medicine supported by public expenditure. The public health doctor offered the local politician a relatively inexpensive way to deal with some of the problems of industrializing Canada. Despite its occasional failures, the quarantine service did seem capable of protecting Canada against disease. Immigration law itself reflected a growing concern with health matters and incorporated new medical standards defined by the new doctors. Health Boards were conceded to be exclusively medical bodies. By the end of the century 'regulars' had triumphed in Canada as they had in the United States.

NOTES

1. Ronald Hamowy, *Canadian Medicine: A Study in Restricted Entry* (Vancouver: The Fraser Institute, 1984), 21. McGill's first medical graduate was refused a licence by the Medical Board of Lower Canada in 1833 for reasons explored in Barbara Tunis, 'Medical licensing in Lower Canada: the dispute over Canada's first medical degree', *Canadian Historical Review, 55* (1974), 489–504.

2. Joseph F. Kett, 'American and Canadian medical institutions', *Journal of the History of Medicine and Allied Sciences, 22* (1967), 343–56; Jacques Bernier, 'François Blanchet et le mouvement réformiste en médecine au debut du XIXe siécle', *Revue d'histoire de l'Amérique Française, 34* (1980), 223–44; Geoffrey Bilson, *A Darkened House* (Toronto: University of Toronto Press, 1980), 146.

3. Barbara Tunis, 'Medical education and medical licensing in Lower Canada: demographic factors, conflict and social change', *Histoire sociale/Social History, 14* (1981), 67–92; Fernand Ouellette, *Lower Canada, 1791–1840* (Toronto: McClelland & Stewart, 1980), 335–6.

4. Jacques Bernier, 'L'integration du corps médical québecois', *Historical Reflections/Reflexions historiques, 10* (1983), 91–111. Claudine Pierre-Deschenes, 'Santé publique et organisation de la profession médicale au Québec 1870–1918', *Revue d'histoire de l'Amerique Française, 35* (1981), 355–75.

5. Heather MacDougall, 'Epidemics and the environment: the early development of public health activity in Toronto, 1832–72', in R.A. Jarrell and A.E. Roos (eds), *Critical Issues in the History of Canadian Science, Technology and Medicine* (Thornhill and Ottawa: HSTC Publications, 1983), 137. 'Walter Telfer,' *Dictionary of Canadian Biography, 8* (Toronto: University of Toronto Press, 1985).

6. Bernier, op. cit., n. 4 above, 109.

7. Charles E. Rosenberg, 'The therapeutic revolution: medicine, meaning and social

change in nineteenth century America', in Morris Vogel and Charles Rosenberg (eds), *The Therapeutic Revolution: Essays in the Social History of American Medicine* (Philadelphia: University of Pennsylvania Press, 1979), 3-25.

8. R.D. Gidney and W.P.J. Millar, 'The origins of organized medicine in Ontario, 1850–1869', and Colin D. Howell, 'Elite doctors and the development of scientific medicine: the Halifax medical establishment and 19th century medical professionalism', in Charles G. Roland (ed.), *Health, Disease and Medicine: Essays in Canadian History* (Toronto: Clarke Irwin for The Hannah Institute, 1984), 65-95, 105–22.

9. Bilson, op. cit., no. 2 above.

10. MacDougall, op. cit., n. 5 above, 137.

11. Editorial, *British American Journal of Medical and Physical Sciences, 4* (1848–9), 220; *Memorandum on the Cholera* (Ottawa: Bureau of Agriculture, 1866, 1873), 23.

12. Bilson, op. cit., n. 2 above, 150.

13. Rainer Baehre, 'Joseph Workman (1805–1894) and lunacy reform' (unpublished paper presented to Canadian Historical Association, June 1980); J. Workman, *On Asiatic Cholera* (Montreal, n.p. 1835).

14. *Dictionary of Canadian Biography, IX*, 595–7.

15. A. von Iffland, 'The Quebec Board of Health, the cholera at Beauport and its treatment', *The British American Journal of Medical and Physical Sciences, 5* (1849), 199-200, 108.

16. Heather MacDougall, 'Health is wealth: the development of public health activity in Toronto 1832–1890' (Unpublished PhD dissertation, University of Toronto, 1981).

17. Wolfred Nelson, *Practical Views on Cholera* (Montreal: n.p. 1854), 1, 6–7.

18. Gidney and Millar, op. cit., n. 8 above, 84–7. Hamowy, op. cit., n. 1 above, 108, argues that in practice the amalgamation of 'regulars' and 'irregulars' allowed the 'regulars' to limit entry of 'irregulars' to practice.

19. H.E. MacDermott, *One Hundred Years of Medicine in Canada, 1867–1967* (Toronto: McClelland & Stewart, 1967), 54–5; Hamowy, op. cit., n. 1 above, ch. 3.

20. Paul Starr, *The Social Transformation of American Medicine* (New York: Basic Books, 1982), 102–12.

21. Bernier, Pierre-Deschenes, op. cit., no. 4 above, 91–111, 355–75.

22. Jacques Bernier, 'La standardisation des études médicales et la consolidation de la profession dans la deuxieme motié du XIXe siècle', *Revue d'histoire de l'Amérique Française, 37* (1983), 51-66.

23. G.G. Roland, 'The early years of antiseptic surgery in Canada', *Journal of the History of Medicine and Allied Sciences, 22* (1967), 380–91; MacDermott, op. cit., n. 19 above, 28–9.

24. This statement is based on an assessment of the number of papers published by medical faculty at the two universities.

25. Abraham Flexner, *Medical Education in the United States and Canada* (New York: Carnegie Foundation, 1910; reprinted New York: Arno Press, 1972), 150, 326; Charles Godfrey, *Medicine for Ontario* (Belleville: Mika, 1979), 249.

26. MacDermott, op. cit., n. 19 above, 58. Heather MacDougall, 'Enlightening the public — the views and values of the Association of Executive Health Officers of Ontario 1886-1903', in Roland, op. cit., n. 8 above, 436–64.

27. Geoffrey Bilson, 'Dr. Frederick Montizambert: Canada's First Director General of Public Health', *Medical History, 29* (1985), 390; Neil Sutherland, *Children in English Canadian Society* (Toronto: University of Toronto Press, 1976), Part II; Pierre-Deschenes, op. cit., n. 4 above. Paul Starr suggests that an attraction of the new scientific public health for politicians was that it made cheaper solutions possible for public health problems, Starr, op. cit., n. 20 above, 189–94.

28. Geoffrey Bilson, 'Towards selection: public health and Canada's 1906 Immigration

Act' (Unpublished paper presented at ACSANZ Biannual Conference, Brisbane, 14 May 1986).

29. Barbara Lazenby Craig, 'State medicine in transition: battling smallpox in Ontario 1882–1885', P.A. Bator, 'The health reformers versus the common Canadian: the controversy over compulsory vaccination against smallpox in Toronto and Ontario, 1900–1920', *Ontario History, 75* (1983), 319–47; 348–73.

9

'Our salubrious climate': attitudes to health in colonial Queensland

Helen R. Woolcock

Imperial experience in tropical countries confirmed the belief that Europeans had difficulty surviving, let alone working in hot climates. So when Queensland became a separate Australian colony in 1859, serious doubts were raised concerning her future. The new outpost occupied the north-eastern sector of the island continent and covered an area eleven times that of England and Wales;[1] its white population numbered only 25,000, most of whom lived in the southern half of the colony; the northern, unexplored half lay in the tropics. Yet, rather than consider the odds against them, Queensland's founders saw the untapped potential and determined to 'civilize' the land in the name of progress. From the outset the climate was regarded not as an impediment but as an asset, fundamental to the colony's viability and prosperity.

The conviction that Queensland possessed a healthy and health-giving climate persisted throughout the colonial period (1859 to 1900) and until the present. This conviction rested on the assumption, supported and sustained by medical evidence, that any country which offered a variety of climates, unlimited space, fresh air, pure water, warmth and sunshine must be healthy. Nineteenth-century colonial literature — official records, travellers' accounts and books of advice for immigrants — detailed these features, noting their effect on Queensland's progress. Although certain drawbacks were mentioned, the impression remained that the climate was not only conducive to healthy living, but could also prevent, alleviate or even cure disease. Moreover, the belief that hot climates were inimical to the health of the white race gradually eroded when it was demonstrated that Europeans could live and work in the north 'without loss of energy', and that pathological microbes, rather than the heat, caused tropical diseases. Thus the idea emerged that colonists, by their hard work and perseverance and spurred on by medical achievements, were able to prove that the white man could 'triumph in the tropics'. This concept dominates twentieth-century surveys of Queensland's development and suggests that the challenge of the climate, as much as its salubrious nature, contributed to colonial prosperity.[2]

More critical studies which investigate the role of the environment and its relation to health illustrate the enormous range of factors involved, but they deal only with the Australian scene in general and the tropical north in particular.[3] This study therefore seeks to explore attitudes to health by focusing on the almost obsessional belief in the salubrity of Queensland's climate, its roots, and how it was vindicated. To achieve this object, we will consider the impact of the climate on the colony's progress, the influence of contemporary medical theories and practice, and evidence from the colonial health records.

CLIMATE AND COLONIAL PROGRESS

Captain Cook's reports of eastern Australia in 1770 were the first to draw attention to the potential and excellent climate of the great southern land; he found 'all such things as nature hath bestowed on it, in a flourishing state'.[4] Fifty years later, development of the more northerly regions of the eastern seaboard began with the establishment of a convict colony on the banks of the Brisbane river, some 500 miles north of Sydney. When transportation ceased in 1840, the whole area opened up rapidly, and within two decades the northern settlers proclaimed their independence from New South Wales. Undaunted by the task ahead, Queensland's early leaders tackled the most urgent needs — capital and labour — by turning to the mother country to raise loans and by launching a vigorous immigration programme. During the next forty years, as governments rose and fell, Queensland survived three major boom-bust cycles in which the climate played a key role. Although British institutions and ideas were transplanted, British methods often failed to adapt to colonial conditions and new arrivals had difficulties adjusting to an unfamiliar environment.

Sufficient inducements were therefore needed in order to recruit immigrants and encourage them to settle. Promotional activity relied heavily on the offer of generous land grants, the prospect of material prosperity, and the attraction of a sunny and healthy climate. There were also negative factors to counteract — misconceptions, adverse criticism of the colony and perceived threats to progress. In 1860 the pundits asserted that

> The tropical climate of the northern coast lands was . . . deadly to members of the white races; the interior was declared to be almost entirely devoid of surface water — for the greater part of the year a fiery furnace, and at intervals of capricious periodicity ravaged by destructive floods. It was assumed to be a country where the white man would wither and the coloured man thrive . . . a land wholly unfit for the home of civilised peoples, and only adapted to the wants of the degraded aboriginal native. It was ignorantly affirmed that the sheep stations intended to be formed in the far western country must be failures, and . . . that under the tropical sun the sheep, if it could live in Queensland at all, would soon carry hair instead of wool. Even in Southern Queensland the agricultural possibilities of the land were sadly unappreciated.[5]

Despite these dire predictions and a distance of 12,000 miles from Britain, there was never any question that the colony would be developed as a civilized land. Such countries were, after all, the most progressive. The rise of social Darwinism underscored this belief.[6] Although it was generally agreed that the task of colonization should be entrusted to the 'fittest' (or the most civilized), it had been shown that the white races were constitutionally unsuited for survival in the tropics. Here they could exert only a 'civilizing influence' and leave the actual development of such lands to people who were physically adapted to them. Since Queensland's native population would not co-operate in this task, it was thought necessary to introduce 'less degraded' and more amenable coloured labour for the establishment of a plantation and pastoral economy.

Within weeks of his arrival, the first governor informed the Colonial Office that an Asiatic workforce would be required for 'the tropical districts . . . where the climate is unfavourable to European fieldwork on large plantations'; in the temperate regions production could be managed on 'small farms occupied by English migrants and their families'.[7] This decision satisfied colonial entrepreneurs. Since a cheap workforce would enhance profit margins, it was in their best interests to support the tropical theory. An Act, allowing for the introduction of Indian coolies, was passed by the colonial legislature in July 1862 but met with such opposition, particularly from the south, that it was never enforced. However, Polynesians were brought in from the south Pacific islands on fixed-term contracts and employed first on the cotton and later on the sugar plantations. This controversial practice continued for more than thirty years and was resolved only as sugar production methods changed and federation approached. Colonists resented their wages being undercut, were threatened by alien diseases,[8] and decided that, in the Australian Commonwealth, there would be no place for outcast and degraded or uncivilized humanity.

An alien presence, and not the climate, was increasingly seen as the major obstacle to progress. It was one thing to have barbarism on their doorstep, but within their midst proved too threatening. Moreover, colonists were trying to eradicate the taint of convictism. Queensland was particularly vulnerable; she was located closer to the 'barbaric hordes' than the other colonies, had housed some of the worst convicts, and possessed a climate which the 'experts' maintained was a danger to civilized man. It is therefore not difficult to appreciate why, from the beginning, colonial advocates endeavoured to establish that Queensland's climate was equal to, if not more favourable than, that in most parts of Australia. The authorities also insisted that only morally and physically fit Europeans be encouraged to settle permanently.[9] It became a truism that, if healthy people lived in a healthy environment with good prospects, they would survive and prosper.

White settlers spread out rapidly from the south-eastern districts, up along the coast and into the interior. By 1865 some were staking out their claims on the shores of the Gulf of Carpentaria in the far north. Squatters and cattle 'kings' appropriated large inland tracts, agriculture developed and coastal plantations thrived. With each new mineral discovery white men — and the Chinese — poured into the colony. The sudden appearance of Cooktown, some 1,000 miles north of Brisbane, was typical. One morning, soon after the Palmer River gold strike was announced in October 1873, a ship from the south dropped anchor in the Endeavour estuary. 'The miners rushed ashore, tents were put up, cargo unloaded and by evening the life of the town was in full swing.'[10] Cooktown became a tropical city with an estimated white population of 35,000 in its hey-day. European immigrants seemed more than ready to cope with the consequences of living in a hot climate.

By the close of the colonial era, it was evident that Queensland had made substantial progress. The rate of population growth had outstripped that for any other Australian colony, Europeans were established — and thriving — in every part of the country, the alien problem had been resolved, and annual exports were growing. This Cinderella colony had become a jewel in the crown of Empire. Queensland entered the twentieth century confident that her reputation as a promising and healthy land had stood the test of time.

Any review of the colony's progress usually considered the various climatic zones, 'from the most temperate to the most torrid.'[11] The coastal plains and ranges, stretching for some 1,550 miles along the eastern seaboard, produced 'anything from tobacco to alligators, from oranges and sugar cane to turtles and sea slugs'.[12] Increasing heat and rainfall towards the equator encouraged such growth. The vast inland tablelands and plains to the west of the Great Dividing Range were generally hot and dry; only the southern districts experienced frosts and cold winds. Although most accounts pointed out these differences and admitted that the summer heat could be trying, they also stressed the equable nature of the climate. In his 1864 report the Registrar-General provided statistics showing that variations in 'temperature, humidity, and salubrity' throughout Queensland were definitely less than in countries of a comparable size.[13] The climate in the south was said to resemble the 'warm, luscious' atmosphere of southern Europe.[14]

Such favourable reports, however, did not always hold true; the climate could be variable and unpredictable, even brutal. Brisbane may have been likened to Madeira or Sicily, but it was not without its 'vicissitudes', as an article in one of the British medical journals indicated; in the summer of 1884 the temperature fell one day to 60°F. and rose the next to 90°F. in the shade.[15] A point in Queensland's favour during the first few years was the apparent absence of hot winds, but this reversed. In November 1865 the colonial governor wrote to his sister in England:

> A 'hot wind' is blowing from the west, parching up everything . . . day after day the brazen sky is almost unclouded except for a white haze round the horizon. Water is becoming very scarce . . . serious loss of life and property will I fear attend a long continuation of this drought.[16]

Cycles of drought and floods, the latter often accompanied by 'terrific storms', gales and cyclones, were regular climatic events that had devastating economic consequences for a primary-producing and pioneering land. Colonists had to come to terms not so much with the tropical heat, but 'good' and 'bad' seasons, too much or too little water. Furthermore, variations between the different localities led to conflicting opinions. A person arriving in Brisbane on a sunny winter's day might well believe he had discovered 'an earthly paradise',[17] while descriptions of life 'up country' — the 'unbearable' heat and 'wet', the dust and flies — often depict a hell on earth.[18]

In order to reconcile such conflicting and depressing reports, correct misconceptions and dispel ignorance, it was necessary to persistently push the image of a land 'most generously endowed by nature'. Thus, colonial leaders may have bowed to economic interests which supported the tropical theory, but they fully endorsed the healthy-climate theme. The first Registrar-General's report asserted that the climate of the new colony retained its 'healthy character' as far as the northern limits of exploration.[19] Four years later, when the territorial survey was complete, he declared the environment, from north to south, to be 'well-suited to European constitutions', adding that at Cape York (the most northerly point) 'the healthiness of the European inhabitants [was] remarkable'.[20] With each successive report he emphasized how 'blessed' the colony was; even 'the sweet-smelling Eucalyptus' was said to 'exhale a health-giving principle'.[21]

Other government publications repeated the theme; an 1891 *Handbook*, for example, pointed out that 'although the heat makes out-door work arduous and uncomfortable, such work can nevertheless be carried on throughout the summer without injury to men of steady and temperate habits'.[22] Indeed, the heat became a sensitive subject. To refer to it in a host's home was, according to Anthony Trollope who visited the colony in 1871, as indelicate as alluding to 'a bad bottle of wine or an ill-cooked joint of meat'.[23] And as far as working in the heat was concerned, this is what one colonist of twenty years' standing had to say: 'the whole of my observation and experience goes to form the solid conviction that all that has been said, or that can be said, about the unsuitability of the climate of Queensland for Europeans . . . is only so much rotten rubbish'.[24] Both official and lay opinion often went further and claimed that the climate, far from being detrimental, actually promoted health and longevity.[25] This continuing emphasis on the benefits of the climate not only derived from a need to promote the colony, but was also firmly rooted in nineteenth-century medical thought and practice.

CLIMATOLOGY AND CLIMATE THERAPY

Colonial Queensland was dominated by the mother country; British concepts directed her policies and immigrants outnumbered the native-born.[26] Not surprisingly, western medicine was transplanted with little or no thought that it might need to be adapted to the new environment. Also, medicine itself was changing;

the centuries-old qualitative, holistic and relatively static view of disease (humoral pathology) was being replaced by a more localized, dynamic and quantitative approach. Investigators, rather than describe symptoms, had begun to isolate specific causes and processes — biological or chemical, constitutional or environmental.[27]

Disease theories reflected these new lines of inquiry and were incorporated in nosologies or classifications used for the registration of deaths. Vital statistics — births, marriages, deaths and causes of death — served as an index of the health of a nation and its 'progress . . . in the march of civilization.'[28] The establishment of a Registrar-General's Department for England and Wales in 1837 led to the creation of a similar office in most British colonies. Thus, at the time of separation the Queensland government made provision for the compilation of records which would furnish information on 'the effects of the climate in different parts of the Colony on the constitutions of our countrymen, the length of life, the prevailing diseases, the sanitary condition of the towns, and the increase of the population, from natural causes'.[29] The colony generally followed the format of the English Registrar-General's reports, including the Meteorological Report and Farr's tables for classifying causes of death.[30] A revised nosology, to accommodate 'the remarkable strides made in medical science', was first introduced in 1881 in England and three years later in Queensland.[31]

Since the new disease theories were not sufficiently verified or accepted until the 1890s, differences between the two classifications involved no major structural changes; they merely highlighted shifts in medical thinking. Both schemes contained a category for deaths of which the cause could not be defined or specified, and another for deaths due to violence, either accidental or intentional. Fatal diseases linked with developmental problems such as congenital abnormalities and old age were classed together, and a fourth category, by far the largest, included diseases of localized origin, classified according to the affected system — nervous, circulatory, respiratory, etc. Aetiology for this group was vague and largely depended on signs and symptoms associated with a particular organ or tissue. In the class designated as 'Constitutional Diseases', we find gout, rheumatic fever, diabetes mellitus, and all forms of tuberculosis. It was believed that some 'tendency' or alteration in a person's constitution gave rise to such conditions.

The final category (this was listed first in each classification) contained zymotic diseases ('zymotic' referred to the fermenting action of yeast). These generally affected the whole person and were considered preventable since they had an external cause. The category was divided into several sub-groups — miasmatic (epidemic and contagious diseases like measles, smallpox, typhus and typhoid fevers), diarrhoeal (diarrhoea, dysentery, cholera), malarial (ague and remittent fever), zoogenous (hydrophobia, for example), venereal and septic diseases. Two further classes (parasitic and dietic) which were included under zymotic diseases in Farr's scheme became separate categories in the revised classification since distinct and definable causes for these had been determined. Such changes reflected the genesis of a new medical paradigm. How did this evolve, and where did climatology fit in?

From antiquity environment was understood to play a vital role in health and disease. *Airs, Waters and Places*, one of the Hippocratic texts, correlated a variety of symptoms and symptom clusters (diseases) with the geographical and meteorological features in different localities; malaria, catarrh and diarrhoea, for example, were said to be due to the effect of seasonal changes on stagnant water or marshy places. Such concepts survived, and in time consolidated in the belief that a pathological state of the atmosphere, associated with certain climatic and local conditions, was responsible for outbreaks of infectious disease. This line of thinking developed into the miasmatic theory of contagion; air became contaminated with miasmas, poisonous vapours given off by putrifying organic matter, and a person fell victim to disease when miasmas attacked the body and disturbed its vital functions.[32] If local conditions could be controlled by the provision of adequate ventilation, clean water and the proper disposal of human waste and decaying material, then the atmosphere would remain pure. Nineteenth-century sanitary reform was based on this assumption. The climate, or a change in weather pattern, exerted both a negative and positive effect. An 'unhealthy' climate intensified the miasmatic content of the air, enhanced the spread of disease, or rendered a person more susceptible to attack, whereas a 'healthy' climate so altered the state of the atmosphere and a person's constitution that the air was purified and resistance to disease increased. Such a climate was a decided advantage for any locality or country.

Although the notion of a living contagion — a pathogenic organism found in air, water, or other media — had surfaced periodically over the centuries, the miasmatic theory was firmly entrenched by the mid-1800s. Apart from contagious diseases such as smallpox which were known to be transmitted by a specific 'poison', many other infections, particularly the 'filth' diseases (typhus fever, cholera, dysentery, etc.), were attributed to a general atmospheric impurity. However, before the turn of the century, the germ theory was rapidly eroding belief in miasmas. The gradual trend to move away from a symptom-orientated to a specific-agent aetiology had improved disease differentiation and definition. Then, as technology advanced, scientists isolated organisms visible only under the microscope and held each responsible for a discrete disease. The tide of discovery began slowly, had gathered pace by 1875, and by the 1890s was rolling in, bringing with it a new understanding of diseases and their transmission, as well as possible cures.[33] The new climatology which had assumed such prominence under the miasmatic theory, far from fading with it, retained a significant place in both pathology and practice. Climatic influences on the growth of pathogenic micro-organisms were recognized early in the development of the germ theory, and were believed to 'constitute the principal conditions under which the germs develop, grow, multiply, and diffuse themselves, thus becoming of nearly equal importance to the germs'.[34] When bubonic plague reappeared in the late 1890s, no one questioned its microbial origins, but its spread was attributed to the effect of temperature on 'pestilential emanations from polluted and waterlogged soil'.[35] Even climate therapy — the change to a more healthy environment

— received a boost from the recognition that a patient was removed from the locus of infection.[36]

Curative medicine in the middle decades of the nineteenth century had reached an impasse; traditional heroic measures — bleeding and blistering, purges and emetics and a wonderful range of pharmacological concoctions — were being questioned, and only a handful of specifics — vaccination as a preventive for smallpox, quinine for malaria and mercurial compounds for venereal diseases — was available. During this period sanitary science and a rising standard of living and personal hygiene statistically demonstrated the benefits of preventive medicine. Well before the era of specific remedies, epidemic diseases had been brought under control and mortality rates were declining. 'Natural cures' — sea voyages and spas, health resorts and open-air sanatoria — became fashionable prescriptions. Every aspect of climate was investigated and exploited. 'The study of climate has from time immemorial engaged many and skilful workers, and our knowledge of meteorology has made special strides in the last half century', a leading authority on chest diseases observed in 1875. He defined the 'exact relations' of climate to pulmonary tuberculosis

> Firstly, as a direct cause of the disease.
> Secondly, as affording immunity from the disease.
> Thirdly, as ameliorating and curing it.

and gave a detailed account of 'some practical results of climatic treatment'.[37]

Numerous articles appeared in the *British Medical Journal* and the *Lancet* between 1860 and 1900 dealing with climate and its importance not only for medicine, but also for imperial expansion and social progress. Endless publications relating to the subject rolled off the regular press, special societies sprang up, conferences and congresses were convened, and a world-wide health industry flourished. Climatologists studied 'The air . . . its temperature, humidity, pressure, and purity, the amount of sunshine . . . the winds . . . [and] the nature of the soil',[38] and compared hot and dry, cold and moist, elevated and sea-level, inland and coastal climates. Medical men correlated these features with diseases, noting harmful and beneficial results. Evidence continued to come forward in support of the 'immunizing' properties of climate and its power to modify certain diseases.[39] Also, the relationship between climate and health, though 'difficult to establish' often because of biased perceptions, generated theories concerning the rise and fall of civilizations and the evolution of racial and constitutional characteristics. It was claimed that peoples living in countries with an 'optimum temperature' were the strongest, that 'no potent and conquering race' had ever arisen in a hot, moist region, that acclimatization depended primarily on heredity and the human constitution and that, at its most basic level, climate affected 'the feelings and the whole mental disposition of man'.[40] Climatic theories pervaded the entire fabric of western civilization.

Although a 'change of climate', from a less to a more healthy region, was regarded as 'one of the most powerful remedial agents in existence', medical proponents agreed that professional ignorance of its potential resulted from 'the paucity of accurate and definite data'.[41] Many descriptive accounts were superficial and included real geographical blunders. Medical schools, by and large, gave scant attention to the subject, and all too often climate was used as a convenient panacea.[42] As a consequence, doctors frequently wrote to the medical journals seeking advice for themselves and their patients. A typical case was the 'phthisical practitioner', aged 25 years, who asked which would be better, the climate of Australia or Colorado, for the treatment of his illness.[43] Since much of the information relating to Australia was based on hearsay and shrouded in ignorance, no one could give a reliable answer. In 1860 it was correctly noted that mortality increased in the summer, while 'the unusual amount of insanity' was attributed to 'the great consumption of ardent spirits in a climate unfavourable to such indulgence'.[44] Those who had been 'cured', or who knew of such instances, claimed that the Australian climate 'often worked wonders'.[45] On the other hand, less enthusiastic and more informed opinion pointed out that the effect of the climate on 'morbid conditions' had not been fully explored and that any discussion which failed to compare the different climatic zones was 'unpardonable'.[46] Nevertheless, the consensus seemed to be that many parts of Australia possessed a healthy climate, the chief advantages of which were warm temperatures, relative dryness, sunshine and an open-air life. As Queensland became better known, certain areas, like the Darling Downs (the great southern tableland), were included in Australia's list of therapeutic locations.[47]

Guidelines for climate therapy were simple enough for ailments such as gout, bronchitis, dyspepsia and 'nervous affections', but increased in complexity for phthisis (pulmonary tuberculosis or consumption), the disease which, more than any other, provided a rationale for this form of treatment.[48] Although phthisis death-rates had been declining in England since the 1820s, it remained a major killer, especially among those in the prime of life. With the discovery of the tubercle bacillus in 1882, understanding of the disease and its contagious nature grew, replacing the belief in its constitutional and environmental origins. The adoption of isolation measures, evidence that exposure to sunlight reduced the virulence of the infection, and an awareness of the implications of bovine tuberculosis, introduced new controls. But when a specific cure failed to materialize,[49] climate (a cool, dry and 'pure' atmosphere) coupled with appropriate hygienic and dietary arrangements kept its place as the primary remedy for the disease in its early stages; the benefit of any form of treatment for advanced consumptives was questioned. Samuel Dougan Bird's book, *On Australian Climates, and their Influence in the Prevention and Arrest of Pulmonary Tuberculosis*, appeared in 1863 when interest in and migration to the Antipodes was growing. Thereafter, increasing numbers of 'phthisical sufferers', desperate for a cure, sailed south and the great debate over the remedial value of the voyage and the Australian climate intensified.[50] The colonies allegedly became a dumping ground for incurables, the incidence of tuberculosis rose, and it had to be admitted that no climate offered *the* cure. Without a viable alternative, the Australian climate retained its reputation as a therapeutic agent for consumption. At least Queensland had no shortage of the best natural remedy — sunshine.

The colony's climate offered many advantages, but critics always pointed to the tropical north. Years of colonization had shown that protracted residence in hot and moist climates impaired the function and physique of Europeans.[51] The body's 'power of adaptation' might be 'marvellous', but there were limits; in the tropics 'flexibility' became 'extinct' after two or three generations.[52] Although opinions differed over constitutional requirements and the role of heredity, few questioned the belief that the heat was responsible for the high incidence of and fatalities from miasmatic and diarrhoeal diseases, to say nothing of sunstroke and sun fever.[53] Yet, as white colonists paid more attention to sanitation and hygiene, these conditions proved less fatal. Then ideas changed rapidly with accumulating evidence that 'the causes of disease, deterioration and deaths in the tropics are due not so much to the influence of the climate as to pathogenic germs'.[54]

Even so, as late as 1893, the case of Queensland's sugar plantations was cited to illustrate the futility of Europeans attempting to work in 'damp heat'.[55] A more astute observer, however, suggested that 'the assertions of the advocates of coloured labour' perpetuated the myth, since the facts indicated that 'Farm labour was carried on by the white man . . . in tropical Australia . . . with no worse consequences than in temperate regions.'[56] Indeed, as early as 1861, the following comment relating to 'the alleged unsuitableness of the climate to European labourers' appeared in an Irish journal:

> I can hardly believe it [the objection] to be seriously intended for the ears of any one personally acquainted with the country. The colonists have always been accustomed to engage in the severest kinds of work without injury to health, in all seasons; and they would, doubtless, be very much astonished at being told they were unequal to cotton-hoeing and cotton-picking.[57]

Twenty-five years later, it 'continue[d] to be accepted' that Australia's 'great heat' was less injurious than in other countries and rarely produced sunstroke.[58] The healthy-climate concept gained ground as the hot-climate theory lost support.

By the turn of the century the exciting possibilities of disease control had almost eliminated the threat of 'unhealthy' climates, acclimatization no longer meant 'survival of the fittest' but 'control of the tropics', the future of the empire seemed assured and the experience of Europeans in tropical Australia could become the norm. Recognizing Queensland's success with white settlement and the need for systematic research *in situ* of ongoing problems in this area, the Australian government in 1909 established an Institute for Tropical Medicine at Townsville (North Queensland). Here 'useful work . . . bearing on the acclimatisation of the white man was accomplished'.[59] Although its functions were transferred twenty years later to the School of Tropical Medicine at the University of Sydney, the challenge of the north has continued to extend man's knowledge and control of conditions in the tropics. It is clear that medical evidence sustained and vindicated the belief in a healthy climate, but could the same be said for the colony's health record?

QUEENSLAND'S HEALTH

The official health record for colonial Queensland appeared annually in the Registrar-General's reports.[60] When compiling these he had access to similar documents from the sister colonies and the mother country, for he not only commented on their content and compared vital statistics, but interpreted the Queensland statistics using the same conceptual framework.

In mid-nineteenth-century England sanitary reform based on climate-related theories was seen as the key to the nation's health. The most recent reports (1857 and 1858) for England and Wales were available by 1860. In the former the mortality rate (21.2 deaths for every 1,000 of the population) was attributed largely to very high temperatures in July and August. 'A summer of unusual warmth . . . promotes growth [and] is probably salutary to the human frame where the land is drained, decaying refuse is buried . . . and cleanliness is observed,' the English Registrar-General wrote; but where these conditions were lacking, fever, ague and especially diarrhoea prevailed.[61] Dr Farr explained in his supplement to the report that high temperatures associated with 'stagnancy of air', over crowded, and filthy cities gave rise to diarrhoea. The wind, he noted, had an important sanitary effect; it was 'capable of bringing and of carrying away the organic elements which are the seeds sometimes of zymotic diseases'.[62] An above-average mortality for the following year was said to be due to severe pressures on the poor and aged, impure water, an increased incidence of respiratory diseases caused by extremely cold weather, and a diphtheria epidemic: 'Each epidemic has its own congenial climate.'[63]

When Queensland's Registrar-General compiled the first report, he considered the new colony — the scattered population, its few old people, freedom from pauperism and epidemics, as well as its warmth, sunshine and sea breezes — and concluded that the climate was 'decidedly healthy'.[64] A death-rate of 18.6 confirmed his assessment. The rate (16.02) was even more gratifying for 1861, but an examination of the causes of death raised the first warning signal. Juvenile mortality was too high and the growing population, though 'blessed with a healthy climate . . . all the necessities and most of the luxuries of life', needed protection from disease; sanitary controls were required to maintain a wholesome environment.[65] He was right. In 1862 the death-rate rose sharply to 20.6, the increase being concentrated chiefly among children and in the seaport towns during the hot months. New arrivals suffered greatly through 'exposure to the summer heat', and a worsening drought aggravated difficulties with acclimatization. Only 29½ inches of rain fell in Brisbane compared to 69½ inches the previous year. Although the high mortality was associated with 'the peculiar state of the atmosphere', there appeared no hint that the climate was anything less than healthy.[66]

Then in 1863, as the influx of immigrants increased, Queensland experienced the worst floods on record. The death-rate jumped to 23.9 and exceeded the average mortality for England. This was most disturbing, particularly when the colony's natural advantages were compared to conditions 'back home'. The Registrar-General, believing that 'negligence' accounted for many of the deaths, urged that colonists be more careful of both human life and health principles.[67] The idea that man must co-operate with nature to combat disease surfaced regularly in the English reports of the 1860s, and was typically expressed in the remark that 'Favourable weather often has to contend with ignorance and neglect.'[68] The colonial death-rate reached an all-time high (25.7) in 1866, a year of heavy immigration, severe flooding following another drought, and total economic collapse. During these early years 'convulsions', 'wasting diseases' in children and diarrhoeal complaints were the most common causes of death, along with accidents (many were drowning victims) and phthisis. Pioneer living, unfamiliar weather conditions and growing 'sanitary evils' took their toll. Although the death-rate fell in the late 1860s (immigration was greatly curtailed), mortality patterns did not change.

By the end of the first decade Queensland's health record revealed three particular trends which recurred during the remainder of the colonial period. First, sanitary reform, despite the government's recognition of its importance, seemed to be regarded as a private rather than a public responsibility. Colonists were expected to adjust to the climate and not presume upon its benefits by disregarding the basic precautions for healthy living. Thus the Registrar-General noted with satisfaction in his 1869 report that, in the process of acclimatization, new settlers had tried to improve their sanitary arrangements.[69] Second, the incidence of phthisis deaths was exaggerated by terminally-ill consumptives arriving from the southern colonies in a last-ditch attempt to find a cure. Imported diseases became an increasing problem. And third, the climate apparently did little or nothing to reduce mortality. In England the dangers of a hot season had diminished with progressive public health reform, while the high death-rate from respiratory disorders indicated that the cold weather proved 'more fatal'.[70] Such reports squared with the Queensland experience and not only raised doubts concerning the curative properties of the climate, but undermined belief in the lethal effects of heat. These shifts of opinion, however, did not weaken the claim that the climate created an atmosphere conducive to health.

The 1870s began with 'an exceptionally healthy year' which registered the lowest death-rate (14.59) since separation. Several features of the mortality attracted attention.[71] Only four deaths from sunstroke were recorded for the whole colony; the increase in miasmatic diseases suggested that, apart from a few rudimentary improvements in Brisbane, 'everything [had] yet to be done' elsewhere in order to raise public health standards; Queensland, like Madeira, could become the 'Grave of the English' on account of the number of phthisis cases sent there; and accidents, many of which were preventable, remained a significant cause of death. But the juvenile mortality, a most 'painful' subject, dominated the statistics; 46.56 per cent of the total deaths for 1870 were under 5 years of age. Although the colonies to the south recorded a similar rate and the latest returns for England were only slightly less (42.26 per cent), the proportion for Queensland ought to have been lower. The inference was clear: with such a climate, the colony had no excuse for an unnaturally high mortality.

During the 1870s public health legislation and quarantine sparked off a controversy that achieved no satisfactory resolution until the following decade. The debate clearly demonstrated the political implications of the belief in a healthy climate.[72] On the one hand the government boosted the colony's image by emphasizing its favourable environment, and on the other excused their parsimony and lack of effective law-enforcement by placing the blame for continuing sanitary abuses on the local authorities or the colonists themselves. The death-rate rose to a high of 23.8 in 1875, new mining centres became hotbeds of typhoid fever and dysentery, and the incidence of phthisis increased; weather patterns and economic conditions fluctuated. Each year the Registrar-General read reports from England of the 'salutary effects' of sanitation,[73] compared statistics from the other colonies, and came to the conclusion that Queensland seemed to be one of the most unhealthy parts of Australia; even the 'health-generating gum-trees' had been wantonly destroyed.[74] Again he urged that steps be taken to provide for a clean environment and to improve personal hygiene. Soap was the 'great civilizer'; uncleanliness was 'a relic of barbarism'.[75] The 1879 report recorded with some frustration that it was 'frightful to think' how sanitary science 'in its present advanced state' could be so neglected in a climate that was 'perhaps equal in healthfulness to anything known in the world'.[76] This asset was deliberately being ignored to the detriment of colonial progress.

Other concerns also came to a head during this decade. In his 1874 report the Registrar-General went to considerable lengths to correct the impression that Queensland's climate was 'exceptionally unfavourable to children'.[77] Certainly infant mortality was high, but no more so than that for England and the older Australian colonies; 'true' infant mortality (the proportion of deaths under one year to the number of live births) for Queensland between 1865 and 1874 averaged 12.57 per cent compared to 16.0 per cent for England in 1870. He also stressed that the colony's unusually large juvenile population made the problem seem worse than in countries with a more evenly distributed age structure.[78] The other problem was the phthisis mortality; by the late 1870s this disease had become the most common cause of death in Queensland. Not only did late-stage consumptives continue to arrive, but it was found that tuberculosis was spreading with alarming fatality among the Polynesian labourers, the very people who had been brought in because the climate was supposedly unsuited to Europeans.[79]

Pulmonary tuberculosis headed the colony's mortality lists for the last two decades of the nineteenth century. There were several reasons for this. Immigration increased dramatically in the boom conditions of the early 1880s, and would certainly have included a proportion of consumptives among the growing numbers of cabin-class passengers who did not require a health certificate. In 1886 it was estimated that half those who died in Queensland from phthisis had lived there less than five years; this trend continued into the 1890s.[80] In fact, the English Registrar-General in his 1897 report admitted that 'many who became affected . . . remove[d] to other countries to die', and so contributed to the declining mortality for that disease in England and Wales.[81] Also, the exquisite susceptibility to infection among the alien population remained; almost 50 per cent of the high mortality for the Chinese and Polynesians was due to consumption.[82] Yet phthisis fatalities gradually diminished, since immigration almost dried up during the depression years of the late 1880s and early 1890s, the number of aliens decreased with the approach of federation, and measures to control tuberculosis and protect the non-infected were introduced as an adjunct to climate-therapy. The fact that the colony's phthisis mortality was relatively low for long-term residents and the native-born, and that the overall death-rate for the disease, though high, was less than in Britain and Europe, underscored the healthy-climate theme.[83]

Apart from tuberculosis, mortality patterns for Queensland and the mother country showed fewer similarities during the second half of the colonial period. England after 1880 was reaping the benefits of sanitary reform while the colony still grappled with the problem. The English reports also reflected medical advances at an earlier stage. Although the association of respiratory complaints with cold weather and diarrhoeal disorders with high temperatures persisted, the emphasis shifted from 'atmospheric influences' and sanitation to the impact of specific diseases, the role of germs and new methods of prevention such as immunization. Another feature of these reports was a steady decline in the death-rate which reached its lowest point for the century (17.0) in 1896. But infant mortality remained a 'sad reflection' of the health status of that country,[84] as it did in Queensland. However, figures for the latter were comparable to those for England and the older Australian colonies, in spite of the fact that children in the northern districts and on the goldfields suffered more than in other areas. Yet again, ignorance and neglect rather than the climate were held responsible for the higher mortality.[85] By the dawn of the new era (1901) returns for under-five-year-olds in Queensland's northern regions were 'almost the same [as] for New South Wales and Victoria'.[86] Such evidence, it was believed, would surely put to rest fears that the tropical climate was unfavourable to the British race.

After 1884 the colony's death-rate, as a whole, began to show a decided improvement. But in that year the combined effect of a period of heavy immigration (European and alien), economic difficulties, 'glaring sanitary defects' and a drought, produced one of the highest mortality rates (22.97) on record. Dysentery, especially among the Polynesians, replaced phthisis as the primary cause of death, and typhoid fever which had been the twelfth most fatal disorder in 1880, registered third, exceeding by more than 300 per cent the mortality rate for that disease in any of the sister colonies.[87] The evils of the plantation system made Englishmen 'blush', the sanitary condition of Queensland's towns and mining centres became a stench in the nostrils of her politicians, and both adversely affected the colony's image. Then, in the wake of the long drought, severe floods, and economic depression, immigration was reduced to a trickle, Polynesian repatriation began and the government took a more active role in public health affairs. The sanitary scene improved and the death-rate fell rapidly. In 1897 it reached the lowest point for the colonial period (11.38), a figure significantly less than the corresponding rate for England and Wales. In view of the fact that a considerable proportion of the population lived in the tropics, this gratifying trend, as the Registrar-General observed, spoke out 'most emphatically for the natural salubrity of the climate'.[88]

Such a statement had echoed through the colonial years in spite of the tropical theory, 'bad' seasons, difficulties with acclimatization and unfavourable mortality returns. The possibility or suggestion that the climate might be implicated in the colony's health problems was rarely entertained or quickly negated; medical evidence, and the sometimes questionable health record, were both used to support colonial ideology. For a greater part of the period, the official attitude implied that, with such a climate, minimal government intervention was necessary since the population should have been able to maintain its own health standards. Any deficiencies were therefore due to the alien presence or to the colonists themselves who, through ignorance and neglect, had failed to take advantage of, and even abused, one of their greatest assets. A high death-rate was viewed as a blot on civilization and a disgrace. The continuing low mortality returns in the 1890s not only indicated progress in the right direction, but provided the final vindication for the belief in a healthy climate.

This belief grew out of the need, from her inception, to create a positive image of the colony — one rich in potential and resources, a viable outpost of empire. The claim to possess a healthy climate proved politically expedient. It was rooted in, validated and sustained by contemporary medical theory and practice and, despite the drawbacks, Queenslanders generally were convinced of its veracity. The belief persisted because, in the final analysis, positive evidence overruled or cancelled out the negative. Europeans settled and thrived in the tropics, diseases were brought under control and mortality rates declined, the population grew and the colony prospered.

NOTES

1. *Votes and Proceedings of the Legislative Assembly of Queensland* (hereafter *QVP*), 1877, vol. 2, 678. Early descriptions emphasized the immense size of the colony.

2. See, for example, *Our First Half-Century* (Brisbane: Government Printer, 1909); *The History of Queensland: Its People and Industries. An Epitome of Progress*, 2 vols (Brisbane: States Publishing Co., 1921); R.W. Cilento and C. Lack (eds), *Triumph in the Tropics: An Historical Sketch of Queensland* (Brisbane: Smith & Paterson, 1959); and K.B. Fraser, 'Glimpses of yesterday north of Capricorn', *Medical Journal of Australia* (16 September 1967) (2), 531–5.

3. A sample of the literature includes G.N. Blainey, 'Climate and Australia's history', *Melbourne Historical Journal, 10* (1971), 5–9; G.C. Bolton, *Spoils and Spoilers: Australians Make their Environment, 1788–1980* (Sydney: Allen & Unwin, 1981); and P.P. Courtenay, *The White Man and the Australian Tropics* . . . , (Townsville: History Department, James Cook University of North Queensland, 1975, mimeo).

4. Quoted in Cilento and Lack, op. cit., n. 2 above, 31.

5. *Our First Half-Century*, n. 2 above, 16.

6. The notion of 'civilized' man emerged as a consequence of intellectual developments in Europe from the time of the Renaissance. The discovery of 'less developed' lands and 'barbaric' peoples emphasized the 'superior' elements of western civilization; Darwin's *Origin of Species* (1859) provided a theoretical framework for such concepts, and the works of Francis Galton (1822–1911), the English statistician and psychologist, strongly influenced ideas concerning the 'progress' of civilized man. According to C.M.H. Clarke, *A History of Australia*, 6 vols., (Melbourne: Melbourne University Press 1962–88), vol. 4 (1978), 392, 'The proximity of barbarism to civilization had a long history in Australia.'

7. *Twentieth General Report of the Emigration Commissioners* (London: Spotiswoode, 1860), 146.

8. The Polynesians were said to have introduced filariasis (a mosquito-borne disease) and hookworm, and the Chinese, leprosy. See Cilento and Lack, op. cit., n. 2 above, 293.

9. For a full discussion of the selection procedure for immigrants see H.R. Woolcock, 'Health care on Queensland immigrant vessels: 1860–1900' (Unpublished PhD thesis, University of London, 1983), 71ff.

10. N. Phelan, *Some Came Early, Some Came Late* (Melbourne: Macmillan, 1970), 209.

11. See E.M. La Meslée, *The New Australia* (Paris: E. Plon, 1883), trans. and ed. Russel M. Ward (London: Heinemann, 1973), 204.

12. Arthur Temple, *The Making of the Empire: The Story of Our Colonies* (London: Andrew Melrose, 3rd edn, 1898), 223.

13. *QVP* 1865, 863.

14. John Foster Fraser, *Australia: the Making of a Nation* (London and New York: Cassell, 1911), 240. For a typical description of the climate see S.W. Silver & Co., *Handbook for Australia and New Zealand* (London: S.W. Silver, 1888), 244–6, esp. 245.

15. *Lancet* (17 May 1884), 924.

16. ' "My Dear Janey": a letter from R.G.W. Herbert to his sister', *Queensland Heritage, 2*, (6) (May 1972), 35.

17. La Meslée, op. cit., n. 11 above, 71.

18. See Hector Holthouse, *Up Rode the Squatter* (Adelaide: Rigby, 1970).

19. *QVP* 1861, 907–8.

20. *QVP* 1865, 863.

21. *QVP* 1882, vol. 2, 153.

22. Extract from *Queensland Handbook* (1890) in Josiah Hughes, *Australia Revisited in 1890* . . . (London: Simpkin, Marshall, Hamilton, Kent, 1891), 355.

23. Hume Dow (ed.), *Trollope's Australia* (Melbourne: Nelson, 1966), 23.

24. Silver & Co., op. cit., n. 14 above, 244.

25. See Thornhill Weedon, *Queensland Past and Present. An Epitome of its Resources and Development, 1897* (Brisbane: Government Printer, 2nd issue, 1897), 124.

26. The aboriginal population of Australia was not enumerated until the 1901 census.

27. For a classic and detailed interpretation of these changes see Richard H. Shyrock, *The Development of Modern Medicine* (New York: Alfred A. Knopf, 1947).

28. *QVP*, 1861, 871.

29. ibid.

30. William Farr (1807–83), an English physician, was appointed as compiler of

abstracts in the Registrar-General's office in 1841. His pioneer work in vital statistics greatly extended the scope and influence of the annual and census reports for England and Wales. Farr's disease classification appeared in 1853.

31. The revision was carried out by a Committee of the Royal College of Physicians, London, headed by Dr William Ogle. For details of the changes and an outline of the Ogle classification, see *QVP* 1885, vol. 2, 559–60 and 1886, vol. 2, 375.

32. This theory and its history are summarized in W.F. Bynum, E.J. Browne, Roy Porter (eds), *Dictionary of the History of Science* (London: Macmillan, 1981), s.v. 'Contagion'.

33. See Erwin H. Ackerknecht, *A Short History of Medicine* (Baltimore: Johns Hopkins University Press, rev. edn, 1982), 175–85, esp. 180.

34. *Lancet* (2 June 1894), 1357; see also *Lancet* (24 January 1885), 173. Later studies confirmed that many parasites, bacteria and their insect vectors survived only under particular climatic conditions; see R.W. Cilento, 'The conquest of climate', *Medical Journal of Australia* (8 April 1933) (1), 421–32, esp. 428.

35. *Lancet* (30 December 1899), 1851.

36. *Lancet* (17 May 1890), 1079.

37. *British Medical Journal* (8 January 1876), 38–9. Such claims were supported with ample and convincing illustrations. The author later embraced the germ theory, but his emphasis on the role of climate remained; see *Lancet* (2 June 1894), 1357–60.

38. *Lancet* (27 September 1890), 676.

39. See *Lancet* (11 September 1897), 673, and *British Medical Journal* (8 May 1880), 713–14.

40. *British Medical Journal* (25 August 1860), 659–60. Numerous articles illustrating these ideas appeared in the medical journals; see, for example, *British Medical Journal* (12 September 1896), 682, and *Lancet* (27 May 1893), 1268, (15 August 1891), 404, and (27 May 1899), 1440–1. See also Lewis B. Flinn, 'Reflections on the relationship of climatology to Medicine', *Transactions of the American Climatological Association, 79* (1968), 146–56. Even the determination of life assurance and superannuation depended on climatic theories.

41. *Lancet* (6 August 1864), 167, and (27 September 1890), 676.

42. Medical climatologists objected to doctors leaving the selection of the resort to the patient. See *British Medical Journal* (21 November 1885), 979–80.

43. *British Medical Journal* (15 September 1888), 647.

44. *Lancet* (11 August 1860), 144.

45. See, for example, *Lancet* (7 February 1863), 163.

46. Following each glowing report of the Australian climate, there usually appeared a more balanced article or negative opinion.

47. See *Lancet* (27 September 1873), 474, and (15 September 1888), 552.

48. Dr Herman Weber, an 'acknowledged master' of the subject, along with others established rules of treatment. See *British Medical Journal* (3 June 1899), 1321–4.

49. Robert Koch (1843–1910), a German physician, isolated the tubercle bacillus in 1882. His announcement of tuberculin in 1890 suggested that this was the cure; but he was premature. Tuberculin proved of value in diagnosis.

50. This debate has been dealt with at some length in J.M. Powell, 'Medical promotion and the consumptive immigrant to Australia', *Geographical Review, 63*, (4) (1973), 449–76, and K.B. Thomas and B. Gandevia, 'Dr Francis Workman, emigrant, and the history of taking the cure for consumption in the Australian colonies', *Medical Journal of Australia* (4 July 1959) (2), 1–10.

51. *Lancet* (18 January 1873), 105–6.

52. *British Medical Journal* (8 September 1860), 697–700, esp. 697.

53. The journals are peppered with articles on sunstroke and sun fever. No consensus

was reached as to whether the direct rays of the sun or high temperatures were responsible.

54. *British Medical Journal* (24 September 1898), 912.

55. *Lancet* (27 May 1893), 1268.

56. *British Medical Journal* (30 April 1893), 1167–8, esp. 1168.

57. E.G. Mayne, 'Remarks on the colony of Queensland as a field for emigration', *Journal of the Royal Dublin Society*, *3* (1860–1), 343.

58. *British Medical Journal* (21 August 1886), 363.

59. A. Balfour and H.H. Scott, *Health Problems of the Empire: Past, Present and Future* (London: Collins, 1924), 172. E.M. Derrick in 'Medical research — a continuing challenge', *Medical Journal of Australia* (25 April 1970) (1) 829–32 outlines further investigation into tropical diseases in Queensland.

60. Reports for 1860 to 1900 were published in *QVP* 1861–1901.

61. *British Parliamentary Papers* (hereafter *BPP*) 1859 (Cd. 2559), Sess. 2, vol. XII, 34.

62. ibid., 219.

63. *BPP* 1860 (Cd. 2712), vol. XXIX, 566.

64. *QVP* 1861, 907.

65. *QVP* 1862, 447.

66. *QVP* 1863, 365; see also 371.

67. *QVP* 1864, 893.

68. *BPP* 1868–9 (Cd. 4146), vol. XVI, 55.

69. *QVP* 1870, 357.

70. See, for example, *BPP* 1866 (Cd. 3712), vol. XIX, 50.

71. See *QVP* 1871–2, 427–30.

72. For a full discussion of this controversy see E. Barclay, 'Fevers and stinks: some problems of public health in the 1870s and 1880s', *Queensland Heritage*, *2* (4) (May 1971), 3–12.

73. See *QVP* 1877, vol. 2, 648; and 1879, vol. 1, 1192.

74. *QVP* 1877, vol. 2, 681, and 1876, vol. 2, 469.

75. *QVP* 1877, vol. 2, 681, and *BPP* 1860 (Cd. 2712), vol. XXIX, 569.

76. *QVP* 1880, vol. 1, 153.

77. *QVP* 1876, vol. 2, 399. Regular reports in the British medical journals relating to the colony's health commented on the high infant mortality.

78. *QVP* 1877, vol. 2, 667 and 681.

79. See *QVP* 1879, vol. 1, 1189–90, and 1880, vol. 1, 147–8.

80. *QVP* 1887, vol. 3, 336.

81. *BPP* 1898 (Cd. 9016), vol. XVIII, 32.

82. *QVP* 1884, vol. 2, 154, and 1886, vol. 2, 372.

83. *QVP* 1883, 360, and 1891, vol. 3., 683, and 1896, vol. 3, 999.

84. *BPP* 1905 (Cd. 2618), vol. XVIII, 3.

85. *QVP* 1896, vol. 2, 904 and 1001.

86. *Our First Half-Century*, n. 2 above, 232.

87. *British Medical Journal* (24 November 1883), 1032.

88. *QVP* 1896, vol. 3, 988–9.

10

The medical profession in colonial Victoria, 1834–1901

Diana Dyason

INTRODUCTION

In many ways, Australia's medical experience is not readily comparable with that of other British colonies in the nineteenth century. As other essays in this book have shown, the heavily populated colonies of India, Africa, and the West Indies presented medical problems and diseases which were unknown in temperate Australia. On the whole, Australian doctors considered themselves part of the British medical profession, sharing similar professional education and objectives, but they brought with them a determination to implement the medical reforms of a common register, equal legal rights for all qualified practitioners, and restrictions on those not qualified. In the senior colonies of New South Wales and Victoria, the profession was part of a larger imperial scene. However, their professional interests were by no means identical with those of their metropolitan colleagues. The locus of the profession in Australia was the 'colony', not the empire. Metropolitan examples and achievements were faithfully reported, noted, sometimes envied and occasionally emulated. But local institutions were sooner or later established to deal with local concerns: professional societies and journals, hospitals and medical schools with which to protect and promote colonial interests, and from an early date in Victoria these took on a specifically Australian character. The differences between the colonies reveal in many ways the independent political, institutional, and economic development of each.

The history of the medical profession in Australia reflected the central role of medicine and medical men in colonial public life, especially in Victoria, which had the highest *per capita* income in the British Empire. Concentrating on Victoria, this essay will characterize the medical profession in that colony — its dimensions, its preoccupations, and its institutions — and will outline certain factors relevant to its place in colonial and imperial affairs.

THE DOCTORS

From the early 1840s, Victoria was highly attractive to immigrants from the United Kingdom. It was British, it was new, it was not a penal colony, its climate was generally clement and, unlike India or the West Indies, it was almost free of 'exotic' diseases and high mortality epidemics.[1] Above all, fertile land was there for the taking, as the colony's indigenous people, animals and plants were unable to compete with the exploitative imports.[2] By 1850, more than 47,000 unassisted and 28,000 assisted immigrants had come to Victoria. The gold rushes between 1851 and 1859 encouraged a further 460,000 unassisted immigrants to Victoria, creating a rapidly expanding medical market.[3] At least that was the way the colony appeared to many doctors who, faced with extreme competition at home, determined to establish themselves in colonial practice.

The first permanent settlers in Victoria arrived in 1834 from Van Diemen's Land under the leadership of Edward Henty and with John Pascoe Fawkner in 1835.[4] Henty's party included Dr Alexander Thomson and Dr Barry Cotter. Thomson took up land in the Geelong area and became the first government medical officer in Victoria, but he soon relinquished his post, which was taken over first by Cotter and then by Dr Patrick Cussen.[5] Only Cussen's name appears on any of the Medical Registers. The first advertisement for medical practice appeared in the *Port Phillip Gazette*, 15 June 1837, when Dr David Patrick and Dr Wilke announced their partnership.[6]

Following them came approximately 2,494 registered practitioners in Victoria between 1838 and 1901. For 2,438 the qualifications and period of registration are known.[7] To even the most casual of nineteenth-century observers, Victoria's medical profession would have appeared predominantly 'British', at least until the last two decades of the century when the graduates from Melbourne University became numerically significant. The qualifications of all nineteen United Kingdom licensing bodies were represented in the colony. The 2,494 colonial doctors had between them 5,286 qualifications of which 3,807 or 72 per cent were issued by the British institutions (most of the remainder were Melbourne degrees).[8] For the period 1838–1901, only 136 doctors (5 per cent) had other than United Kingdom or Australian qualifications; and eighteen of these were Canadian. (See Table 10.1) Even allowing for multiple qualifications, it is plain that graduates of Scottish institutions made the largest contribution to Victoria's medical profession and to the pool of graduates in the general community.[9]

T.S. Puschmann has provided the number of qualifications granted by each British licensing body from 1876 to 1880 (inclusive).[10] Of these, between 2 and 3.5 per cent appeared on the Victorian Registers.[11] By the mid-1880s, university graduates comprised more than 50 per cent of the Victorian profession; between 1890 and 1901, graduates increased to 61 per cent and the single licentiates dropped to 10 per cent of the profession. Most of this change is attributable to the Melbourne University Medical School.[12] For the period 1850–1901, the medical profession in Victoria collectively held 645 Scottish, 92 Irish, 68 English and 525 Melbourne

Table 10.1: Qualifications from British institutions held by doctors registered before 1901 in Victoria

Institution	*Licenciates, Members, Fellows*	*Degrees*
Royal College of Physicians, London	122	–
Royal College of Surgeons, England	719	–
The Apothecaries Society of London	347	–
University of London		28
University of Oxford		3
University of Cambridge		13
University of Durham		24
Royal College of Physicians, Edinburgh	592	
Royal College of Surgeons, Edinburgh	594	
University of Edinburgh	13	301
Faculty of Physicians and Surgeons, Glasgow	215	
University of Glasgow	1	207
University of Aberdeen		86
University of St. Andrews		51
Kings and Queens College of Physicians, Ireland	188	
Royal College of Surgeons, Ireland	202	1
The Apothecaries Hall of Ireland	56	
University of Dublin	2	78
The Queen's College, Ireland	1	13
Totals	3052	755 (25%)

Source D. Dyason, 'The medical profession in Victoria, 1834–1901' (paper presented to the Australian Historical Association Conference, Melbourne, 1984).

degrees, together with 1,145 Scottish, 1,188 English and 449 Irish licences. Forty-seven (18.5 per cent) of our 1876–80 sample had qualifications from more than one country, the most common combination being an English and a Scottish licence, or a Scottish degree with an English licence. The sixty-four Australians graduating between 1876 and 1880 contributed to the relative decline in licences.[13] Thus for the colonial period approximately a quarter of the medical immigrants from the United Kingdom, and half the total Victorian profession, were university graduates.[14] These figures were not equalled elsewhere in the Empire during the nineteenth century. Obviously Victoria was not merely a dumping ground for Britain's incompetents. A lower doctor:patient ratio resulted in financial benefit to the practitioners who remained behind, but Victoria gained much more than Britain from this imperial 'brain drain'.

Many of Victoria's pioneer doctors were involved with pastoral ventures. The 1973 *Victorian Year Book* noted that prior to 1851, 'many of the squatters were Scottish farmers' sons', most of them of some education and standing. A strong group of Anglo-Irish gentry migrated in the 1840s, including William Stawell (later Attorney General) and Redmond Barry, the first Chancellor of the University of Melbourne.[15] Paul de Serville's study lists a total of 406 'gentleman colonists', that is those who were 'members of titled, landed or armigerous families' or who were 'gentlemen by profession, education, commission and upbringing, prominent in society and noted by contemporaries'. His three lists together include twenty-four medical men, or approximately 4 per cent of the total. Possibly the *Victorian Year Book* understates the situation, because at least twenty-four of the eighty-three doctors in Victoria prior to 1851 belonged to the gentry as de Serville defines it. Certainly, as K.S. Inglis has found, 'colonial doctors assumed a social status which was more than a reflection of conditions at home [England]. Their activity in the public affairs in Victoria was remarkable.'[16] Members of the medical elite figured largely in the development of most of the scientific and cultural institutions of the colony, including the University of Melbourne, the Botanical Gardens, the Herbarium, the Observatory, the Museum of Natural History, and the Philosophical Society — later the Royal Society — of Victoria. All were founded between 1853 and 1854, followed by the State Public Library in 1856 and the Art Gallery in 1861.[17] Medical men served as Provisional Municipal Officers of the newly incorporated town of Melbourne (1842) and on other local councils. Doctors were prominent in Masonic and church circles, and as founding members of the Port Phillip and Melbourne Clubs. Dr George Arden produced the colony's first newspaper, the *Port Phillip Gazette*, in 1838.[18]

Doctors were also reasonably well represented in the colony's parliaments.[19] Dr (later Sir) Francis Murphy, MRCS, was a member of the Legislative Council, 1851–5, and speaker of the Legislative Assembly, 1856–71. Sir James Palmer, F.R.Med.Ch.Soc., was Speaker of the Legislative Council, 1851–6. In 1890 William C. Little, a Canadian practising in Warracknabeal, wrote to a Canadian colleague that — in spite of unqualified, alcoholic, and incompetent doctors — 'a medical man is looked up to much more than at home [Canada]. The doctor ranks first here [Victoria] or equal and the lawyer third'; and again in 1891, 'A doctor [here] is much more respected than at home.'[20] These early doctors helped make Victoria as Sir Charles Dilke found it in 1890, 'most interesting, energetic and a pioneer in many fields'. They also illustrated his claim that Victoria had 'few people with cultivation and experience, so that those that have them rise to great powers'.[21]

MAKING A LIVING

Throughout the colonial period, and particularly from the late 1880s, Victorian doctors complained of the difficulties of earning an adequate living, and of the oversupply of doctors. Although no action was taken, in the 1890s there was talk of reducing the intake of Melbourne University's Medical School. From registration and census data, it appears that before the gold discoveries of the 1850s, the population per doctor in Victoria was 800 in 1850, and increased to 943 in 1851. The major gold rushes over, the population per doctor returned to 838 in the 1860s, but increased to 1,550 by 1871, and peaked at 1,639 in 1881, declining to 1,269 in 1891, and to 1,130 by 1901. At no time, however, did Victoria's *maximum* equal Britain's *minimum* of 1,721 persons per doctor in 1881.

Ivan Waddington argues cogently that both the intent and the effect of the United Kingdom Medical Act of 1858 had been to limit entry into the profession and to raise the status and earning power of its members.[22] Despite its more favoured status, Victoria's medical profession adopted similar goals. Experiences during the gold rushes had highlighted the overcrowding of the profession, particularly in the gold districts. For example, K.M. Bowden lists 380 different doctors on the Ballarat and Mt Alexander (the Castlemaine and Bendigo) goldfields with a combined population for the three areas of approximately 110,000, or one doctor for every 300–400 people.[23] These were hardly profitable arrangements even if the majority of the diggers had had the money to pay for medical services. In fact, most were too poor. George Wakefield, LSA, like many other members of the Apothecaries' Society, imported and sold drugs and proprietary lines, along with over-the-counter advice, to augment his practice and his not always successful speculations in land and mining.

Goldfields and declining gold towns were not the only factors causing the maldistribution of medical services. For most of the colonial period, Melbourne's population was less than two-thirds that of rural Victoria, yet the ratio of population per doctor in the country was consistently one and a half to two and a half times greater than that in the capital. By 1881, Melbourne-based doctors outnumbered those in the rest of the colony. Then, as now, the cultural and intellectual attractions of city life outweighed the possible advantages of a larger and often more lucrative practice outside the colony's capital.

Professional status, earning capacity, the climate and the vigour and freedom of the colony persuaded many a goldrush doctor to convert his planned stay of 'just a year or two' into a lifetime commitment. William Little's career at Warracknabeal (1889–1910) serves as an archetypal success story. Within four months of his arrival in the colony he was earning £250–375 a month. This was, by his own account, much more than he would have earned in Canada. His practice was profitable because he was prepared to work hard and had tremendous enthusiasm. He likened 'beginning practice' to 'newly married life, wonderfully interesting and exciting'. Although interested in a Melbourne practice, Little found the cost of setting up in the city (estimated at £2,000) prohibitive[24] and as an ex-agricultural student recognized the virtues of the developing agricultural districts. As surgeon to the Warracknabeal hospital, he was paid £100 p.a. and £50 as Shire Health Officer, and was paid a fee for each free vaccination he performed under the compulsory vaccination Act.[25] In addition, he had a hospital to which he sent his private patients and 'it paid him well'. His fee for major surgery — such as the amputation of a limb — was £200, including attendance. Through hard work, Little's earning capacity was above the average, but it could so be drastically reduced by a slack locum tenens as to curtail his holiday (losing up to £400 in three weeks).[26] Although he did not practise during the last few years of his life, his will specified *inter alia* bequests of cash totalling £13,450 and three properties in Toronto. The remainder was to be distributed amongst his relatives in Canada.[27]

George Wakefield, less successful than Little, also remained in the colony but was much more ambivalent about colonial life.[28] He swung between enthusiasm for and criticism of the colony, interspersed with nostalgia for England. 'I prefer this [Victoria] infinitely before England in many respects', he wrote in May 1865. And again in January 1862,

> There is a certain charm to colonial life, a kind of independence which is not met with at home and which suits me wonderfully well. The business I do is more an amusement than a trouble . . . I should have to work much harder at home [to make £1.5]. I have no rent or taxes to pay.

He added, however: '[i]n fact it is everyone's desire to return to England but few can raise the necessary funds to enable them to do so'.[29] By June 1862 Wakefield was persuaded that 'There are far better countries than this, British Columbia for instance . . . I am convinced I could do better in any other country than this. It is too overstocked, especially with doctors.' Still, Dr Wakefield, like many migrants, was determined 'never to return to England until I can do so in better circumstances than I left'. In the event he remained in Victoria, mainly because things were worse financially in England than in Victoria, and he could not stand the English climate. But mostly he lacked the money for his fare and to re-establish himself in England.

Ludwig Bruck reported that the average yearly earnings of Victorian doctors in the 1890s were between £350 and £1,200 — with perhaps 7 per cent (170 throughout Australasia) earning between £1,000 and £2,000 and 2 per cent between £2,000 and £4,000. A small minority earned between £4,000 and £6,000.[30] A recent study of the Victorian probate records by Ray Duplain puts the average values of medical estates in nineteenth-century Victoria between £2,000 and £6,000, with extremes of more than £90,000 (for example Dr G. Le Fevre and Dr G.A. Syme) and less than £100.[31] But these fortunes resulted from investments, not professional fees. In England, but not in Australia, the specialists at the major teaching hospitals often earned in excess of £10,000 a year from student fees, consultancies and private practice.[32] The few teaching positions in Victoria were not lucrative.[33] The hospital honoraries did benefit significantly from patients referred by former students. Nevertheless, there was sufficient poverty amongst its members for the profession to establish a Medical Benevolent Society in 1864.

Rather surprisingly, William Little's letters do not mention Friendly Societies or Lodges. Yet these provided medical services for up to half the population in some of Melbourne's suburbs and in numerous country towns. Many a colonial doctor started his career with a Lodge, and a few did very well indeed, earning £10,000 a year. Most Lodge doctors earned between £500 and £1,999 p.a., which compared favourably with the average medical income of £359 to £1,299. Many Lodges allowed their doctors the right to private practice and to charge extra for vaccinations (2s 6d), midwifery cases (2–5 gns) and for travelling time.[34]

Friendly Societies fitted in well with the democratic and egalitarian beliefs and independent attitudes of many colonists. But they did not suit a profession bent on controlling all areas of health care, and which made fee-for-service a matter of principle, treating a salaried position as a threat to the sacrosanct 'doctor/patient relationship'. The objective of the ensuing 'Battle of the Clubs' waged by the British Medical Association branches and in Victoria by the Medical Defence Association was not just to end the much complained of 'sweating', but also to remove the power of 'their inferiors' to hire and fire them.[35] Complaints against club practice and low fees were common but ineffective from the 1860s. Even in 1895, at a conference of all Australian professional medical associations, only 25 per cent favoured the fee-for-service payment in the British Medical Association and Medical Defence Assocation platforms.[36] The British Medical Association state branches and the Medical Defence Association paraded all the attitudes and tactics associated with militant trade unions — boycotts, blacklisting, strikes and heavy pressure on members. The public expressed its dislike of the tactics employed, and the profession suffered somewhat in terms of the respect and status it was traditionally accorded. But the doctors had gained a model agreement for the terms of their employment which virtually eliminated competitive tendering; imposed an income limit for the Lodge members of £400 p.a. which rendered approximately 10 per cent of them ineligible for medical benefits; and limited Lodge practice to a General Practitioner type of service which resulted in the salaried doctor becoming a rarity.[37]

REGISTRATION

The fight for reform of the medical profession in the United Kingdom had waxed strong for over fifteen years when the first settlers arrived in Victoria in 1834. Consequently most of the doctors coming to the colony were already prepared to implement reform programmes. There was no attempt to recreate Royal Colleges or their equivalents in Victoria; the common register and equal legal rights for all qualified practitioners were the accepted norm.[38] Nevertheless, there was a hierarchy within the profession erratically related to the flexible divisions within colonial society which changed with social, financial, and political fortune. Qualifications, skill, or status acquired abroad were often ignored in the election of hospital honoraries and Medical Society presidents, which were generally accepted as evidence of professional eminence. However, the honoraries were not *necessarily* the best-qualified candidates.

Whilst the United Kingdom Medical Acts of 1858 and 1886 allowed long-standing unqualified practitioners to continue in practice, Victorian legislation accepted only those who 'had passed through a regular 3-year course of instruction and had practised regularly in the colony' since 1853.[39] Only nine men took up this option. Following the passage of the British Medical Act of 1858, it was revealed that 'out of 33,339 physicians practising in the United Kingdom, 21,531 [64.5 per cent] were found to have no academic qualifications whatsoever'.[40] There was no equivalent of this in Victoria. As editorials on medical reform and medical legislation in the *Australian Medical Journal* and the lay press show, doctors envied lawyers their right to full professional self-regulation, particularly the power to deregister members.[41]

For doctors, the most important medical institution was the Medical Registration Board. This defined the profession and limited paid medical practice and public appointments to men with 'recognized' qualifications. Only practitioners with recognized qualifications were considered 'professional'. The first register of medical professionals in the Australian colonies was established under the New South Wales Medical Witnesses Act of 1838.[42] Registration was voluntary and only twelve doctors — seven physicians and five surgeons — from Victoria are listed. In 1844, in response to logistic problems and separatist sentiments, Victoria was granted its own three-member Medical Board and a separate Register, which was first published in 1845 and listed twenty-five doctors. Of the eighty-three doctors known to be in Victoria prior to 1851, seventy had registered at least once before 1901.

When Victoria passed its first Medical Registration Act in 1854, it was essentially a copy of the old Medical Witnesses Act and continued voluntary registration. But competition for patients and propaganda within the profession rapidly increased the percentage of registrants. Registration became mandatory under the Victorian Medical Registration Amendment Act of 1862.[43] The first Medical Register under this Act consisted of a Part I, listing 335 doctors who had re-registered or were newly registered; and a Part II, listing 358 doctors who had registered previously but who had not re-registered and were given twelve months' grace. By 1864, all but six names had vanished from Part II.[44] Annual re-registration became mandatory under the 1865 Consolidating Act which remained in force until the Medical Act of 1890.[45] This Act also limited government-financed medical positions — such as coroners, vaccinators and medical officers in public hospitals and asylums — to registered doctors.

Women doctors were few in colonial Victoria. The Medical Board was slow in granting registration to women and the University of Melbourne even tardier in admitting them. Only nineteen women — of whom twelve had overseas qualifications — were registered before 1901, and all of these after 1887.[46]

In theory, the 1862 Act gave the Medical Board of Victoria the necessary powers to weed out unqualified practitioners. And indeed, of the thirty-two doctors registered prior to 1850 who gave no qualifications, eleven had disappeared by the 1863–4 register. However, there is little reason to suppose that all the others lacked genuine qualifications because a number reappeared in later registers.

Nevertheless, the 1862 Act was not a strong piece of legislation. A drafting deficiency which was not fully corrected until the twentieth century prevented the Medical Board of Victoria from deleting the name of anyone found guilty of a misdemeanour, a felony or grossly improper conduct, or presenting false credentials. Its counterparts in New South Wales and in Britain had such power. Both the public and parliament were loath to grant Victorian practitioners an absolute monopoly. Nor was there a valid political reason to prevent people attending alternate practitioners such as herbalists if they so chose, provided no claim for 'medical' fees was made by the alternate practitioner.[47]

There were cases of fraudulent practice (e.g. using the qualifications of a deceased doctor), just as there were qualified pracitioners who covered for and were paid by 'quacks'.[48] Whilst not devoid of 'quacks', Australia, unlike North America, saw little of sectarian medicine, and of the unorthodox medical systems, only homeopathy[49] gained any measure of coherent public support. Although many men with no more than an apprenticeship came to the Australian colonies to practise medicine, relatively few stayed in Victoria, and New South Wales became the 'paradise of quacks'. Bruck's list of unregistered practitioners in 1886 included one 'Yandell of Castlemaine' who was described as a former plasterer turned herbalist, while a James Lamsey was 'said to have the most lucrative practice in Sandhurst' despite being a 'Chinese doctor'; but Bruck could identify only thirteen such individuals in Victoria compared with 183 in New South Wales.[50] 'Quacks' became one of the longer entries in the index of the *Australian Medical Journal*. However, the anti-quack diatribes delivered by the Victorian medical establishment were often excessive, sometimes misdirected, and strongly influenced by the false assumption that if quacks were suppressed their erstwhile clients would automatically transfer to qualified men.

HOSPITALS AND A MEDICAL SCHOOL

Victoria's colonial medical profession became organized in a period when, in England, under the influence of new techniques including anaesthesia and antiseptic surgery, and the mushrooming of new hospitals, the practice of medicine was being irrevocably altered. However, true specialization, within the traditional fields of surgery, medicine, or obstetrics and gynaecology, was very slow to develop in Victoria. This delay in specialized practice reflected the structure of the University of Melbourne Medical School. Although a five-year course was offered from its commencement in 1862, it was staffed by only one professor, G.B. Halford, who taught anatomy, physiology, surgery, and pathology; and by six lecturers, in medicine, obstetrics and the diseases of women and children, materia medica, forensic medicine, chemistry, comparative anatomy and zoology. A second chair (pathology and anatomy) was not created until 1882, and chairs in obstetrics, surgery, medicine, pediatrics, and biochemistry were not founded until well into the twentieth century. In addition, Melbourne's two major public hospitals, the

Melbourne (1846) and the Alfred (1871), which with the Women's Hospital provided the clinical teaching, were tardy in appointing specialists to their staffs.[51]

Until the establishment of Sydney University's Medical School in 1883, Melbourne University provided the only medical school in Australia. A further half century was to pass before all the symbols of specialization already familiar in the United Kingdom were developed.[52] Certainly financial problems facing both the University and the hospitals retarded the development of new disciplines, but there was also an underlying egalitarian ideology which favoured general practice and held that true specialization was inappropriate, and uneconomic outside Melbourne. The majority of doctors did not want to replicate England's two-tiered profession, with highly paid consultants reaping all the rewards. Although most doctors working in Victoria's rural areas were forced to be general practitioners, many of them tried to keep up with advances overseas. Lister's papers on antisepsis, for example, were reported to the Medical Society of Victoria just months after their publication in the *Lancet*, and were put into practice in both Melbourne and the Western District very shortly afterwards.[53]

The concepts of voluntary or charity hospitals and benevolent societies were part of the cultural baggage accompanying all British immigrants. Melbourne's first and only *true* charity or subscription hospital, not to be confused with *the* Melbourne Hospital (1846), was established in 1840, and by 1842 had twenty beds, an outpatients' clinic, and was staffed on an honorary basis by four doctors.[54] Unlike their British counterparts, Victoria's charitable institutions received government support. This was essential because the colonists had unanimously rejected the notion of an English Poor Law system. Thus, only charitable institutions were available to care for the destitute, when sick, aged or orphaned, and the government subsidized the charities to provide most of the benefits of the English Poor Law Institutions.[55] The pattern of matching government grants with funds raised by charitable institutions was introduced with the establishment of the Melbourne Hospital (1846), and generalized thereafter. But even though the Melbourne Hospital was close in its ideals and its organization to the English voluntary hospitals, nevertheless 'the peculiarities of Australian society prevented it from being an exact copy'.[56]

The Melbourne Hospital was the first of more than forty-three public hospitals established in Victoria between 1837 and 1901. In a new colony, whose population was largely deprived of family support groups, both hospitals and benevolent asylums took on a special importance and were established in most towns of any size.[57] By the end of the century, few Victorians lived more than 15 or at most 25 miles from a hospital. This fact helped foster a sense of local responsibility. For the profession, each hospital and each benevolent asylum meant at least one honorary medical position with salaried appointments (mainly residential) at the larger institutions. The hospitals used various procedures in selecting honorary staff, ranging from election by lay governors, with or without assessment by a medical committee, to appointment by an all-medical committee. In some country towns, virtually every registered doctor in the area had, at one time another, held an appointment at the local hospital.

Victoria's charity hospitals played a social role similar to their English counterparts in that they both emphasized the stratification of society and offered opportunities for social recognition and advancement across the strata.[58] Like any new colony, Victoria had to develop new social structures, but without the army and a large bureaucracy such things as land, wealth or professional institutions became the determinants of social status. Like the London Hospital, the Melbourne Hospital played a very important role in the city's social and political life in the nineteenth century. Sometimes the elections of its honoraries rated more column space in the Melbourne press than did those of the colony's parliamentarians.[59] Membership of the Committee of Management of the Melbourne Hospital was one form of social advancement, and an honorary position at the Melbourne not only increased a doctor's social and professional status, but also his income. Honorary appointments at the Melbourne and other public charities (all tacitly rank-ordered) were important in determining the hierarchy of the profession, as well as in offering unequalled access to clinical material, particularly for surgeons. But the overriding attraction for many honoraries was the consequent increase in their private practice.

Of the medical staffs at the Melbourne and the Alfred, 87 per cent of the honoraries and residents at the former and 83 per cent at the latter had higher qualifications.[60] Each had one or more university degrees or a Fellowship from one of the Royal Colleges, while only 5 per cent (at the Melbourne) and 4 per cent (at the Alfred) had the minimal qualification of a single non-university licence. The remainder of the staff had two or more licences. At Bendigo (founded 1853) the figures were 73 per cent higher, 11 per cent minimal; Ballarat (1856) 67 per cent higher, 13 per cent minimal; Mooroopna (1878) 58 per cent higher but no single licentiates; Swan Hill (1860) 38 per cent higher, 15 per cent with minimal qualifications.[61]

At least 9 per cent of the total colonial profession was at one time or another connected with the Melbourne and/or the Alfred Hospital and over 5 per cent were associated with the four country hospitals. Very conservatively, given the turnover in honorary staff, this suggests that at least a quarter of the colony's medical profession had at some time in their careers provided free medical services in one or more of the colony's charitable institutions. Bruck claimed that, in 1898, 228 honoraries in Victoria's hospitals were providing free medical services to the value of £52,640.[62] To reduce this 'imposition' he recommended mandatory signs on every hospital saying 'For the sick poor' and over the Outpatients' Department a notice reading 'For the destitute only'. Bruck's Chadwickian suggestions ignored the increasing role of the hospitals as centres of teaching, clinical expertise and new technologies, and falsely assumed that a significant majority of hospital patients could afford private medical care.[63] He also ignored the legislation governing charitable institutions which had been amended in 1884 to allow space to paying patients. Bruck contended that the doctors were 'altogether too eager to have hospitals established in the districts in which they resided'. Many cases, especially accidents, 'are admitted to these institutions who, if there were no hospitals in the district, would become private patients of the doctor'. Thus the doctors were reducing their own incomes.[64] In criticizing the exploitative hospitals, Bruck recognized that hospital appointments attracted public confidence and hence increased income for the few to the detriment of the majority. But he failed to acknowledge that the hospitals also determined the very structure of the profession.

MEDICAL SOCIETIES

The establishment and maintenance of appropriate and acceptable qualifications and work practices go only part way to defining a profession. Victoria's practitioners took a further step towards professionalization in founding and continuing medical societies and a successful medical journal. Both were meant to bind members with a sense of shared values and knowledge, to provide a means by which professional ideas could be defined, enforced and reinforced, to establish a code of conduct for practitioners, and to introduce peer review.

Victoria was the only Australian colony able to maintain at least one medical society and one continuing medical journal for most of its history. The first medical society, the Port Phillip Medical Association, was established with sixteen members in 1846, just twelve years after the first settlement. The minutes of the Society, which set out its constitution on 6 October 1846, claimed 'this Association has derived no assistance whatever from previously existing Associations'. The Port Phillip Medical Association constitution predated those of the American Medical Association (1847), although not, of course, the several colonial American medical associations which began in the late eighteenth century. Britain's Provincial Medical and Surgical Association had begun in 1832, and metamorphosed into the British Medical Association in 1856. The Port Phillip Medical Association's purposes and objects were set out in forty-nine Rules and Regulations. The Association was to consist of legally qualified practitioners 'residing within the Town of Melbourne'. Its primary objects were 'the promotion of medical knowledge and more free professional intercourse; also the formation of a medical library and a museum, to be funded from the subscriptions'.[65] The regulations established ethical rules governing transactions between doctors and set a scale of fees which remained largely unchanged until the last decade of the century.[66]

The Minutes of the first of the three Victorian societies reveal little evidence of 'cultural cringe' or dependence upon the United Kingdom. Indeed, the Association's founders hoped that it would 'lead the way to a better state of things in the medical profession at large'. Just thirteen months after its inauguration, the Port Phillip Medical Association was petitioning the House of Commons in favour of Wakely's Medical Bill and requesting 'that the privileges and protection' it would afford to qualified practitioners be extended to members of the profession in the Australian colonies which as yet had no adequate legislative powers of their own.[67]

Ironically the application of the Association's ethical rules led to its demise in November 1851; but its objectives were carried on. On 7 May 1852, some of the members of the Port Phillip Medical Association called a public meeting to reconstitute it as the Victorian Medical Association. This time there were fewer rules (only thirty-nine) and those dealing with ethical issues did not induce self-destruction. Again, great emphasis was placed on the library.[68] In August 1854, the Victorian Medical Association and the smaller Medical Chirurgical Society (based at the Melbourne Hospital) met to consider amalgamation. This was achieved by 19 July 1855, with the foundation of the Medical Society of Victoria. Again the objectives of the society emphasized not only the library, but also the delivery of scientific papers and promotion of professional interests.[69] The Medical Society of Victoria remained the only viable association in the Australian colonies until 1879 when Dr Louis Henry returned from England with authority to establish branches of the British Medical Association in Australia. The first, founded in 1879, was the British Medical Association (Victorian Branch), the third overseas branch of the British Medical Association. There was considerable overlap of membership between the two societies, as their purposes were rather different. The Medical Society of Victoria promoted scientific programmes whilst the British Medical Association (V.B.) dealt largely with political and disciplinary issues. The British Medical Association was attractive to country doctors who could not attend the Medical Society of Victoria meetings; the member's subscription to the *British Medical Journal* was an added drawcard. Nevertheless, not until after the turn of the century did the Medical Society of Victoria attract more members than the British Medical Association (V.B.). The two societies were affiliated in 1907, but the Medical Society of Victoria maintained its separate identity, and, despite the 'fusion', was still the legal entity responsible for assets, which included the Hall and Library.[70]

There is no doubt that the creation of the overseas branches of the British Medical Association was an example of professional imperialism which benefited the parent body. The British Medical Association saw itself as 'an Imperial institution extending its ramifications to all parts of the Empire and linking together the members of the profession', in one body '[for] the advancement of scientific medicine and the social well being and dignity of its associates'.[71] The colonial membership increased both the status and power of the Association, so that in England it was acknowledged as the voice of the profession on most matters. It negotiated with the Colonial Office and the India Office for better working conditions and remuneration for their doctors, but this capacity was of little relevance to Victoria. The British Medical Association was effective in many colonies in achieving an improved reputation and statutory rights for the profession. In Victoria, these goals had been achieved by 1862 without its help, which partly explains the rather slow development of the British Medical Association

(V.B.) and the continued popularity of the Medical Society of Victoria. In the other Australian colonies the BMA branches played a much more significant role in nineteenth-century medical politics. However, their real power was exhibited in the twentieth century.

In the Australasian colonies, the energies of the British Medical Association were directed to increasing membership and dismantling the contract system of the Friendly Societies. These campaigns were influenced by the ideology being promulgated by the British Medical Association and the American Medical Association. However, the local campaigns were not directed from London but were the independent efforts of the state branches, with the more radical New South Wales branch setting the pace.[72] The influx of unqualified practitioners onto the goldfields led to the formation of local associations of qualified men. The objectives of such societies were clearly set out in the motion creating the Ballarat Medico-Chirurgical Society, whereby 'all legally qualified medical practitioners within the District [were] organised for the mutual protection of their rights and privileges, the diffusion of professional knowledge and the discouragement by every just and constitutional means, of all classes of unqualified practice'.[73] The most effective action of these associations in maintaining professional standards were standing advertisements in local newspapers giving the names and qualifications of their members. When registration became compulsory in 1862 the emphasis of these societies shifted to less political areas, and after 1879 one or two became unofficial local chapters of the British Medical Association (V.B.).

The medical profession supported its professional associations. The Medical Society of Victoria attracted 31 per cent of Melbourne's doctors in 1867 and 77 per cent in 1881, before declining to 53 per cent in 1891. Because meetings were virtually inaccessible to country doctors, the percentage of all doctors registered in Victoria who belonged to the Medical Society of Victoria was only 5 per cent in 1861; 15 per cent in 1871; 31 per cent in 1881; 46 per cent in 1891. When one considers the distances and transport problems, the Victorian situation compares very favourably with that in the United Kingdom, where the British Medical Association in 1870 attracted 28 per cent of the doctors in England and Wales, but only 5 per cent of doctors in Scotland and 12 per cent of those in Ireland.[74]

In 1891, Melbourne University medical graduates, feeling theatened by increasing competition in the profession and an economic depression, formed the Melbourne Medical Association to promote the interests of the Melbourne graduates. In 1895, this group revived the defunct (1879–84) Medical Defence Association, and by the turn of the century it had 331 members, compared with 280 in the Medical Society of Victoria and the 248 in the British Medical Association (V.B.).

One of the global aims of the British Medical Association had been to corner medical markets for British-trained doctors. This had been a reality in Australia from the beginning of settlement, but in Victoria by the 1880s the rising tide of Melbourne graduates had changed the situation. In spite of valued rights and facilities offered to Victorian members visiting London, the British Medical

Association did not dominate the Victorian medical scene until the twentieth century.

MEDICAL JOURNALS

Arguably the greatest achievement of the Medical Society of Victoria was to found the *Australian Medical Journal* in 1856, and then in 1859 to convert it to a proprietary body formally independent of the Society's political and financial fortunes (even though the majority of the subscribers and contributors were Medical Society of Victoria members). Given Australia's small population and the fate of most nineteenth-century medical journals the world over, the essential continuity (in spite of changes in name) of the *Australian Medical Journal* from 1856 with today's *Medical Journal of Australia* is an indication of a long-standing dedication to medical science, and the sense of professionalism and of the joint purpose shown by Victoria's registered doctors.

In his annotated bibliography, Bryan Gandevia provides a useful table of the dates of foundation, demise and amalgamation of medical journals in Australia.[75] Only the *Australian Medical Journal*, 1856–96 (not to be confused with the New South Wales journal of the same name, 1846–7), the *Australasian Medical Gazette*, 1881–1914 (which became the official organ of the British Medical Association in Australia), and the *Intercolonial Medical Journal of Australia*, 1896–1910, survived more than five years.[76]

As a critical study of the *Australian Medical Journal* will shortly reveal, its survival and achievements have been seriously underrated.[77] This is in spite of its favourable reception by its British counterparts. The *Medical Times and Gazette* welcomed 'a new contemporary', and took it as evidence of 'a flourishing state of medicine in the Antipodes'.[78] The *Lancet* categorized the *Journal* as a 'most able attempt', and in 1860 congratulated it on surviving and noted that it contained 'chiefly original matter' which was found 'fresh, practical and good'.[79] The range, quality and content of its best articles were very similar to, and sometimes better than, the average found in the *Lancet* or the *British Medical Journal*. Overall it compared more than favourably with colonial journals in other parts of the Empire. Canada, with its more populous and very much older colonies, produced sixty-one medical journals before 1900, but only six of these, all established after 1870, survived for as long as twenty years.[80]

Prior to 1880, over 650 items referring to Australia appeared in a variety of British medical journals and 101 colonial doctors had contributed articles, reviews or news items to these journals.[81] Victoria figures in the title of seventy-six items (excluding 'personal' notices), compared with Tasmania (thirty-three), New South Wales (twenty-nine), South Australia (five) and Western Australia (three). There is no evidence to suggest that Victoria's medical problems were intrinsically more interesting than those of the other colonies, so we may take these figures as demonstrating the self-confidence and greater professionalization of the Victorian medical community, and their belief that their reports and statistics were genuine contributions to medical knowledge. Although the *Australian Medical Journal* carried reviews, notices, and comments on, and some extracts from, the overseas medical press, these did not dominate the journal and it never became merely a collection of borrowed writings as did some of its contemporaries.

CONCLUSION

From the 1840s the medical profession in Australia generally, and in Victoria particularly, exhibited many of the colonial features described by Roy MacLeod. With autochthonous societies, and a zeal for 'responsible government',[82] the profession was geared to a local colonial market. By the end of the century, not only were the Australian colonies federating, but federation was on the agenda of the state branches of the British Medical Association as well. Intercolonial medical conferences were flourishing, and the medical profession in other colonies joined Victoria in looking for recognition in the wider community.

Doctors fulfilled important social and practical roles in the Australian colonies. They treated the sick in Victoria; they successfully developed a journal and societies to promote their profession's image, and to 'professionalize' their members. They disseminated scientific knowledge, and were prominent in colonial government and public culture. From the fifth decade of the nineteenth century, editorials and leading articles in the *Australian Medical Journal* were publicly accepted as the 'voice' of medicine. Other journals became significant in the 1880s and 1890s. From the foundation of the University of Melbourne Medical School in 1862, doctors were trained in courses that were more demanding, or at any rate longer, than most medical courses in the United Kingdom.[83] In 1890, with the acceptance of Melbourne degrees for Registration in the United Kingdom, Victoria's medical profession felt itself to be fully independent and on an equal footing with its British counterpart. Colonial it might have been; whinge it did; but cringe it manifestly did not.

NOTES

I would like to express my gratitude to Richard Gillespie, Trevor Holland, Elaine Counsell, Barry Butcher, Caroline Clark, Judith Quilter, Gregory Tunchon, and Ann Tovell for their invaluable help in researching this paper, and to Rita Hutchison for her skill and patience in preparing the original typescript. I would also like to thank the editors, Roy MacLeod and Milton Lewis and their assistants, who are largely responsible for the final form of this paper. Unless otherwise stated, figures relating to the various categories of qualifications and doctors are derived from work done under an ARGC Grant.

1. Statistical information for Victoria is plentiful. The first population census was taken in 1836 in the Port Phillip District (as the colony was known until separating from New

South Wales in 1851). The Victorian Registration Act of 1853 made registration of births, deaths, and marriages compulsory. *Year Books* published from 1873 provide informative details on the health of the colony and its disease environment. While they appear to have inflicted a devastating toll upon the aboriginal population by diseases carried with them, European settlers encountered few indigenous health problems. During the early years of settlement, however, smallpox, venereal disease, and tuberculosis created particular problems and by the mid-1860s most of the common diseases in the United Kingdom were established in the major settlements. Compulsory vaccination, introduced in 1854, effectively limited all smallpox outbreaks in the colony. Like most pre-industrial economies, Victorians also suffered their share of ghastly and often fatal accidents.

2. A.W. Crosby, *Ecological Imperialism: The Biological Expansion of Europe, 900–1900* (Cambridge: Cambridge University Press, 1986), 295ff.

3. *Victorian Year Book, 1973*, Centenary Edition, no. 87 (Melbourne: Victorian Office of the Commonwealth Bureau of Census and Statistics, 1973), 31ff. But the main force driving the flood of emigrants was food, not gold: the belief that life would be better in the new land, a belief that 'The labouring man, let his labour be what it may, eats meat three times a day in the colonies, and very generally goes without it all together at home.' P.D. Edwards and R.B. Joyce (eds), *Anthony Trollope in Australia* (St Lucia: University of Queensland Press, 1967), 284.

4. Edward Henty (1810–78) was the fourth son of Thomas Henty of Sussex, an immigrant farmer in Van Diemen's Land. Edward established the first permanent settlement in the Port Phillip District in 1834, and was later joined by other members of his family. The Henty brothers became major land holders and prominent public figures. See Marnie Bassett, 'Henty, Thomas *et al*', *Australian Dictionary of Biography*, vol. 1 (Melbourne: Melbourne University Press, 1966), 531–4. John Pascoe Fawkner (1792–1869) was the son of a convict sentenced to transportation to Van Diemen's Land. As a young man Fawkner was himself in trouble with the law, but he was a man of many skills and abounding energy. In 1835 he founded the first settlement in the Hobson Bay (later Melbourne) area of Port Phillip. He started the *Port Phillip Patriot* after his first newspaper was suppressed, because unlicensed. Fawkner served on the First Legislative Council (1851–6) and as an elected member from 1856 to 1869. He became the 'grand old man of contemporary Victoria'. See Hugh Anderson, 'Fawkner, John Pascoe (1792–1869)', *Australian Dictionary of Biography*, ibid., 368–71.

5. Dr Thomson was appointed from Sydney by Governor Richard Bourke to attend the thirty soldiers, three surveyors, one constable, and one customs officer all dispatched with Captain William Lonsdale, the magistrate sent to administer the newly gazetted Port Phillip District. The first census of 1836 detailed the population of the District as 142 males, 35 females, and 26,000 sheep, sundry horses and cattle. Dr Cotter in 1837 entered into partnership with Dr McCurdy and advertised 'a large and valuable supply of the best medicine, [and] every kind of cattle remedy'. Cussen was also a foundation member of both the Port Phillip Medical Association (1846) and the Medical Society of Victoria (1854), and was listed as 'gentleman' in Paul de Serville, *Gentlemen of Port Phillip* (Melbourne: Melbourne University Press, 1980), 160–90. See also E.A. Mackay, 'Medical practice during the goldfields era in Victoria', *Medical Journal of Australia* (26 September 1936) (2), 421–8, esp. 422; and E.A. Mackay, 'Medical men as pastoral pioneers', *Medical Journal of Australia* (13 October 1934) (2), 476–83, esp. 476, 481.

6. Mackay, op. cit., no. 5 above, 422.

7. Before 1854, not all the doctors on the registers stated their qualifications and many, particularly those newly arrived or newly graduated, gave their address as Melbourne, although shortly afterwards they might have moved elsewhere.

8. Specialist diplomas are not included because they were few in number and irrelevant for registration. Some Melbourne graduates when visiting Britain acquired further qualifications.

9. Economic conditions in Scotland were seriously depressed. There were few opportunities for Scottish graduates in English hospitals; often considerable antipathy was shown them. Indeed, England had its own over-production problems. Rapidly increasing student enrolments reached 1000 per year in England for the period 1890–4. See M. Jeanne Peterson, *The Medical Profession in Mid-Victorian London* (Berkeley: University of California Press, 1978), 237–9, 249.

10. T.S. Puschmann, *A History of Medical Education* (facsimile of 1891 edn, New York: Haafner, 1966), 495ff, esp. 520–3. To reconcile Puschmann's figures with his summarizing claims, it is necessary to omit Fellows from the calculations (a reasonable procedure in that many Fellows were elected, not examined).

11. Altogether 7.8 per cent of the Royal College of Physicians (Edinburgh) licences and 5.5 per cent of the University of Glasgow's total qualifications (including 3.7 per cent of its MDs) came to the colony. Puschmann's figures show that from 1876 to 1880, the United Kingdom awarded 2435 medical degrees and 4936 licences. Of the latter, 2116 (43 per cent) were from the Royal College of Surgeons (England) and 1275 (26 per cent) were from the Society of Apothecaries. For the period 1876–80, nine of the forty-one categories listed by Puschmann were unrepresented in Victoria. However, several of these were conjoint licences whose individual elements were represented. Both the MB and the MD degrees from Oxford, the MD (Cambridge), the MS and MD (Durham) and the MD BS and MS (London) were also unrepresented in the 1876–1880 Victorian sample. The absence in Victoria of Oxford and Durham medical degrees (1876–80) is not significant; a single medical graduate from either source is equivalent to more than 2 per cent. However, only two (0.86 per cent of the 231 degrees granted by the University of London) were registered in Victoria. A 2 per cent quota requires another three degrees. The variation may be due to chance, but the prestige of the University of London Medical School and the demand for its graduates is a more likely explanation.

12. Melbourne medical degrees increased from a maximum of seven in any one year and a total of fifty-three graduates in the period prior to 1880, to a total of 458 (twenty to thirty-seven per year) for the 1880s and 1890s. K.F. Russell, *The Melbourne Medical School, 1862–1962* (Melbourne: Melbourne University Press, 1977), 218–56, provides the names of the Melbourne medical graduates in each year between 1862 and 1962. The number of colonial doctors with two or more licences varied between a high of 33 per cent in the 1850s and a low of 28 per cent in the sixties. The MRCS Eng. with a LSA or a LRCP Eng. were the most common combinations.

13. Thirty-five (81.4 per cent) of the doctors qualifying in the 1876–80 Victorian sample had only Australian degrees (thirty-four from Melbourne and one from Sydney). The University of Sydney Medical School (established 1883) and the University of Melbourne Medical School were empowered by their charters to grant MD degrees a.e.g. and by examination.

14. The Scottish universities produced four degrees for every three licences from the non-university bodies, but in Victoria the ratio of Scottish degrees to licences was 1:2, with ratios of 1:3 for Ireland and 1:17 for England.

15. *Victorian Year Book*, n. 3 above, 425.

16. K.S. Inglis, *Hospital and Community: A History of the Royal Melbourne Hospital* (Melbourne: Melbourne University Press, 1985), 28.

17. This gallery, later the National Gallery of Victoria, was the first public Art Gallery in Australia.

18. P.L. Brown, 'Arden, George (1820?–1854)', in *Australian Dictionary of Biography*, n. 4 above, 26–7.

19. Kathleen Thomson and G. Searle, *A Biographical Register of Victorian Parliament, 1859–1900* (Canberra: Australian National University Press, 1972).

20. Margaret Gillet, *Dear Grace: A Romance of History* (Melbourne: Melbourne

University Press, 1986), 84, 162. Little's correspondent, Octavia Grace Ritchie (the Grace of the title) was one of the first women graduates of McGill University, taking her BA in 1888 and MD from Bishops College, Montreal, in 1890.

21. Sir Charles Wentworth Dilke, *Greater Britain* (London: Macmillan, 1868); and *Problems of Greater Britain* (London: Macmillan, 1890), esp. 111–13, 128.

22. From 1861 to 1881 the number of British males in employment rose by 24 per cent but the number of doctors increased by under 5 per cent. See Ivan Waddington, *The Medical Profession in the Industrial Revolution* (Dublin: Gill Macmillan, 1894), 140, 148–9. The number of Licentiates of the College of Surgeons had increased from 5000 in 1824–5 to 8125 in 1833–4, i.e. a 60 per cent increase in ten years. Similarly the number of licences issued by the Society of Apothecaries rose from 214 in the period 1815–20 to 408 between 1825 and 1830.

23. K.M. Bowden, *Doctors and Diggers on the Mount Alexander Goldfields* (Maryborough, Victoria: Bowden, 1974), 197; K.M. Bowden, *Doctors at Ballarat* (Balwyn, Victoria: Bowden, 1977), 195. Interestingly, only eleven doctors appear on both lists.

24. Gillet, op. cit., n. 20 above, 82.

25. ibid., 149. See also author's comment, 122. For another view of country practice, see Joan Gillison, *The Colonial Doctor and His Town* (Melbourne: Cypress Books, 1974), 46, 51, 264–8.

26. Gillet, op. cit., n. 20 above, 176.

27. Little's wealth derived at least in part from investments in land and from his hospital. Nevertheless, he seems to have dealt successfully with the non-payment of fees which bedevilled so many doctors, particularly in country practices. His will is lodged at the Public Records Office, Laverton, Victoria.

28. George Wakefield, 'L.S.A. Letters (edited)', in K.M. Bowden, *Goldrush Doctors at Ballarat* (Balwyn, Victoria: Bowden, 1977), 89–98; original held in Australian National Library Archives (Canberra), MS 684/1 (hereafter ANLA 684/1).

29. ibid. It is possible that the P.S. which contains this last sentence has been attached to the wrong letter. The writing is very different from that of 28 October 1854 but is consistent with 1 May 1856.

30. Ludwig Bruck, 'The present state of the medical profession in Australia, Tasmania and New Zealand', *Australasian Medical Gazette* (March 1893), 97.

31. Ray Duplain of Deakin University, private communication to author.

32. Waddington, op. cit., n. 22 above, 28–31, 50–1, 149ff. An enquiry into the shortage of British military surgeons was told that a medical man in civil life could expect £300 within five years of commencing practice, and £500 after ten years, gradually rising to £800 or £1000. However, doctors trained at St Bartholomew's or St Thomas' were earning £500–£1500 ten years after graduation. See *Report of the Committee appointed by the Secretary of State to enquire into the Causes which tend to prevent Eligible Sufficient Candidates from Coming forward for the Army Medical Department*, 1878–79 (C. 2200), xliv, 257.

33. The foundation Professor of Anatomy, Physiology *and* Pathology was paid £1000 p.a., and foundation lecturers £500 p.a. each.

34. David Green and Lawrence Cromwell, *Mutual Aid or Welfare State: Australia's Friendly Societies* (Sydney: Allen & Unwin, 1984), 96–7, 121; Bruck, op. cit., n. 30 above, 97.

35. For detail on the battle, see Green and Cromwell, ibid., 101–29. Ludwig Bruck, *The Sweating of the Medical Men by the Friendly Societies in Australia* (Sydney: L. Bruck, 1896). The Medical Society of Victoria launched the first of many attacks on Lodge practice with R.T. Tracy, 'Presidential address', *Australian Medical Journal* (1861) 6, 60–9, esp. 64.

36. The first, short-lived Medical Defence Association was established in 1879, the second (still extant) was created in 1895 by the British Medical Association (Victoria

Branch), the Medical Society of Victoria, and the Melbourne Medical Association (the last restricted to Melbourne graduates). The Medical Defence Association was limited to protecting the 'economic and political interests of its members'. See T.S. Pensabene, *The Rise of the Medical Practitioner in Victoria* (Canberra: Australian National University Press, 1980), 109–11.

37. Green and Cromwell, op. cit., n. 34 above, 123–9.

38. The constitutions of the Port Phillip Medical Association, the Victorian Medical Association, and the Medical Society of Victoria provided fully democratic procedures for the election of office-bearers, and the Presidential terms were fixed. The Minutes Books of these societies are in the Australian Medical Association Archives (Parkville, Victoria).

39. Following United Kingdom practice, commissioned officers in the services lacking formal qualifications were covered by special clauses in the Victorian 1854 and 1862 Medical Acts.

40. C. Lloyd and J.L.S. Coulter, *Medicine and the Navy, 1200–1900*, vol. 4 (London: Livingstone, 1957), 24. *Bulletin of the History of Medicine, XXX* (1957), 151.

41. See Medical Society of Victoria, card index to the *Australian Medical Journal*, Australian Medical Association, Parkville, and see also *Ballarat Star*, 8 October 1857; 'Editorial', *Australian Medical Journal*, 4 (1882), 238; 'Editorial', *Australian Medical Journal, 9* (1864), 158; 'Quackery and distortion', *Australian Medical Journal, 10* (1865), 181–91; 'Editorial', *Australian Medical Journal, 11* (1866), 283.

42. The New South Wales Medical Registers appeared either in the *New South Wales Government Gazette* (1839–41) or in the *Port Phillip Government Gazette* (1845–51). Of the twenty-four doctors mentioned by de Serville only eight appeared on the registers.

43. Victorian Medical Registration Amendment Act, 1862. 25 Vic. 158.

44. The majority had probably left the colony — returned home, followed other gold or land rushes, or departed as ship's surgeons. Until a detailed study of the shipping lists is undertaken, it will be impossible to settle the question. Many pastoralists, including doctors, left Victoria during the depressions of the 1840s and 1860s.

45. Medical Act, 1890. 54 Vic. c. 1118. For the texts of Acts relevant to medicine in the various Australasian colonies, see Ludwig Bruck (ed.), *The Australasian Medical Directory and Handbook* (Sydney: The Australasian Medical Gazette Office and London: Ballière, Tindell, 1883), 1–57; for Victorian Acts, 23–5. As late as 1925, the Medical Board wrote to the Chief Secretary urging amendment of the Medical Act on the ground that Victoria lacked an improper conduct clause in its legislation. An amendment to this effect was finally passed in 1933. Pensabene, op. cit., n. 36 above, 131.

46. Ailsa Zainu'addin, 'The admission of women to the University of Melbourne 1869–1903', in S. Murray-Smith (ed.), *Melbourne Studies in Education 1973* (Melbourne: Melbourne University Press, 1973), 50–106, esp. 96ff; M.H. Neave, *This Mad Folly: The History of Australia's Pioneer Women Doctors* (Sydney: Library of Australian History, 1980); D. Dyason, 'James Jamieson and the Ladies' in Harold Attwood and R.W. Home (eds), *Patients, Practitioners and Techniques*, 2nd National Conference on Medicine and Health in Australia, 1984 (Medical History Unit, University of Melbourne, 1985), 1–19; K.F. Russell, *The Melbourne Medical School, 1862–1962* (Melbourne: Melbourne University Press, 1977), 74–77. The first woman to graduate from Melbourne University was Bella Guerin, with a Bachelor of Arts in 1883. In 1891 Grace Stone became Melbourne University's and Australia's first woman medical graduate. In 1896 she co-founded the Queen Victoria Hospital for Woman.

47. The profession resented the amount of community support for alternative practitioners, particularly homeopaths. When a new Medical Practitioners Bill was being debated in 1892, a petition in support of alternative practitioners, signed by 4,000–5,000 people, was presented to parliament. (See T.S. Pensabene, op. cit., n. 36 above, 126). The Victorian parliament was, as a matter of tradition, anti-monopoly. Pensabene argues that

doctors' status was low until the end of the nineteenth century. As scientific medicine became effective, the orthodox profession's control of new knowledge critically assisted its rise to power (ibid., chs 1 and 11). I believe Pensabene overstates his case.

48. William Kelly, *Life in Victoria or Victoria in 1853 and Victoria in 1858 Showing the Improvement made by the Colony within those Periods, in Town and Country, Cities and Diggings*, Historical Reprint Series, no. 6 (Australia: Kilmore Lowden Publishing Co., 1977), 71; *Australian Medical Journal, 11*(1866), 283; 'Illegal practice', *Australian Medical Journal, 16* (1871), 85–7.

49. Bruck, op. cit., n. 45 above, 94–8, esp. 95.

50. L.Bruck, *The Australasian Medical Dictionary and Handbook . . . 2nd Issue* (Sydney: The Australasian Medical Gazette Office, 1886), 259ff.

51. Russell, op. cit., n. 12 above, chs 2 and 3, esp. 12, 30–4. The Melbourne Hospital made its first specialist appointment — a pathologist, in 1870; a new outpatient department of skin diseases in 1885; an honorary anaesthetist in 1895. In 1896, the Melbourne Hospital appointed a skiagrapher (radiologist). See Inglis, op. cit. n. 16 above, 71. For an account of the deficiencies of clinical teaching see Russell, op. cit., n. 12 above, 66–71, and Ann M. Mitchell, *The Hospital South of the Yarra* (Melbourne: The Alfred Hospital, 1977), 114, 212ff, who attributes low standards of clinical teaching to the lingering 'apprenticeship tradition' (even though apprenticeships had never been recognized in Victoria). The Alfred opened without any specialist appointments but established medical pathology in 1885; ear, nose and throat, eye, skin in 1886; a chloroformist in 1888; a skiagraphist in 1898.

52. For the situation in England, see Peterson, op. cit., n. 9 above, chs IV and V, esp. 138, 141, 148–53, 187. Victoria's specialist hospital were the Women's Hospital (1856) (originally the Lying-in Hospital); the Children's Hospital (1870) (originally The Hospital for Sick Children); the Eye and Ear Hospital (1869) (originally the Melbourne Institute for Diseases of the Eye and Ear); and the Mental Asylums at Yarra Bend (1848) and at Ararat and Beechworth (late 1860s). Because of their charitable function, the hospitals were not available to the financially secure who, except in some cases of emergency, were treated in private hospitals or in their own homes. The public mental asylums were govenment institutions, admitting both paying and pauper patients.

53. D. O'Sullivan, 'William Gillbee (1825–1885) and the introduction of antiseptic surgery to Australia', *Medical Journal of Australia* (11 November 1966) (2), 871–7, and 'The introduction of antiseptic surgery to Australia, *Medical Journal of Australia* (5 November 1967) (2), 896–902. D. Dyason, 'William Gillbee and erysipelas at the Melbourne Hospital: medical theory and social actions', *Journal of Australian Studies, 14 (1984), 3–28, esp. 4–6.* B. Gandevia, 'A history of general practice in Australia', *Medical Journal of Australia* (12 August 1972) 2, 381–5. See also Gillett, op. cit., n. 20 above, part III; Gillison, op. cit., n. 26 above, 263, 280–1.

54. H.B. Graham, 'Happenings of the now long past: the centenary of the Medical Society of Victoria', *Medical Journal of Australia* (16 August 1932), (2), 213–47, 217; Inglis, op. cit., n. 16 above, 6–7.

55. R.E.W. Kennedy 'The charity organisation movement in Melbourne 1887–1897' (Unpublished MA thesis, University of Melbourne, 1966), 40–55.

56. Inglis, op. cit., n. 16 above, 10, 16.

57. Forty public hospitals, outside the Melbourne area, were established between 1846 and 1898. The first hospital in the colony was established in Melbourne, a small government hospital for the convicts sent as labourers for the government administration (est. 1837); The Charity Hospital, Melbourne (est. 1840); The Melbourne Hospital (est. 1846); Port Fairy; (for some years the second busiest port in the Port Phillip District) (est. 1846); Geelong (est. 1852); Bendigo, Castlemaine (est. 1853); Maryborough, Warrnambool (est. 1854); Kilmore (est. 1855); Ballarat, Beechworth, Kyneton, Portland (est. 1856); Ararat,

Heathcote, Maldon, Stawell (est. 1859); Amherst, Dunolly, Swan Hill (est. 1860); Daylesford (est. 1862); Creswick, Inglewood (est. 1863); Hamilton (est. 1864); Woods Point (est. 1865); Sale (est. 1866); Mansfield (est. 1870); The Alfred Melbourne (est. 1871); Clunes (est. 1871); Wangaratta (est. 1872); Alexandra (est. 1873); Horsham, St Arnaud (est. 1874); Mooroopna (est. 1878); Colac, Echuca (est. 1882); Nhill (est. 1883); Bairnsdale (est. 1888); Warracknabeal (est. 1891); Mildura, Walhalla (est. 1892); Omeo and Williamstown (est. 1894); Whycheproof (est. 1898). See n. 52 above for the list of specialist hospitals.

58. A.E. Clarke-Kennedy, *The London — a Study in the Voluntary Hospital System*, 2 vols (London: Pitman Medical, 1962), vol. 1, 79ff.

59. Inglis, op. cit., n. 16 above, 133–41. See also 'Press Cuttings', Melbourne Hospital archives.

60. It was not feasible to determine the relative academic value of a qualification; therefore 'higher' does not imply *necessarily* better training or higher competence, but United Kingdom social values treated any university degree or a senior collegiate qualification as vastly superior to even a multiplicity of licences. In Victoria, this attitude helped Melbourne graduates obtain hospital appointments.

61. This information comes from the hospitals' annual reports and from my prosopographical study of the Victorian medical profession.

62. L. Bruck, *On the Uses and Abuses of the Public Hospitals in Australia, Tasmania and New Zealand with Thirty-two Practical Suggestions for Reform* (Sydney: L. Bruck, 1899), 13. For the whole of Australia he calculated the value of the honoraries' services at £625,742 p.a.

63. ibid., 68; Mitchell, op. cit., n. 51 above, 190ff, 245–9. Bruck recognized pay wards could not cover the true costs, and that problems would arise over the doctors' fees and medical access to the wards by private doctors.

64. In support of his claim, Bruck cites the case of a woman who became gravely ill in an area without a public hospital and was looked after by the local doctor. The doctor recovered fees of more than £300 from the government.

65. Port Phillip Medical Association, n. 38 above.

66. Australian Medical Association Archives, n. 38 above, Port Phillip Medical Association Minutes, 4 September 1846. The scale of fees was three-tiered, 10s 6d, 5s, or 3s per consultation, varying according to the patient's estimated income. Home visits were one guinea, available at half price for the middle-income group, but not available to the third category. Standard midwifery fees were five guineas, three guineas and from two to one guinea. The mileage fee varied from 10s 6d to 7s 6d. In the 1880s, fees for the category-three patients increased to 5s and rates for night visits and travelling also increased. Clauses 29 and 35–9 of the rules were directed to eliminating any personal, hostile or disparaging remarks reflecting on members.

67. Graham, op. cit., n. 54 above, 222.

68. Under rule 29, in the event of the demise of the Association its property (viz. the library) was to be 'given in trust to the Committee of Management of the Melbourne General Hospital' until such time as a new medical Association should be formed. When this happened a similar clause regarding property was included in the next Society's constitution.

69. Graham, op. cit., n. 54 above, 215.The rules were again reduced, this time to fifteen.

70. The president of the joint association was designated president of the Medical Society of Victoria and the British Medical Asssociation (V.B.) until 1952, when the Australian Medical Association was created from a merger of the Medical Society of Victoria with all the British Medical Association state branches. Maintaining a medical society for all but thirteen years of the colony's existence was unique in Australasia, and, I believe, in the British Empire.

71. Editorial, 'The B.M.A. and its colonial branches', *British Medical Journal* (1885)

(ii), 882; T.J. Johnston and Margorie Cargill, 'The British Medical Association and its overseas branches: a short history', *Journal of Imperial and Commonwealth History, 3* (3) (1973), 303–8.

72. Green and Cromwell, op. cit., n. 34 above, ch. 6, esp. 111–12, 115, 120–9.

73. The Castlemaine Medical Association (1853) started with eighteen members, the Mount Alexander Medical Association in April 1854 with twenty-five and the Bendigo District Medical Association in July 1854 with nineteen. Bowden, op. cit., n. 28 above, 191–2. The Ballarat Medico-Chirurgical Society (January 1855) begun with sixteen doctors. By March 1856 the membership had risen to thirty; Bowden, op. cit., n. 23 above, 102–3.

74. *British Medical Journal* (8 July 1876) (ii), 35. The area of Victoria is only 2,237 sq. km less than the total area of England, Scotland and Wales.

75. Bryan Gandevia, Alison Holster, and Sheila Simpson, *Annotated Bibliography of the History of Medicine and Health in Australia* (Sydney: Royal Australasian College of Physicians, 1984), 120. This work lists 2,760 items. B. Gandevia, 'A review of Victoria's early medical journals', *Medical Journal of Australia* (9 August 1951), 184–8.

76. The *Intercolonial Medical Journal of Australasia* resulted from the merger of the *Australian Medical Journal* with the *Intercolonial Quarterly Journal of Medicine and Surgery* (1894–6). The *Intercolonial Medical Journal of Australasia* reverted to the *Australian Medical Journal* (1910–14) which in turn merged with the *Australian Medical Gazette* to form the current *Medical Journal of Australia*, the official organ of the Australian Medical Association. Other Victorian journals were: *Medical Record of Australia* (1861–3); *Medical and Surgical Review* (Australasian) (1863–5); *Australian Medical Gazette* (1869–71); *Melbourne Medical Record* (1875–7); *Intercolonial Quarterly Journal of Medicine and Surgery* (1894–6).

77. Judith Quilter, a graduate student in History and Philosophy of Science at Melbourne University, is preparing a critical history of the journal and I am most grateful to her for her assessment of the journal's position on the world scene.

78. *The Medical Times and Gazette, 13* (1856), 420.

79. *The Lancet* (1856) (ii), 515; (1860) (i), 201–20.

80. *Canada Lancet* (1870–1922); *Canada Medical Record* (1872–1904); *Canadian Journal of Medicine and Surgery* (1897–1936); *Maritime Medical News* (1888–1910); *Union Médicale de Canada* (1807–) *Montreal Medical Journal* (1888–1910). For medical journalism in Canada see C.G. Roland and P. Potter, *Annotated Bibliography of Canadian Medical Periodicals, 1826–1975* (Toronto: The Hannah Institute, 1979); C.G. Roland, 'Canadian medical journalism in the nineteenth century', *Canadian Medical Association Journal, 128* (1983), 449–59, esp. 464.

81. Ann Tovell and B.Gandevia, *References to Australia in British Journals prior to 1880* (Melbourne: Museum of Medical History, Medical Society of Victoria, 1961).

82. Roy MacLeod, 'On visiting the "moving metropolis": Reflections on the architecture of imperial science', *Historical Records of Australian Science, 5* (1982), 1–16, esp. 7.

83. The Victorian Registration Act of 1862 specified, but had not limited, registration to native-born or naturalized British subjects. As a consequence the Privy Council refused, until 1890, to extend the British Medical Act to cover Melbourne degrees, despite there being a clause allowing for the registration of foreign Diplomas. See Russell, op. cit., n. 12 above, 35–6, 79.

Part III

Crises of Empire: The Politics of Race and Epidemic Disease

11

'The dreadful scourge': responses to smallpox in Sydney and Melbourne, 1881–2

Alan Mayne

Nineteenth-century Australian urbanization was a product of British marketplace growth and imperial expansion. Colonial cities such as Melbourne and Sydney boomed and stagnated according to their usefulness to British private capital formation. This utility and hence their continuing growth were dependent upon the extent of their integration into an evolving global network of regional economies and trade routes which serviced the metropolitan centre. As mediums for British economic expansion, they functioned also as cultural transmitters of British custom and social organization for the new settler societies in south-eastern Australia. They were recreations and bastions of the parent culture, and acted as bases for the cultural as well as the economic redefinition of their hinterlands from 'wilderness' into jewels of empire.

Analysis of developing colonial sanitary practice during the last quarter of the nineteenth century confirms the interlocking functions of Melbourne and Sydney as commercial sorting-houses and as cultural transmitters of empire. Both roles are highlighted by responses in the two cities to the appearance of smallpox in 1881–2. Neither role was without ambiguity and tension, as the disease crises attest. Smallpox interrupted regional trading networks, and the dynamics of the international market system clashed with the quarantine restrictions imposed in the periphery; the slum-disease, smallpox, by focusing attention upon the inner-city poor, underscored the primitive rhythms of the local labour and housing markets which underpinned developing capital accumulation within the colonies. The smallpox emergencies of 1881–2 demonstrated not only the economic but the cultural hegemony of empire. The periphery sought overseas reference points to shape its discourse and social policy: public knowledge of smallpox derived from images of London slums, and evolving sanitary administration copied British blueprints. Yet the process of cultural transmission, like the expansion of market exchange, was characterized by tension and change within the periphery: British custom became modified to suit the different social realities of the less sophisticated colonial economies. The social history of disease and medicine in colonial Australia reveals the social structures and the cultural conflicts generated within the imperial periphery by the political economy of empire.

I

European settlement in Australia occurred through its port cities: they acted as gateways to new regions. Permanent settlement began with the founding of Sydney (from Botany Bay) in 1788, and Hobart (Tasmania) in 1804 as penal repositories and maritime outposts for the British Crown. It was, however, the economics of the British private marketplace which determined the subsequent pattern of colonial settlement. Sydney, well placed to service a rich and expanding hinterland, developed into a bustling port city as British shippers, merchants, and financiers sought profits in New South Wales. Hobart, a model state prison but a paltry prize for British investors, stagnated after the cessation of convict transportation in 1853. Across the Bass Strait, however, private enterprise tapped new marketplace potential in the south-eastern regions of the mainland with imperial authorities reluctantly playing second fiddle. A new gateway city, Melbourne, had prospered from 1835 as the linchpin in the economic development of what in 1851 separated from New South Wales to become the new colony of Victoria.

Its growth propelled by the goldrush of the 1850s and by the subsequent proliferation of global trade links, Melbourne eclipsed Sydney to become for a time the largest colonial capital in nineteenth-century Australia. By the early 1880s Melbourne boasted a population of some 268,000, or 31 per cent of the total Victorian population. This marketplace metropolis eagerly embraced the epithet of a passing English tourist; 'Marvellous' Melbourne. The 225,000 population of Sydney, 30 per cent of the New South Wales total, sneered. In the middle 1890s they would be gratified in turn when another English visitor styled their city, by then numbering well over 400,000 people and gaining on its larger southern rival, 'the queen of the Southern Hemisphere, and the centre of commerce for this vast continent'.[1]

The rapid growth of Melbourne and Sydney in the 1880s underlined their accumulating commercial functions. They were service centres to their regions, handling rural production for export to world markets, and supplying overseas credit and imported goods to their hinterlands in turn. The coastal shipping network around south-eastern Australia, already by the 1880s dominated by steam, converged on the two capitals. Heavy public investment in railway construction during the 1870s and 1880s tied rural hinterland closer to port metropolis. Reductions in overseas shipping charges, technological advances in telegraphic communication and marine engineering, and the concomitant crystallizing of regular and reliable overseas shipping services, embedded both capitals in the world trading network. By the 1880s, too, Melbourne and Sydney had in themselves become major sites for profitable private investment: British capital financed a roaring house boom and the provision of basic urban services and amenities.[2]

In proportion to the development of Melbourne and Sydney as commercial centres within an empire marketplace, there evolved in both cities a social structure dominated by elites whose strength and prestige were founded on the handling of goods, investment, and information. A self-conscious and confident urban bourgeoisie had by the 1880s taken to themselves the local direction of economic, cultural, and political affairs in the two colonies. Colonial culture reflected the seemingly smug 'certainties' of the overlapping business-political-professional leadership concerning the achievements and further potential of the British Empire in Australia.[3]

Four of these elite 'certainties' received particular emphasis in the contemporary print medium, in public festivities, trade exhibitions, and in urban design and architecture. These were, first, the assertion of colonial and civic progress, in terms both of past achievements and the promise of continuing growth; second, confidence in scientific and technological innovation; third, the concept of a community of wealth and interest; and fourth, belief in trusteeship by cautious managerial government. Cross-factional competition within the colonial bourgeoisie, by regularly using the four themes as rhetorical contexts for conflict, had the effect of entrenching these 'certainties' even further in colonial culture.

Colonial and civic material progress received constant emphasis. City guidebooks drew proud attention to the symbols of successful membership in a global economic system: the trade exchange, complete with telegraph facilities, hourly telegram postings of shipping movements, and newspaper room stocked with colonial, English, and 'foreign' journals; the busy wharves and warehouses; the commercial clubs; the handsome headquarters of banks and insurance companies; the well-stocked shops of the central retailing thoroughfares. In Sydney, the imposing headquarters of the Australian Mutual Provident Society was adorned with the sculptured representation of 'Australia receiving the gifts of peace and plenty'.[4] These colonial achievements were couched in terms of the reassuring bonds of empire: finance institutions emphasized in their names and their boards of directors their links with the London money market; the Italianate façade of Sydney's new General Post Office displayed allegorical representations of the four quarters of the globe with which regular communication was now carried on. In both statistical comparisons and architectural equivalents, the new urban elite expressed their hopes and claims by reference to the economic trends and the urban blueprints of the mother country. Asserting Sydney to be the greatest port in the southern hemisphere, the NSW statistician in 1887 made grand comparisons with the ports of London and Liverpool.[5]

Elite certainties were also expressed in the emphasis given to science and technology as vehicles of material progress. Newspapers stressed their conquest of distance with up-to-date information from Britain, Europe, and the west coast of the USA. International exhibitions at Sydney in 1879 and Melbourne in 1880 sought to educate audiences in the new technologically based community of interest sustained by information exchange and commerce between the Empire and other European powers. The exhibitions, by proudly asserting colonial inventiveness and innovation in speedily adopting the latest overseas technologies, sought also to demonstrate the integral role enjoyed by the Australian colonies within this sophisticated global structure. With local branches of the British Medical

Association (BMA) established in Melbourne and in Sydney during 1880, local medical science could similarly trumpet the end of Australian isolation from international scientific research and debate. Meanwhile newspapers quoted regularly from English sources the advances speedily being made by scientific medicine in the reduction of sickness and death. Predicting confidently 'a complete revolution' thereby in the treatment of infectious disease, Dr J.E. Neild, President of the Victorian branch of the BMA, contended in 1882 that 'the progress of medical science was never so apparent as at the present time'.[6]

Medical advances, technological achievements, and the material progress which both had made possible among British people and their European trading partners, were optimistically claimed in Melbourne and Sydney to have produced in the Australian colonies a social structure characterized by general prosperity and by social consensus. It was claimed that no entrenched class barriers soured community life here. Rather, elite rhetoric about colonial social progress found regular expression in the concept of Australia as a 'Working Man's Paradise', where working people had opportunities to 'enjoy a multitude of comforts which they never possessed before'. Marking the annual celebration of British settlement, the *Sydney Morning Herald (SMH)* in 1876 could think of

> no community that has better means of living than that of New South Wales. . . . . The many have plenty as well as the few. Provisions are for the most part cheap, and labour generally brings its price. If elsewhere there is a possible danger of people getting too little, we are not entirely free sometimes from the danger of having too much.[7]

Such social progress and social cohesion, it was comfortably predicted, were guaranteed by the English model of parliamentary and municipal government. Parliamentary government, enshrining manhood suffrage and the secret (or Australian) ballot, extended from the mother country 'the fundamental principles of public policy in the light of which alone large communities can be widely governed'. Wise government sought to underwrite 'the stability and prosperity of the country', which meant preserving and extending the dynamics of the private marketplace, and defending from unnecessary public interference the rights of individuals to accumulate private property.[8] The requirements of private property, and the provision of public services in support of private property, were the further responsibility of municipal government which, introduced in Sydney in 1840 and Melbourne in 1842 with a restricted property franchise, sought to apply the English urban marketplace model of 'good rule and government' in the new cities of the colonial periphery.

II

The appearance of smallpox in Sydney and Melbourne was a severe jolt to the marketplace elite. In mid-June 1881 an editorial leader in the Sydney *Daily Telegraph* announced the outbreak of 'the dreadful scourge' in one of the most thickly populated districts of the inner city.[9] Alarm had previously been raised in May, when a case of suspected smallpox had been detected amongst the inner-city's Chinese community; but just as this case was pronounced convalescent, reports of fresh smallpox outbreaks throughout the inner city proliferated. Houses were hastily disinfected, their occupants isolated, and confirmed smallpox cases were evacuated to the quarantine station at the North Head of Port Jackson. By the end of July however, as fresh cases continued to appear, overcrowding the quarantine station and prompting the colonial government to appoint a Board of Health and to establish a permanent isolation hospital for infectious diseases, the *Daily Telegraph* concluded that 'no longer [was there] room to doubt that the outbreak of small-pox in Sydney will assume the form of an epidemic'.[10] The disease, in fact, waxed and waned into the new year, provoking initial panic but then, increasingly, indifference as it became evident that the disease was not especially virulent and was confined to the poorest working-class sections of the inner city. The majority of Sydney's population, living in the suburbs, remained immune. Government medical authorities pronounced the epidemic officially ended in February 1882.

Melbourne health authorities were by then in the midst of a smaller smallpox emergency of their own. The southern city had found much to fault in the handling of the Sydney smallpox crisis. The Melbourne *Argus* contended that the outbreak had 'found the authorities totally unprepared.' Subsequent actions, sneered the Melbourne *Age*, amounted 'to . . . nothing but blundering from first to last'.[11] Victorian medical circles were still more damning. The Melbourne-based *Australian Medical Journal* maintained in September 1881 that the Sydney authorities' initial 'neglect was followed by a period in which quarantine was wildly and cruelly enforced, and now has come a state of despairing apathy; all hope of stamping out the plague seems to have been abandoned'. Sydney's poor example was exemplary: Melbourne should 'learn from the shortcomings of our neighbours'.[12]

That lesson had to be learned quickly. Melbourne newspapers in early January 1882 carried news that the Orient Line steamer *Garonne*, bound from Plymouth via the Cape, had arrived in Adelaide with smallpox on board and was now proceeding to Melbourne. Emergency measures were immediately set in train to cleanse the ship, its mails and cargo, and to isolate the 205 passengers disembarking in Melbourne at the Portsea quarantine station in Port Phillip Bay. Arrangements were simultaneously made by the Central Board of Health, Melbourne City Council, and the metropolitan police to combat the spread of smallpox into the city.

Notwithstanding one death and the intermittent announcement of a handful of fresh cases amongst passengers at the quarantine station, community alarm gradually diminished and preparations were being made late in the month for the release of the *Garonne*'s passengers, when the over-strained quarantine service was burdened with another smallpox emergency. This time, disease was detected aboard the P&O steamer *Mizapore*, bound from London via Bombay, Perth, and Adelaide.

Warning that the new danger was worse even than that posed earlier by the *Garonne*, an editorial leader in the *Age* predicted 'that we must prepare ourselves for a still more serious struggle with the small-pox fiend than we have yet passed through'. With the passing of the weeks, however, such language appeared over-dramatic, and in late February, with returning confidence, the rival *Argus* announced that with the release from quarantine of most passengers there were 'now only a few passengers on the station, and they are in the convalescent hospital'.[13]

In Britain, the isolated Australian smallpox incidents of 1881–2 deservedly received scant notice. In Melbourne, only one mild case of smallpox had been detected in the city as a consequence of the *Garonne* and *Mizapore*, a trivial result if compared with the fifty cases in Melbourne which were to spread from the steamer *Rome* in 1884. The Sydney crisis, arguably the most serious outbreak of smallpox among Europeans ever recorded in Australia, none the less caused a mere forty deaths and totalled only 154 reported cases.[14] Both smallpox incidents were yet remarkable for the community alarms which they caused in Sydney and Melbourne. Contemporaries spoke of widespread panic in both cities. In Sydney, this took the form of wild rumours about the imagined spread of smallpox from neighbourhood to neighbourhood, and allegations of healthy people dragged from their homes by government officials, harshly treated at the quarantine station, and infected with smallpox or other loathsome diseases by impure vaccination supplies. In Melbourne, community obsession with images of inmates crawling through the scrub from the quarantine ground to spread infection in the city, led to the clearing of a wide no-man's-land around the ground, the stationing of special police, and plans for a high perimeter fence.

The disproportion between the scale of the smallpox outbreaks and that of community reflexes is interesting in three respects. First, the outbreaks were blown out of proportion because the colonial periphery borrowed from the mother country an inappropriate cultural framework of reference for comprehending smallpox, which was unrelated to local realities. Second, panic was fuelled by, and served to highlight, the primitive nature of colonial administrative structures and procedures for protecting community health. Third, community fears found expression in a search for scapegoats, focusing upon the Chinese and the inner-city poor, as social intercourse degenerated into typecasting and victimization of those less socially articulate and economically powerless.

Sydney and Melbourne, as trade and information exchange points in a network radiating from Britain, drew much of the information for their social discourse from that same network. The language of epidemic disease, its causes and consequences, was drawn pre-eminently from Britain. Hence the Melbourne *Argus*, warning in July 1881 that the 'small-pox epidemic is beginning to assume disquieting proportions in Sydney', described 'the nature and possible results of the malady' by reference to medical discourse in the *Fortnightly Review* and the *North American Review*.[15] Even the colonial spelling of 'small-pox' echoed British idiom. Colonial medical circles, without experience in the treatment of epidemic diseases, also turned for information to English medical sources and to expatriate doctors with working experience from the mother country. Dr C.K. Mackellar, President of the NSW Board of Health, took pages of notes from English texts to guide his colleagues in 1881.[16] At a protracted debate by the Medical Society of Victoria in 1882 over the difficulties of distinguishing smallpox from chickenpox, doctors conceded their lack of expertise: 'few practitioners in this colony, and especially graduates of our own University, have seen, or will see, cases of small-pox'. Participants in the debate deferred to those few who could claim to have 'seen a very great deal of small-pox, having been in practice in London during the severe epidemic of 1870–71'.[17]

British precedents and comparisons thus dominated colonial thinking. The resulting images of wholesale slaughter were shaped, in particular, by reference to the great British smallpox epidemic of 1870–3, and to the London epidemic of 1880–1. Tapping reports of the London outbreak from the *British Medical Journal*, its colonial namesake warned of the threat to Australian ports on the eve of the outbreak in Sydney. Commenting upon the disease's subsequent spread in Sydney, the journal cautioned 'we know too well what to expect; in London alone, in the small-pox outbreak of 1871–2, we learn that fifty thousand cases occurred; an epidemic of similar proportions in Melbourne would mean between three and four thousand cases'.[18] The *Evening News*, as it announced the appearance of smallpox in Sydney, predicted that they might be on the threshold of an epidemic as great as that already raging in London.[19] Community attitudes were shaped as much by imperial images as by local realities.

The NSW Board of Health, in a subsequent review of the Sydney smallpox crisis, concluded that public panic was mainly due to the colony's lack of preparation and organization for containing the spread of infectious diseases.[20] Intercolonial quarantine practice was uneven and uncoordinated. At each colonial port of call for the *Garonne* and *Mizapore*, local authorities made only piecemeal arrangements for their consignment of passengers, mails, and general cargo, and then shunted the ships off to their next port of call. Although in Melbourne the *Argus* trumpeted the efficacy of Victorian quarantine and pointed the finger at NSW for quarantine 'laxity',[21] the Portsea quarantine station was in fact itself without basic facilities and could not accommodate passengers from the *Mizapore* until the *Garonne*'s passengers had been released. In Sydney, the NSW Treasurer wrote with wry amusement to the Premier, recalling how

> When we were in our troubles about the Smallpox, the Melbourne press used to cry us down, and say what they would have done, and how they were prepared for such a contingency, but now it turns out, notwithstanding the warning they had, that they are quite unprepared, and the scenes being enacted

at the Melbourne Quarantine Ground, are worse than we had here, when we were taken unawares.[22]

Sanitary arrangements for combating infectious diseases among the general community were just as primitive. The outbreak of smallpox in Sydney found the city with no general Health Act, no co-ordinated public health administration and no infectious diseases hospital. In the resulting chaos, patients and journalists complained of cruelty, mismanagement, and neglect, prompting two censure debates in parliament and the appointment of a Royal Commission.[23] In both cities, newspapermen, politicians, doctors, and bureaucrats grasped instinctively for precedents and models in curative medicine from the mother country: a board of health in Sydney, and an ambulance corps, an infectious diseases hospital, and comprehensive vaccination and compulsory notification of infectious disease in both cities.

The NSW press and parliament initially blamed the spread of smallpox on Chinese immigration, and on the 'seed-plots of disease' produced in the city's Chinese quarter by immoral and overcrowded living.[24] Chinese market-gardeners and hawkers were ostracized; Chinese were barred from public transport, abused and assaulted in the streets. Increasingly, however, the European poor of the inner city became identified with smallpox in Sydney, and were blamed for perpetuating it. Again, the colonial periphery based its assumptions upon the orthodoxies of sanitary science in the major centres of the urban trading system. The *SMH* cited the *Scientific American* and the example of downtown Chicago to argue that smallpox was associated with 'filthy places'. The *Daily Telegraph* was guided by the recent experiences of the 1880–1 epidemic in London, where 'small-pox seems to have taken up its home in the poorer districts, the residents of the West End and the more respectable suburbs being almost entirely free from its ravages'.[25] Overseas sanitary experience had demonstrated that smallpox was 'a filth disease . . . spread . . . by overcrowding, by defective drainage and ventilation, by stagnant and polluted water and air, by ignorance and dirt'. It had taught, moreover, that the 'germs of disease that are [thus] generated in back-slums will travel to broad thoroughfares . . . and in this way the unhealth of the few becomes that of the million'. Guided by these principles, sanitary precautions and systematic house inspections in Sydney were therefore begun in 'the lower quarters of the city'.[26]

Local developments confirmed the overseas predictions. The smallpox epidemic was concentrated in dilapidated pockets of the inner city where, as the Board of Health noted, it 'principally attacked the labouring classes'.[27] The 'other half' and the 'back slums' of Sydney, both of them images transcribed from the different social and spatial context of nineteenth-century Britain, were therefore condemned by colonial image makers and their suburban audience for nurturing disease and thus endangering the health of all.[28] The poor stood condemned, neatly and simplisticly, for '*packing themselves* in small and dirty tenements, as sardines are packed in a tin' [my italics]. The *Daily Telegraph* attacked 'the lower strata of society' for their 'inordinate, unseemly, and perverse fondness for dirt and . . . daily defiance of sanitary laws'.[29] The City Health Officer drew attention to lack of co-operation by the inhabitants of the infected city districts, noting 'the filthy state of premises even only a day or two after being thoroughly cleansed'.[30] Angry correspondents wrote to the newspapers to urge the sweeping away of the inner city's 'closely packed network of lanes and rookeries'. The Sydney City Council, with the encouragement of the Board of Health, embarked upon a comprehensive programme of slum clearance to rid the city of 'hovels and nests ripe for the development of the germs of disease'.[31] This initiative sparked proposals for the Melbourne City Council, likewise, to clear 'the overcrowded and filthy dwellings existing in some portions of the city . . . which are not only a disgrace to Melbourne, but a positive danger to the public health'.[32]

III

The smallpox traumas in Sydney and Melbourne challenged the publicly expressed 'certainties' of the colonial marketplace elite. In every instance, however, their assumptions and priorities were successfully reasserted in imitation of British cultural models, but modified by the local realities of colonial market structure and cultural custom. Challenge and response highlights the socio-economic structures of private capital accumulation, and the inequalities and tensions inherent in the political economy and culture of empire.

Smallpox challenged elite expectations about colonial and civic progress, by interrupting the trading networks upon which their prosperity was based. Quarantine restrictions announced by the other Australian colonies against shipping from Sydney, and sanitary inspection of railway traffic on the NSW-Victorian border, interrupted free trade. In Melbourne, all vessels arriving from NSW ports were detained until examined and cleared by port health officers. Upon the outbreak of smallpox in Sydney the NSW government, anxious to minimize such interruption to trade, had telegraphed all the Australian colonies with assurances that all necessary precautions were in train, and later telegraphed again to announce prematurely the ending of the epidemic.[33] The government prodded the Board of Health hopefully for relaxation of quarantine restrictions, and when the Board eventually agreed in February 1882 the Treasurer joyfully telegraphed to the Premier, then travelling to New York and London, announcing that the port of Sydney at last had a clean bill of health from the other colonies.[34]

The beginnings of Australian quarantine regulation had been based on English precedent. The NSW Quarantine Act of 1832 was hurriedly modelled on the English statute of 1825, so as to guard the colony from the cholera epidemic then raging in the mother country. Colonial authorities could thus proclaim any overseas areas as infected places, and all ships arriving from proclaimed ports or having experienced disease during passage were liable to be placed in quarantine for as long as might be directed.[35] In Britain, medical criticism of the contagionist assumptions underpinning indiscriminate quarantine of ships from infected areas combined with the commercial considerations of growing international trade to prompt the gradual discontinuance of blanket restrictions on vessels from infected ports. The continuation of the older system across the Channel, in the Mediterranean and the Black Sea, came to be damned as medically ineffective and as a means merely 'of official exaction and commercial loss'.[36]

The older quarantine system, which was none the less perpetuated by the International Sanitary Conference of 1886, convened at Constantinople by the French in response to the cholera threat then posed to Europe, was increasingly attacked by British commerce and sanitary science as being founded on 'altogether retrograde and impractical' scientific principles which served only to act 'to the great prejudice of trade'.[37] At the 1874 International Sanitary Conference in Vienna, a split occurred between the comprehensive quarantine system championed by France and Turkey, and the practice which had evolved in Britain of port medical inspection and selective detention. By 1881, as the Australian colonies confronted smallpox, the scale and momentum of British commerce had rendered quarantine there an anachronism. The English Local Government Board condemned the 'utter futility'[38] of comprehensive quarantine, and in the following year, influenced by the protests of British steamship companies at the delays and losses caused by 'the vexatious and redtape quarantine regulations' enforced at Port Said, the British government proposed a fresh international conference to ensure that British shipping should no longer be hampered by what the *British Medical Journal* termed 'the somewhat antiquated continental school of hygiene'.[39]

Quarantine practice in Melbourne and Sydney was considerably influenced by these English developments. In the NSW capital, port health authorities from 1876 followed the model of medical inspection and selective detention begun formally in England during 1873.[40] In Melbourne, the practice of sending a health officer onto each ship before it berthed was discontinued in 1880; henceforth a pilot notified the health officer if disease had been reported on board. Justifying this change, the Victorian government argued that the new procedure 'closely follows . . . that which is adopted with safety in the immensely more crowded port of London'.[41]

Colonial quarantine none the less differed from Britain's in retaining the practice of regularly proclaiming overseas ports infected places. Australian ports simply did not handle the same volume of commerce as that which had forced modifications in the quarantine administration of the biggest English port cities. The smaller commercial scale of Australian ports however provides only a partial explanation for differing quarantine practice. Significant variations are evident in the ways colonial quarantine proclamations were enforced. Although in 1881 under Victorian quarantine, all ships from NSW were detained by Victorian authorities, they were not subjected automatically to prolongued quarantine detention. The ships were individually inspected and released if free of infection. Similarly in

NSW, when San Francisco, or the Queensland ports, or cities in France, Spain, or Portugal were proclaimed as infected areas in the 1870s and 1880s, shipping from these ports was only *liable* to quarantine after individual inspection.[42] By contrast, Victoria in 1881 announced the quarantining of *all* vessels from China, and in NSW, government ministers were likewise 'agreed that all vessels with Chinese on board should be stopped as far as we can — and at once'.[43] Thus quarantine practice was influenced by Australian racial prejudice to become an instrument of immigration restriction. Again in 1888, ordering that its proclamation of 1881 against Chinese ports be strictly enforced, the NSW Board of Health required that all vessels from China and Hong Kong be placed in quarantine.[44] Colonial cultural imperatives, bound up with distance, isolation, and racial consciousness, combined with local marketplace conditions to preserve quarantine strategies which contrasted with those of Britain.

Local commercial growth was none the less modifying colonial quarantine in the direction of British practice. The Victorian Board of Health concluded during 1881 that the volume of land communication with NSW was such to make 'any system of inspection and fumigation . . . inoperable'.[45] Complaints in the same year by Melbourne shipowners at the 'inconvenience and delay' caused to intercolonial trade by port quarantine precautions led to the easing of Victorian restrictions.[46] P&0 representatives in Melbourne caused officials 'considerable perplexity' by exerting pressure in 1882 to have the detention of the *Mizapore* altered so as not to disrupt its cargo schedule and, more important, its overseas timetable, fixed by government contract as a mail steamer. The global flow of goods, finance, and information through the urban marketplace system generated cycles of movement which increasingly subsumed the economic and administrative structures of the two south-eastern Australian capitals.[47]

It is therefore significant that international shipping companies increasingly sought modifications to the restraints upon commerce caused by colonial quarantine regulations. When in January 1882 the *Garonne* sailed north from Melbourne to Sydney, the Orient Line objected to, and sought the easing of, NSW Board of Health rules governing the unloading of cargo. The P&O Company likewise in the following month requested fewer delays to the *Mizapore* in Sydney.[48] The French Compagnie des Messageries remonstrated in 1885 at the 'rather strict' quarantine imposed in Sydney on one of its steamers, and requested the shortest possible detention.[49] Perhaps swayed by these accumulating criticisms, the NSW Board of Health conceded to a request in 1885 by the Orient Line that coaling and the discharge and loading of cargo be allowed to proceed during the quarantine period.[50] The progressive integration of the colonial economies into a single trading system, already evident in the administration of intercolonial quarantine during the smallpox emergency of 1881, was clear to all by the time of renewed smallpox anxieties in 1884. Asked what restrictions were in train to prevent the disease spreading from neighbouring colonies, the NSW Colonial Secretary explained that the 'trade between Victoria and South Australia and this colony is so great that it would result in very great inconvenience if we were to proclaim those colonies infected'.[51] Adding its backing to the intercolonial Sanitary Conference of that year, convened in Sydney on the model of the international sanitary conferences, the NSW Board of Health urged that in the interests of free trade, and

> considering the recent increase in the rapidity of communication with other countries and the very frequent arrival of foreign going steamer-vessels it is very desirable that the Government should take steps to induce the Governments of the other colonies to concur in a general and uniform mode of dealing with cases in which quarantine is required.[52]

IV

The smallpox emergencies in Sydney and Melbourne, as well as interrupting colonial commerce, also challenged elite assurances about science and technology. Marine engineering, which boosted Australian prosperity by taming distance, was also perceived to have brought the colonies into dangerously close contact with overseas ports where smallpox and cholera were endemic. The modern city, a symbol of European technological sophistication, was also a centre of death. In sombre mood, the *SMH* noted how 'Great cities are generally the scenes of great havoc when an infectious disease gets a firm hold.'[53] Primitive statistical comparisons of crude death-rates in Sydney and English cities brought no joy: Sydney's record was worse.

Medical science, and with it the claims of its practitioners to be regarded as an elite profession, were consequently also challenged by the smallpox crisis. The *SMH*, normally a champion of medical achievement, conceded at the epidemic's beginning that the 'origin of small-pox is wrapped in mystery, and the same may be said of the laws by which it does its deadly work. There is perhaps no malady about which even medical specialists are so much in the dark'.[54] When a BMA deputation urged the NSW government to enact compulsory vaccination as in Britain and Victoria, the newspaper questioned whether in fact the deputation could provide 'firm and indisputable' facts about vaccination, as it had claimed. Twisting the knife, the writer noted that 'medical science . . . is so called only by courtesy. Of fixed and irrefragable principles there are none, and hence we see theory and practice so constantly and so greatly changing'.[55] The *Daily Telegraph* remarked at the end of the smallpox emergency that regardless of what 'a select circle of scientists' might say, the epidemic had taught that 'an ounce of fact is worth a ton of theory'.[56]

Community confidence in medical claims to expert knowledge had been shaken by the epidemic.[57] This crisis over the legitimacy of medical certainties focused in part upon diagnosis. As in Melbourne during the smallpox outbreaks of 1869 and 1884, dissatisfaction was widely voiced at doctors' hesitancy, disagreements, and mistakes in diagnosing smallpox. If doctors were unable to distinguish between smallpox and chickenpox, wrote one lay 'observer', then 'what is the good of them I should like to know?'[58] Criticism was also directed at medical treatment. Government medical officers were accused of 'gross blundering and culpable negligence'.[59] Private doctors were criticized for their unwillingness to treat smallpox patients, and reluctance to report cases they did treat to the health authorities: income, it seemed, came before public service. Newspapers in Sydney and Melbourne filled with letters suggesting popular preventives and remedies for smallpox. Doctors sneered with good cause at this 'legion [of lay suggestions] . . . swept up from every possible hole and corner',[60] because the letters underlined the extent to which formal medical training and treatment were discounted in the community.

Manifestly, elite 'certainties' were not the certainties of the whole community. This is perhaps most evident in discussions of vaccination, which was upheld by the medical authorities in both colonies as the best guard against smallpox. Opposition, they claimed, parroting the medical establishment in England, was confined to a few strays in the profession, and to the gullible. However, compulsory vaccination was not enacted in NSW, notwithstanding lobbying by the Board of Health and the BMA. Indeed, so strongly did popular opinion develop against vaccination in NSW that the Victorian Central Board of Health intervened to slate 'the circulation of such fallacies amongst the ignorant and unreflecting part of the community'.[61] The NSW BMA resolved, too, that a response was urgently needed to counteract the 'disastrous effect' of anti-vaccination meetings and literature 'among the simple and half-educated'.[62]

The medical elite in both colonies turned to Britain for statistics and arguments, but so did the NSW Anti-Vaccination League, which modelled itself upon the anti-vaccination leagues in Britain. British medical opinion had been divided over vaccination matters since the epidemic of the early 1870s. Confusion was exacerbated early in 1880 by Sir Thomas Watson, who first repudiated and then reasserted his long-held views on the nature of smallpox, cowpox, and vaccination. The extent of agitation in England against compulsory vaccination and against the use of human vaccine supplies prompted the BMA in 1880 to organize a special conference on the use of calf vaccine instead. Dr Charles Cameron, with BMA support, prepared amending legislation to allay anxieties about the strength and purity of vaccine supplies, and the British government in response announced that it would begin to supply animal vaccine.[63]

Watson, Cameron, and echoes of the English debate on vaccination were reported in the colonial press. One consequence was the strengthening of lay scepticism at conflicting opinion among medical experts. Another was renewed colonial debate about safe vaccines. The BMA and the NSW Board of Health, mimicking their colleagues in Britain, argued that the best defence of vaccination (let alone the best defence against smallpox) lay in a guaranteed supply of fresh calf lymph. Both colonial governments, following the lead of the Local Government Board in England, moved to establish stations for the production and distribution of calf lymph. Anti-vaccinators, inside and outside parliament, mixed Herbert Spencer on race with Thomas Watson on cowpox to counter that humanized lymph was a source of consumption, insanity, syphilis, and leprosy, and that calf lymph was itself nothing more than 'small-pox in a beast', and could moreover introduce 'diseases of the lower animals'.[64]

The colonial medical establishment responded to criticisms by emphasizing yet more medical exclusiveness, coupled with laboratory science and medical technology. In parliament, on government boards, in their societies, and in the press, they lauded medical professionalism and public spirit, while at the same time they turned against lay-appointed salaried doctors as scapegoats to be blamed for the medical mistakes of the smallpox crises. Such 'unreformed' public medicine was savaged by them as the pariah of the profession, where low pay and routinism had secured only 'men who are a disgrace to the profession, and who were wandering about the city unable to obtain a livelihood'.[65] Reformed public medicine required instead direction by medical experts who enjoyed the confidence of the executives of the medical and scientific societies and of the professional journals which they sustained. The formal reconstitution, in January 1882, of the NSW Board of Health from its *ad hoc* beginnings was a partial realization of these ambitions; the subsequent bureaucratic evolution of Australian maritime quarantine as 'a scientifically-based branch of preventive medicine' represented a further victory for their hopes.[66]

Discounting public preventive medicine as it had been developed by low-paid and consequently low-status doctors within the evolving health departments of both city councils, the medical elite called instead for the latest in British medical technology to complement the new dawn promised by reformed state medicine. In Melbourne, the *Australian Medical Journal* and the Medical Society of Victoria looked for defence from smallpox in the building of a scientifically planned quarantine ground, together with a fully equipped infectious diseases hospital and hierarchically arranged medical staff.[67] Just such a hospital was opened in 1883. In Sydney, too, the smallpox epidemic resulted in the construction, after the urgings of the local medical establishment, of an infectious diseases hospital and the rebuilding of the quarantine station. In both cities, however, emphasis was placed upon the isolation of the new hospitals from suburban housing, because smallpox alarms in the two cities had fuelled popular misgivings concerning even these latest medical technologies. Panic and protest had been reported in London during 1881 among residents who feared the spread of infection from nearby smallpox hospitals.[68] In Sydney and Melbourne, subsequently, there were complaints, deputations, and protest meetings by local communities fearful of a smallpox hospital in their areas.[69]

Reflecting the medical establishment's views, the major dailies urged local neighbourhoods to take a less parochial view of community medical needs. Lay people were reassured that new medical technologies, combined with advances in aetiology, would ensure future immunity from infectious disease. While Melbourne watched anxiously the spread of smallpox in Sydney late in 1881, the *Argus* announced that at the recent International Medical Congress in London,

Louis Pasteur had foreshadowed magic bullets 'almost too wonderful to be true', which promised total control over disease: 'microbes, or minute organisms, by which . . . many diseases are caused, can be so cultivated as to make them harmless . . . whilst they will protect animals from the diseases of which they are in the uncultivated state the fatal causes'.[70] Reconfirming its confidence in scientific and technological progress, the *SMH* in 1890 marvelled at the 'extraordinary possibilities' suggested by the new sciences of electricity and bacteriology:

> What EDISON has done in the one, PASTEUR and KOCH and a host of less illustrious followers have been doing in the other; and, if anything, the revelations of the micro-organisns that govern the life and death of all living creatures have been more sudden and more startling, and make us wonder more as to what we are coming to, than the telephone, and the phonograph, and other inventions . . . that are related to . . . electricity.[71]

V

Smallpox had challenged elite assurances about science and technology; it also queried their promises about community and social progress. Pointing to the destitution uncovered in the inner city by the disinfecting staffs, the *SMH* noted that 'the small-pox panic . . . has shown . . . half the world how the other half live'.[72] The symbolism of the 'other half' was imported from overseas cities in the urban network. The considerable attention given subsequently by Sydney newspapers during the 1880s to the issue of working-class housing conditions was also very much influenced by the language of slumming literature and sanitary discourse in Britain. Referring to the inner-city districts where smallpox in 1881 was most entrenched, one letter writer argued that since 'in London especially there is a large population living in the utmost misery in its back slums and rookeries . . . therefore . . . such places must be naturally looked for in a city like Sydney'.[73] English social reform debate, especially as it was stimulated by publication in 1883 of George Sims's *How the Poor Live* and Andrew Mearns's *The Bitter Cry of Outcast London*, was extensively discussed in the colonial press, and was transcribed to local social conditions: for surely, the circumstances 'of those described by Mr. G.R. SIMS in his "How the Poor Live" . . . are paralleled by those of many persons burrowing in the back slums of Sydney and Melbourne'.[74] Newspaper descriptions of sanitary inspections in Sydney during the smallpox epidemic of 1881, and of the City Council's 'Slum Surveying Expeditions' to condemn substandard housing throughout the 1880s, provided ample local detail to support the comparison.[75]

The *SMH* cautioned its suburban middle-class readership against concluding 'that our civilisation is a failure, and that we are going from bad to worse'.[76] Yet the other half, whose existence in Sydney was so starkly demonstrated by epidemic smallpox, were indeed the inevitable social casualties of a city economy based upon trade and the accumulation of private capital. Wharves, warehouses, railway yards, and hauling companies required considerable reserves of floating casual labour. So too did the shipworks, foundries, and finishing works which serviced them. Labour markets reflected the uneven and cyclical nature of these demands: fully extended during the annual wool season as the port supplied international markets, they were none the less still subject to sudden periods of slack, and at other times to seasonal downturns in activity. As one dock labourer explained in 1890, employment was always 'very precarious. I have had sometimes a very good week's work, and then been idle for weeks afterwards.' Another labourer remarked that in the building trades, because of the 'fluctuations in employment and the precarious nature of it, we are just on the threshold of existence'.[77] Housing markets mirrored the contours of the markets for labour: the inner city housed the casual labour tied in close proximity to the sources of potential work. High rents, primitive amenities, and widespread sub-letting expressed both their subsequent exploitation by landlords and their continuing vulnerability to workforce volatility.[78]

Such people were doubly hit by the smallpox epidemic in Sydney. Not only was the disease concentrated in pockets of low-cost housing, but heavy-handed preventive measures by the Board of Health and the City Council were targeted upon entire working-class neighbourhoods. These programmes were based upon the cultural premises of outsiders unfamiliar with, and unresponsive to, the economic and social networks within such neighbourhoods. They reflected a simple and unsympathetic desire by the wider community to rid itself of the sources of disease.[79] Municipal house-to-house inspections to condemn insanitary housing were watched with hostility by local inhabitants, for whom condemnation meant eviction, and disruption of their fragile neighbourhood economy.[80] Disinfecting operations and evacuations to the quarantine station similarly caused emotional trauma and economic loss: furniture and crockery were damaged, clothing and furniture burned, wallpaper torn off, and lime daubed indiscriminately. The Inspector of Nuisances described reassuringly to the wider community how his disinfecting staff were sent 'to clean and scrape'; but houses which he dismissed as 'hovels' were none the less homes to their occupants, and, as visiting newspapermen attested, had been proudly tidied and ornamented.[81] 'The Widow of the late Mr. Lindsay' recalled angrily how 'the ambulance men . . . came to my house and burnt everything in the house, leaving me only a blanket as a bed, without any pillow, and with only a dress to wear'.[82] Another woman, released from the quarantine station, was charged by the landlord for arrears in rent, and only the rallying of friends saved her belongings from the bailiffs. A third woman claimed that quarantine had ruined her business as a common lodging-house keeper and grocer.[83] The government, although offering compensation, alleged that such claims were 'extortionate'. The widowed Mrs Lindsay however wrote of 'very gruff' treatment by Treasury officials, 'who kept me coming day after day' and then heavily discounted her claim. John Hughes, a woolpacker whose family had shared a three-room house in a passageway behind the docks, complained in mid-1882 that he had still received nothing 'but rebuffs from the Treasury officials'.[84]

Hughes' protests were dismissed as the stories of 'a reckless and insubordinate man'.[85] Liberal bourgeois rationalizations quickly masked with platitudes the uncomfortable social realities of the inner city which had been glimpsed during the smallpox emergency. Industriousness and prudence would surely bring long-term security to all respectable working people? Hughes's poverty and his protests could be easily discounted because he was labelled a drunkard. By this argument, the inner-city poor, revelling in dirt and drink, had simply squandered their opportunities. Reformers, attuned to the *Bitter Cry*, suggested that in London the poor were the victims less of structural inequalities in the private marketplace than of their own improvident habits: 'the dwellers in those foul dens are not good workers, and the greater number of them are half idle all their lives'. Evangelical charitable associations, modelled upon parent organizations in England, sought to uplift and integrate the urban lower orders with alms and scripture readings.[86]

VI

State poor relief in this 'Working Man's Paradise' was anathema to colonial electorates. The state was none the less looked to often in other ways to underwrite an infant marketplace society in which private capital accumulation was as yet insufficiently developed to have fully evolved a strong and stable investing and entrepreneurial class. Notwithstanding this time-honoured colonial tendency to defer to state initiatives, the smallpox crises of 1881–2 for a time shook confidence in local 'good rule and government'. Cabinet and bureaucracy in both colonies were censured for their inattention to public health. Local government, unfavourably judged in London during the outbreak of 1880–1, was likewise found wanting in the colonies. Praise of the Sydney City Council's energetic response to smallpox was tempered by comment that this 'white-washing, garnishing, and furbishing up as soon as a germ of disease makes its appearance, is evidence of the neglect that has been chronic for years under the very noses of the Aldermen and their officers'.[87] Municipal sanitary administration was likewise slated in Melbourne, where according to the *Argus*, the City Council's public health record showed it 'completely destitute of the energy and creative power which are essential to the efficient regulation of a great and growing city'.[88] The criticisms of city government in Melbourne and Sydney paralleled the resentment felt by urban patricians in Britain, Europe, and North America at the wresting of local office by new political alignments whose power was based among the urban lower middle classes.

In Melbourne, a stronger Central Board of Health and the forming of a Metropolitan Board of Works were suggested remedies. In Sydney, the appointment of expert central boards with comprehensive powers was canvassed. The smallpox emergency, however, also crystallized misgivings concerning the fettering of private property rights by greater and compulsory state powers. In the NSW parliament, the government faced censure for sanctioning policies which were 'tyrannical and cruel and an infringement of the liberties of the subject'.[89] Protests by passengers from the *Garonne* and *Mizapore* at their 'cruel and unenlightened treatment' raised the worrying issue in Melbourne of 'individual rights [being] set at nought for the public good'.[90] In reflective mood, the *SMH* worried that the tendency in young colonies to rely thus heavily upon state action had produced 'a slavish dependence' upon state administration which now threatened the English principle of good government by shrivelling up the community's 'spirit of self-help'.[91]

Such publicly stated anxieties were doubly overstated. First, the *SMH*'s concerns about insufficient community self-help had more to do with its editors' wish to prompt greater civic engagement by the new urban marketplace elite than it had to do with a genuine resolve to encourage popular participation in government. Thus, too, did William Stead chide the Chicago business leadership for its 'indifference to the responsibilities and obligations of citizenship' and urge upon it the government of City Hall.[92] Editorials in the *SMH* expressed admiration for the progressive civic policies pursued in Birmingham once that city's business elite had stood for local office and had elected Joseph Chamberlain as mayor. Similar admiration was expressed for the London County Council. Subsequent administrative and electoral modifications to city and colonial government sought to entrench ultimate decision-making in the hands of the business elite and its professional allies. Second, the overstated rhetoric about the inherent dangers of centralization and compulsion set down unambiguously the perimeters of legitimate state interference in a *laissez-faire* society. Urban bourgeois culture defined state action in terms of guarantees for, not limitations upon, continuing private enterprise.

VII

Melbourne in 1888 celebrated the Centennial International Exhibition. The Exhibition celebrated 'marvellous Melbourne' and the British commercial system in which it was a cog. The Governor of Victoria formally opened the exhibition on behalf of the Queen, welcoming to 'the great metropolis of Victoria' representatives from the other Australian colonies so that together they could 'observe . . . the first centenary of British settlement upon this great continent . . . and . . . record . . . the progress that these colonies have made during their first centennial of life'.[93] The Governor also gladly acknowledged representatives from the governments of New Zealand, the USA, Germany, Belgium, France, and Austria. Their presence symbolized the imperial and international trading network upon which the prosperity of colonial port cities such as Melbourne and Sydney depended.The exhibits, coming 'from all parts of the world . . . emphasised strongly the great industrial resources of Great Britain and her colonies, and also afforded a striking exposition of the truth that interchange is one of the inevitable conditions of life'. The exhibits, by drawing upon 'the highest branches of art . . . science . . . [and] practical inventions', were also intended to 'teach what cultivated art and skilled science have done for the elevation and solace of man . . . [and to herald man's] further improvement and development'.[94]

The Exhibition, together with its elaborately contrived opening ceremonial, were organized by Melbourne's business-parliamentary leadership to project to a popular audience the continuing 'certainties' of material progress, of scientific achievement, of community, and of good government. In so doing, the Exhibition of 1888, like the smallpox crises of 1881–2, clearly expressed two relationships of economic and cultural power and dependency: by the mother country over its colonies, and by the emergent colonial urban bourgeois leadership over Australian social life. Colonial 'certainties', borrowed from the imperial centre, underscored the evolution in the colonies of class in proportion to the accumulation there of private capital. Melbourne's commercial leadership bought space in the celebratory two-volume centennial publication, *Victoria and its Metropolis*, to tell their individual stories of meritorious self-advancement in association with proliferating imperial trade.[95] Webs of significance that were spun by a dominant but still raw culture, their interpretations and prescriptions jarred continually with the social realities of *laissez-faire* economics in Australia, and with the competing interpretations which these generated. Standing juxtaposed to the carefully rehearsed statements about community and progress that were made in 1888, the reactions in Sydney and Melbourne to the smallpox emergencies of 1881–2 highlight the socio-cultural context and consequences of the political economy of empire in Australia.

NOTES

I am indebted to the following friends and colleagues for their constructive criticisms of earlier drafts of this paper: Stuart Macintyre, Roy MacLeod, Lloyd Robson, and Charles Sowerwine. My work was facilitated by the award of a social history writer's grant from the Division of Cultural Activities in the New South Wales Premier's Department.

1. N. Gould, *Town and Bush* (Harmondsworth: Penguin Colonial Facsimiles, 1974), 73.

2. See J.W. McCarty, 'Australian capital cities in the nineteenth century', in C.B. Schedvin and J.W. McCarty (eds), *Urbanization in Australia: the Nineteenth Century* (Sydney: Sydney University Press, 1974), 9–39; R.V. Jackson, *Australian Economic Development in the Nineteenth Century* (Canberra: Australian National University Press, 1977). See the analysis of the evolving capitalist world-economy in I. Wallerstein, *The Modern World-System II. Mercantilism and the Consolidation of the European World-Economy, 1600–1750* (New York: Academic Press, 1980); and I. Wallerstein, *The Capitalist World-Economy* (Cambridge: Cambridge University Press, 1979), part 1: 'The Inequalities of Core and Periphery'; and see the study of dependent capitalist development in nineteenth-century Australia by M. Berry, 'The Australian city in history: critique

and renewal', in L. Sandercock and M. Berry, *Urban Political Economy: The Australian Case* (Sydney: Allen & Unwin, 1983), 15-33. The capitalist market system and the urban network is analysed in D. Harvey, *Social Justice and the City* (London: Edward Arnold, 1973), ch. 6; and see K. Polanyi, *The Great Transformation* (New York: Octagon Books, 1975).

3. See R.W. Connell and T.H. Irving, *Class Structure in Australian History* (Melbourne: Longman Cheshire, 1980).

4. E. Burton, *Vistors' Guide to Sydney* (Sydney: William Maddock, 2nd edn, 1874), 32.

5. T.A. Coghlan, *The Wealth and Progress of New South Wales, 1886–87* (Sydney: NSW Government Printer, 1887), 248-9, 258–61.

6. *Australian Medical Journal, IV*, n.s. (15 August 1882), 373.

7. *Sydney Morning Herald* (hereafter *SMH*), 1 January 1870, 4; 26 January 1876, 6.

8. ibid., 4 July 1881, 4; 26 December 1876, 4.

9. *Daily Telegraph*, 15 June 1881, 2.

10. ibid., 29 July 1881, 2.

11. *Argus*, (Melbourne) 10 December 1881, 8. *Age*, (Melbourne) 24 August 1881, 2.

12. *Australian Medical Journal, III*, n.s. (15 September 1881), 411; *Argus*, 10 December 1881, 8.

13. *Age*, 27 January 1882, 2; *Argus*, 24 February 1882, 6.

14. See 'Report of the Board of Health upon the late epidemic of smallpox, 1881-2', *Votes & Proceedings of the Legislative Assembly of New South Wales*, 1883, vol. 2, 953–74; J.H.L. Cumpston, *The History of Smallpox in Australia, 1788–1908*, Quarantine Service Publication no. 3 (Melbourne: Government Printer, 1914). The Sydney epidemic receives detailed analysis in A.J.C. Mayne, 'Disease, sanitation and the "Lower Orders": perception and reality in Sydney, 1875–1881' (Unpublished PhD thesis, Australian National University, 1980), 284–312; and P.H. Curson, *Times of Crisis: Epidemics in Sydney 1788–1900* (Sydney: Sydney University Press, 1985), 90–119.

15. *Argus*, 13 July 1881, 5.

16. 'Opinions of medical men on compulsory vaccination', *Votes & Proceedings of the Legislative Assembly of New South Wales*, 1881, vol. 4, 1030.

17. *Australian Medical Journal, IV*, n.s. (15 May 1882), 209, 214.

18. *Australian Medical Journal, III*, n.s. (15 May 1881), 221; (15 July 1881), 313.

19. *Evening News*, 16 June 1881, 2.

20. Report of the Board of Health, n. 14 above, 961.

21. *Argus*, 30 August 1881, 4; 18 January 1882, 4.

22. Parkes Correspondence (Mitchell Library, Sydney), James Watson to Henry Parkes, 25 January 1882.

23. See Mayne, op. cit., n. 14 above, ch. 14.

24. *Daily Telegraph*, 18 June 1881, 4.

25. *SMH*, 19 August 1881, 4–5; *Daily Telegraph*, 22 December 1881, 2; see *British Medical Journal*, (4 December 1880), 892.

26. *SMH*, 27 June 1881, 4; 23 June 1881, 5; see A.J.C. Mayne, ' "The question of the poor" in the nineteenth-century city', *Historical Studies, 20*, (81) (1983), 557–73.

27. Report of the Board of Health, n. 14 above, 953.

28. See A.J.C. Mayne, *Fever, Squalor and Vice: Sanitation and Social Policy in Victorian Sydney* (St Lucia: University of Queensland Press, 1982).

29. *Evening News*, 23 August 1881, 3; *Daily Telegraph*, 11 August 1882, 2.

30. Sydney City Council, Letters Received, 1881, vol. 9, no. 1976 (Dr G.F. Dansey, 1 November 1881).

31. *Evening News*, 13 September 1881, 3. *SMH*, 27 July 1881, 3 (letter from Richard Seymour, Inspector of Nuisances); see the Minutes of Proceedings of the NSW Board

of Health (State Archives of NSW), 29 August 1881, 11 October 1881. The development of municipal slum clearance in Sydney is explored in Mayne, op. cit., n. 28 above.

32. *Argus*, 5 July 1881, 5.

33. *Daily Telegraph*, 18 June 1881, 4; *SMH*, 31 December 1881, 6.

34. Minutes of Proceedings of the NSW Board of Health, 20 December 1881, 3 February 1882; Parkes Correspondence, Watson to Parkes, 14 March 1882.

35. See: 3 Wm IV c. 1; see also J.H.L. Cumpston, D.G. Robertson, and J.S.C. Elkington, *Maritime Quarantine Administration*, Quarantine Service Publication no. 16, (Melbourne: Government Printer, 1919).

36. *Lancet*, (12 May 1866), i, 516.

37. *Lancet* (4 July 1874), i, 20; also (28 March 1868), i, 420; (14 January 1871), i, 63; (11 May 1872), i, 661–2; (18 April 1874), i, 554–5.

38. *British Medical Journal* (25 June 1881), i, 1020.

39. *British Medical Journal* (16 September 1882), ii, 520–1; (4 March 1882), ii, 314; (28 October 1882), ii, 859.

40. *Votes & Proceedings of the Legislative Assembly of New South Wales*, 1875–6, vol. 1, no. 138 (10 August 1876), 553.

41. *Age*, 4 January 1882, 6; also *Australian Medical Journal, II*, n.s. (15 December 1880), 553–4.

42. See, for example, *Votes & Proceedings of the Legislative Assembly of New South Wales*, 1875–6, vol. 1, no. 130 (27 July 1876), 513; Minutes of Proceedings of the NSW Board of Health, 10 August 1885, 15 December 1885.

43. *Victorian Government Gazette*, 1881, vol. 1, no. 57 (20 June 1881), 1775; Parkes Correspondence, J.G. Long Innes to Parkes, 17 June 1881; and see *SMH*, 23 July 1881, 5.

44. Minutes of Proceedings of the NSW Board of Health, 13 March 1888.

45. *Argus*, 30 August 1881, 4; 10 December 1881, 8.

46. *Victorian Government Gazette*, 1881, vol. 2, no. 78 (22 July 1881), 2161; also no. 69 (12 July 1881), 2067; *Echo*, 21 July 1881, 3.

47. *Age*, 27 January 1882, 2; see J. Bach, *A Maritime History of Australia* (Sydney: Pan Books, 1982), chs 7 and 8.

48. Minutes of Proceedings of the NSW Board of Health, 23 January 1882, 30 January 1882, 14 February 1882.

49. ibid., 19 August 1885; see Bach, op. cit., n. 47 above, 143.

50. ibid., 22 April 1886.

51. *NSW Parliamentary Debates*, vol. 14 (12 August 1884), 4832.

52. Minutes of Proceedings of the NSW Board of Health, 2 May 1884.

53. *SMH*, 1 June 1881, 4.

54. ibid., 17 June 1881, 4.

55. ibid., 6 August 1881, 4–5.

56. *Daily Telegraph*, 18 February 1882, 4.

57. See Mayne, op. cit., n. 14 above, 307–11.

58. *Evening News*, 14 June 1881, 3.

59. ibid., 16 August 1881, 2.

60. *Australasian Medical Gazette* (1 November 1881), 30.

61. *SMH*, 30 July 1881, 7.

62. *Daily Telegraph*, 8 August 1881, 3.

63. *British Medical Journal* (1880–2); see R.M. MacLeod, 'Law, medicine and public opinion in the resistance to compulsory health legislation 1870–1907', *Public Law*, part I (Spring 1967), 107–28; part II (Autumn 1967), 189–211; F.B. Smith, *The People's Health 1830–1910* (Canberra: Australian National University Press, 1979), 158–70.

64. *SMH*, 4 July 1881, 8; see *NSW Parliamentary Debates*, vol. 5 (4 August 1881), 478–9.

65. ibid., (31 August 1881), 883.

66. Minutes of Proceedings of the NSW Board of Health, 20 December 1881, 6 January 1882; Cumpston *et al.*, op. cit., no. 35 above, p. iii; see Michael Roe, *Nine Australian Progressives: Vitalism in Bourgeois Social Thought, 1890–1960* (St Lucia: University of Queensland Press, 1984), ch. 5.

67. *Australian Medical Journal, III,* n. s. (15 July 1881), 311–14; *Age*, 17 January 1882, Supplement, 1.

68. See *British Medical Journal* (1 January 1881), 24; (19 February 1881), 283–4; (5 March 1881), 351; (26 March 1881), 474–5; (16 July 1881), 91.

69. *NSW Parliamentary Debates*, vol. 2 (6 December 1881), 2411; *Argus*, 10 December 1881, 8; 21 January 1882, 8–9; *Age*, 20 January 1882, 3.

70. *Argus*, 10 October 1881, 4.

71. *SMH* 22 December 1890, 5.

72. ibid., 27 June 1881, 4.

73. *Daily Telegraph*, 10 August 1881, 5.

74. *SMH*, 25 January 1884, 7; see G. Davison, D. Dunstan, and C. McConville (eds), *The Outcasts of Melbourne: Essays in Social History* (Sydney: Allen & Unwin, 1985).

75. See Mayne, op. cit., n. 28 above, part 5.

76. *SMH*, 14 January 1884, 6.

77. *Report of the Royal Commission on Strikes* (Sydney: NSW Government Printer, 1891), Q. 670, 20; Q. 10592, 403; see J. Lee and C. Fahey, 'A boom for whom? Some developments in the Australian labour market, 1870–1891', *Labour History*, no. 50 (May 1986), 1–27.

78. See S.H. Fisher, 'The family and the Sydney economy in the late nineteenth century', in P. Grimshaw, C. McConville, and E. McEwen (eds), *Families in Colonial Australia* (Sydney: Allen & Unwin, 1985), 153–62; S.H. Fisher, 'An accumulation of misery?', *Labour History, no. 40* (May 1981), 16–28; M. Kelly, 'Picturesque and pestilential: the Sydney slum observed 1860–1900', in M. Kelly (ed.), *Nineteenth-Century Sydney* (Sydney: Sydney University Press, 1978), 66–80; A.J.C. Mayne, 'Commuter travel and class mobility in Sydney, 1858–88', *Australian Economic History Review, 21* (1) March 1981), 53–65; Mayne, op. cit., n. 28 above, ch. 1.

79. Mayne, op. cit., n. 26 above, 562–73.

80. Mayne, op. cit., n. 28 above, 176, 193–4; Mayne, op. cit., n. 14 above, 318–19, Appendices 9 and 10.

81. *SMH*, 27 July 1881, 3; Mayne, op. cit., n. 14 above, 301-2.

82. *Daily Telegraph*, 22 April 1882, 3.

83. *NSW Parliamentary Debates*, vol. 2 (15 December 1881), 2705–6; Petition of Julia Russell, in 'Report of the Board of Health', op. cit., n. 14 above, 975

84. *NSW Parliamentary Debates*, vol. 2 (15 December 1881), 2706; *Daily Telegraph*, 22 April 1882, 3, and 30 May 1882, 3.

85. 'Report of the Royal Commission on the management of the Quarantine Station', *Votes & Proceedings of the Legislative Assembly of New South Wales*, 1882, vol. 2, 1168.

86. *SMH*, 14 January 1884, 5; Mayne, op. cit., n. 28 above, ch. 9; Mayne, op. cit., n. 26 above, 562–8.

87. *Daily Telegraph*, 25 June 1881, 4.

88. *Argus*, 24 February 1882, 4–5.

89. *NSW Parliamentary Debates*, vol. 5 (1881), 815–60, 873–905; Mayne, op. cit., n. 14 above, 296–9, 303–7, 311–12.

90. *Argus*, 4 February 1882, 10; *Age*, 26 January 1882, 2.

91. *SMH*, 23 August 1881, 4; 1 July 1881, 4.

92. W.T. Stead, *If Christ Came to Chicago* (New York: Living Books, 1964), 95; C.W. Dilke, *Greater Britain: A Record of Travel in English-Speaking Countries during*

1866 And 1867 (London: Macmillan, any edition), part 3, ch. 5; A. Trollope, *Australia* ed. P.D. Edwards and R.B. Joyce (St Lucia: University of Queensland Press, 1967), 719–20.

93. *Official Record of the Centennial International Exhibition, Melbourne, 1888–1889* (Melbourne: Sands & McDougall, 1890), 206.

94. ibid., 210, 207.

95. A. Sutherland, *Victoria and its Metropolis: Past and Present*, 2 vols (Melbourne: McCarron, Bird, 1888).

12

Sleeping sickness, colonial medicine and imperialism: some connections in the Belgian Congo

Maryinez Lyons

'Legs were made for trousers.'
Dr Pangloss, in *Candide*

INTRODUCTION

In 1904, sleeping sickness was declared to be epidemic in some parts of the Congo Free State. This was the conclusion of a team of British scientists invited from the Liverpool School of Tropical Medicine to conduct a survey of health conditions in central Africa. They advised the state authorities to take immediate action to control the further spread of sleeping sickness. It was certainly not the first time the disease had been reported. The 'sleepy sickness' had been noted in the region in the early 1880s, and fresh outbreaks were confirmed by missionaries and travellers.[1] But, by 1901, a terrible epidemic had spread around the northern shores of Lake Victoria and neighbouring islands in the region of Busoga, in the neighbouring Uganda Protectorate.[2]

The declaration of an epidemic was a watershed in the history of public health for Africans in the Congo; for, more than any other one factor, sleeping sickness prompted the development of the Belgian colonial medical service.[3] This medical service was consciously used by the Belgians as a form of 'constructive imperialism', with which they hoped to establish European influence. The provision of health services was considered by the Belgians to be a central feature of what they called their 'civilizing mission' in Africa.

In discussing sleeping sickness in Africa in the early twentieth century, three points were to prove decisive. First, there was a direct link between sleeping sickness and the rapidly expanding new field of tropical medicine. Second, the epidemic in Uganda, which began in 1901, alarmed all the new colonial powers who feared the loss of potential labour forces. Finally, the European colonizers in Africa were aware of the propaganda potential of public health.

From the earliest days of colonial settlement, it had not been uncommon to find sleeping sickness cited as the cause of abandoned villages and depopulated regions which Europeans encountered during their push into the interior. By the end of the nineteenth century, both African and European observers believed that the disease had long been present in endemic form in some parts of Lower Congo; but in the 1880s and 1890s, the decades of colonial conquest, the disease had become progressively epidemic. While sleeping sickness was certainly a factor in demographic change, so was the withdrawal of peoples from troubled areas, including the major paths of communication along the rivers. It was along these routes that most European exploration and conquest took place. Often, it was not sleeping sickness itself but other causes which were responsible for the distress of African populations. In European medical thinking, epidemics were ascribed to the arrival in an area of people with the disease-causing pathogens, the trypanosomes, in their blood. But colonial Europeans disrupted African societies to the extent that the delicate balance of natural relationships between indigenous peoples and their disease-causing pathogens were thrown into chaos. Violent changes in the human ecology, including famine, exhaustion, and disease, resulted in increased stress and lowered resistance. When sleeping sickness came, the result for many Congolese was devastating.[4] By late 1902, the situation had become so critical that the Belgian Vice Governor-General of the Congo Free State, Felix Fuchs, warned of the need for urgent public health measures to combat the disease.[5]

TROPICAL MEDICINE IN THE MAKING

While public health was of relatively recent history in western Europe, the field of tropical medicine in 1902 was even more novel. The London and Liverpool Schools of Tropical Medicine had existed only since 1899, and Germany's *Institut für Schiffs und Tropenkrankheiten* was established in Hamburg in 1901, but Belgium did not establish its own school in Brussels until 1906. A new field of scientific endeavour, tropical medicine offered opportunities for bright young men to win international reputations. Thus the young English scientist, John Lancelot Todd, pleased by the opportunity to study sleeping sickness in the Congo Free State, informed his family in Canada: 'Tryps are a big thing and if we have luck, I may make a name yet!'[6] Research in this rapidly growing field took medical scientists far from their urban laboratories to 'exotic' regions of the globe and immersed them in the adventure of safari in the 'bush'. Partly for this reason, tropical medicine was glamorous and idealistic. One specialist found 'Negro lethargy, or the sleeping sickness of the Congo . . . a romantic disease, which provided a subject for graphic clinical descriptions'.[7] As *Punch* rhapsodized:

Men of Science, you that dare
Beard the microbe in his lair,
Tracking through the jungly thickness
Afric's germ of Sleeping Sickness,

Hear, oh hear my parting plea,
Send a microbe home to me![8]

Tropical medicine was also intellectually exciting. Successful researchers had to be open to experimentation, ingenious at problem-solving, and innovative in difficult climates — the 'stuff' of missionary medicine. As tropical medicine gradually became more specialized, it incorporated techniques and theories from a number of scientific disciplines. Investigators required knowledge of medical zoology, protozoology and parasitology, helminthology, entomology, bacteriology, chemistry, and haematology, in addition to traditional medicine and microscopy. In April 1898, Dr Patrick Manson published his manual, *Tropical Diseases*, which contained the first cogent discussion of what came to be known as 'Tropical Medicine' in the English-speaking world. Yet, as recently as 1939, H. Harold Scott admitted that there was still confusion over the definition of the term. Tropical medicine did not develop as a full medical speciality, and as time passed, its development took it further from mainstream western medicine.[9]

Most researchers concurred with the 'father of tropical medicine', Patrick Manson, that tropical diseases were those prevalent in warm climates. As they were often insect-borne parasitical diseases, climate and entomic forms became important pathogenic factors. The exemplar of tropical disease, according to Manson, was trypanosomiasis. But a few argued that many so-called 'tropical' diseases had occurred in previous ages in temperate climates — diseases such as malaria, cholera, plague, relapsing fever, leprosy, ankylostomiasis and other helminthic infestations, smallpox, and typhoid fever. This was, however, a more radical view held by few researchers within the British and European tropical medicine research network, and while it found more support by the 1920s, it has only recently again been seriously discussed. Supporters of this view maintain today that many diseases labelled 'tropical' are in reality diseases of poverty, and when socio-economic conditions are ameliorated, many of these 'exotic' diseases decrease and/or disappear.[10]

SLEEPING SICKNESS

If colonial administrators fretted about the effects of sleeping sickness upon potential labour supplies, the international scientific community wished to solve the tantalizing problem of a mysterious disease. The English scientist, Lieutenant Colonel David Bruce, who in Natal in 1896 had first seen a trypanosome in the blood of a horse, thus discovering the cause of *nagana*, or the animal form of trypanosomiasis, explained in 1908 that

> a few years before the opening up of the Congo territories and Uganda, [sleeping sickness] was looked on more as a pathological curiosity than a

> disease . . . the curiosity is that it *never* spread from sick slaves to their neighbours in America or anywhere else out of its home in West Africa.[11]

Sleeping sickness was a real 'social event', capturing as it did the imagination of colonial authorities in Africa in much the same way that AIDS has today alarmed governments throughout the world.[12]

The London and Liverpool Schools of Tropical Medicine responded by sending research expeditions to conduct studies of the diseases threatening colonial territories. Malaria was the first disease to evoke such a response, but with the news from Uganda, sleeping sickness soon dominated research calendars. The Liverpool School's Sixth Expedition, of 21 September 1901, consisted of Drs Joseph Everett Dutton and J.L. Todd who were sent to Gambia in West Africa to study trypanosomiasis. (At this time, they still doubted any connection between this condition and sleeping sickness.)[13] That expedition actually 'melded' into the School's Tenth Expedition to Senegambia, which began on 21 September 1902, and the Twelfth Expedition to the Congo Free State, beginning 13 September 1903. The London School of Tropical Medicine, under the direction of Manson, had first focused upon the study of malaria in India, and then turned to sleeping sickness in Uganda and later other British colonies, including Northern Rhodesia and Nigeria.

In July 1903, upon his return to England from the Senegambia Expedition, John Todd was amazed to find that what he and Dutton had considered to be 'their' parasite was being studied by so many other scientists. By that time, there was an air of urgency and competition.[14]

POLITICS AND COMMERCE IN TROPICAL MEDICINE

From the beginning, the field of tropical medicine, called 'colonial medicine' on the continent, involved questions both of science and of politics. The connection between medical science and economic development recurs in administrative documents in the Belgian Congo. As one researcher explained, 'the elucidation of [sleeping sickness] has a large bearing upon the development and prosperity of Africa'.[15] Ending such an epidemic disease would assure a fledgling colonial administration not only live labourers, but also international prestige.

Medical researchers were fully aware that 'the future of imperialism lay with the microscope'.[16] Later apologists for colonialism often pointed to the extension of western medicine as being one of the most positive aspects of their administrations. And it was recognized as a powerful asset. In 1924, Todd explained that 'Medicine is now more than the healing of the sick and the protection of the well. Through its control of disease, medicine has come to be a world factor of limitless power.'[17] Good health alone allowed Europeans, unlike their forebears, to be permanent visitors to the tropics.

Scientists and governments were not alone in expressing an interest in tropical

Map 12.1 Distribution of Sleeping Sickness in the Congo Free State, Liverpool Expedition, 1905

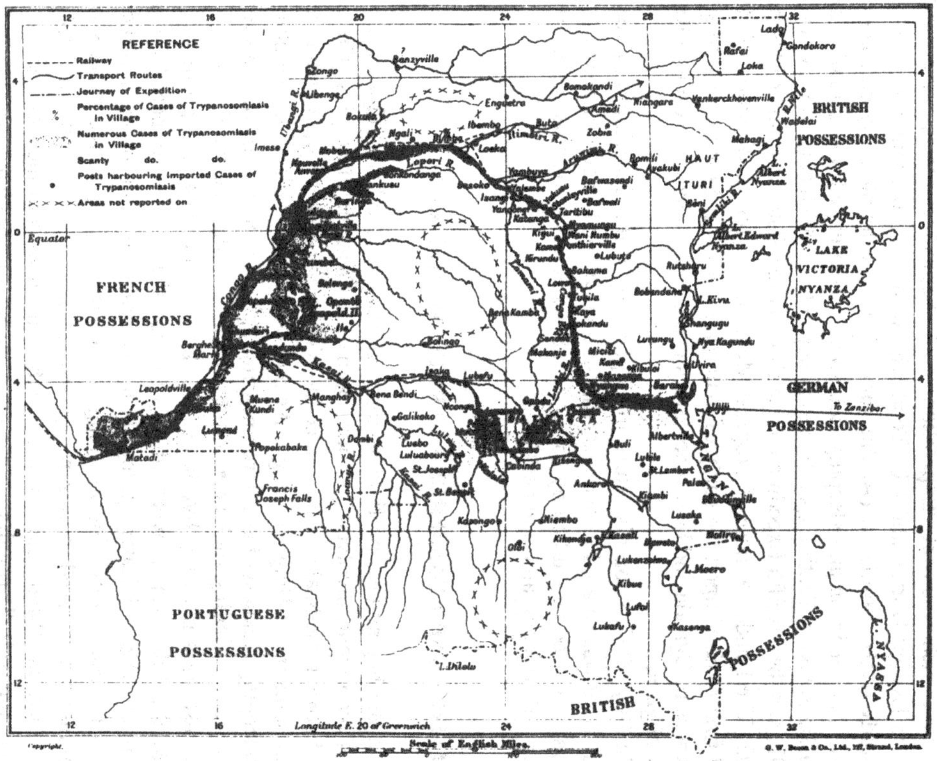

Source: Dutton, Dr J.E., and Todd, Dr J.L., *Memoir XVIII, Reports of the Expedition to the Congo 1903–5*, (March 1906).

medicine. Alfred Lewis Jones, Chairman of the Elder Dempster Shipping Line of Liverpool, was the principal founder and first chairman of the Board of the Liverpool School of Tropical Medicine from 1898 until his death in December 1909. Joseph Chamberlain, Secretary of State for the Colonies, made a plea on 25 May 1898 for the formation of schools in which to prepare colonial officers for the tropics. Jones was quick to respond and in November 1898 he offered the Royal Southern Hospital in Liverpool £350 per annum for three years to promote the special study of tropical disease. He said that 'money spent in our School of Tropical Medicine is an investment, and we expect dividends from it'.[18]

From its inception, the Liverpool School had very close relations with the city's commercial community which had, after all, played a central role in its formation. Jones was well acquainted with the Belgian King Leopold II, whom he called 'Great Chief', and Jones's shipping line was a major transporter of Congo products. His company, Compagnie belge du Congo, possessed the very profitable monopoly of the Congo-Antwerp trade. Chairman of the African section of the Liverpool Chamber of Commerce, Jones was also consul of the Congo Free State in Liverpool, and one of the leading defenders of the state during the great 'Red Rubber' scandal.[19] Edmond D. Morel, the founder and principal force behind the Congo Reform Association in England, said of Alfred Jones, 'Posterity will forget his attitude on the Congo and only remember that he was a powerful captain of industry, a man of great energy and the creator of the Liverpool School of Tropical Medicine.'[20]

THE UGANDA EPIDEMIC, 1899–1905

In the five years between the close of 1900 and the end of 1905, sleeping sickness killed over a quarter of a million Africans in the British Protectorate of Uganda. This tragedy sparked off one of the most dramatic chapters in the history of medicine. Near the end of 1900, Dr Albert R. Cook and his brother, Dr Jack Howard Cook, missionary doctors at the Church Missionary Society's station in Mengo (Kampala), Uganda, observed the first victims of a 'fever' which they soon informed the Ugandan authorities was sleeping sickness — it was, they added, spreading rapidly. Southern Busoga was soon considered the chief focus of the disease, and by the spring of 1902 local African chiefs reported that nearly 14,000 people had died.[21]

News in April 1902 from the Medical Officer at Jinja, Dr A.D.P. Hodges, that 20,000 people had died in the epidemic, increased alarm. The British Foreign Office, urged by Patrick Manson, had already asked the Royal Society to send a special commission to the Protectorate to study the disease.[22] A three-man team — composed of Aldo Castellani, George Carmichael Low and Cuthbert Christy — arrived at Kisumu in July 1902. On 15 October, Low was able to write to Manson informing him that young Castellani had spotted a 'fish-like parasite darting about', and that he believed 'a streptococcus, or an organism resembling it, to be the cause of the disease'.[23]

Combined with Dutton's discovery of the first trypanosome in human blood in December 1901 during the Liverpool School's Expedition to Gambia, Castellani's finding meant that the aetiology of human sleeping sickness was now understood for the first time. The British government took an early lead in sleeping sickness research, an understandable response to the potential threat to their human resources in Uganda. In fact, by 1902, sleeping sickness had become the most important administrative question in Uganda. Unaware at first of the complicated ecological nature of the disease, the British feared that it might spread along the Nile river, even to Suez. There were even fears that the disease might spread to India, with incalculable economic consequences.[24]

Over the next few decades, the Foreign Office, and later the Colonial Office, as well as both Schools of Tropical Medicine, were engaged in research projects and special commissions related to sleeping sickness. Especially important was the establishment of the Sleeping Sickness Bureau in London which collected and published the latest research on the disease. International conferences were held in which Britain, Belgium, France, Portugal, Germany, and Italy participated.[25] Both the Foreign Office and the Colonial Office sent questionnaires to a number of African territories in an effort to discover more about the disease.[26] In fact, it was the Foreign Office from which the Congo Free State government requested information about the disease in late 1902.[27]

From Busoga the disease spread rapidly east and west, and by the end of 1903 there were over 90,000 deaths.[28] By November 1904, it was epidemic as far west as the shores of Lake Albert, which bordered the Congo Free State. Official calculations of mortality rates varied, but, Bruce, a reliable witness, claimed that in Busoga, with a population of 300,000, as many as 200,000 had died! In 1905, one member of the Royal Society Commission estimated that in the past three years sleeping sickness had caused an annual mortality of 100,000 in Uganda.[29] Another reliable source, Brian Langlands, later asserted that between 1900 and 1920, deaths in Uganda from the disease rose to 250,000 and 330,000. All the colonial powers in Africa took note of events in Uganda. We will never know the total mortality for certain, but it is obvious why administrators of all African territories were alarmed.[30]

SLEEPING SICKNESS IN THE CONGO

Glossina palpalis is the particular species of tsetse-fly which transmits the *gambiense* form of sleeping sickness, which was responsible for the epidemics in Gambia and Uganda. Congo State authorities were well acquainted with the fly. It had been first mentioned in 1882 by Gaetano Casati, an Italian cartographer and explorer, while he was in the region which was later to become the Uele district in northern Congo Free State. He reported that 'Cattle cannot be successfully reared by the Mambettu [Mangbetu] on account of a fly called *tsetse*, the stings of which cause death.' And the eminent French parasitologist, Dr Emile Brumpt, accompanying the traveller, Bourg de Bozas, who followed the length of the Uele river in late 1902 and early 1903, had commented upon the ubiquitous *Gl. palpalis* along that river from the Congo State post of Dungu westwards.[31]

The Congo covers an enormous territory of 904, 756 square miles, nearly five times the size of France. The vast tropical rain forest surrounding the Congo river basin is bordered on its northern and southern sides by savannahs. The frontiers between the forest and savannahs are especially important in understanding the epidemiology of sleeping sickness in the Congo, for the *gambiense* form of human sleeping sickness is classically a disease of the 'frontier' in two senses.[32] This is because sleeping sickness is an example of an 'ecological disease'. Early researchers noted that understanding the total biota or ecosystem was crucial to any understanding of the pathology, aetiology, or epidemiology of this disease. The relationship of an individual to the entire ecosystem is a major factor in explaining why he does, or does not, contract the disease. *Gambiense* sleeping sickness typically occurs in transitional regions where forest melds into savannah, and because of the riverine habitat required by the vector of the parasite, the tsetse-fly, *Gl. palpalis*, sleeping sickness most often appears in well-watered areas. Another favoured habitat of this fly are the gallery forests which are long fingers of fringing forest occurring alongside the reaches of water which stretch from their sources in the forested areas out onto the savannahs.

Gambiense sleeping sickness is a 'frontier disease' in a second sense, in that it most often occurs in those regions at the *edges* of human settlement. It is quite literally the frontiers between these settlements and the sylvan forest which provide the ecological setting most likely to favour outbreaks of sleeping sickness. Flies, parasites and their hosts, man, and certain animals, each find suitable environments and, importantly, come into close and continued contact because of their shared need for water.[33]

At the turn of the century, most medical authorities held the view that epidemics of disease erupted under particular conditions; this was the notion of *circumstantial epidemiology*. Thus, after the discovery of the aetiology of the disease in 1902, it was believed that a region containing people, *Gl. palpalis*, and trypansomes, was circumstantially ideal for the outbreak of sleeping sickness. In part, this was accurate. At the same time, contemporary medical experts believed that for a given disease there was a proper medical response. Disease was an invader, medicine was the vanquisher. Experts responded by seeking and then combating the 'germ' with an appropriate weapon in the form of chemotherapy, or medicine. Congo State administrators believed that some regions, like the northern Uele district, with their still uninfected populations, frequent movements and the presence of *GL. palpalis*, were severely threatened and required prompt, preventive action.

SLEEPING SICKNESS AND PROPAGANDA

But there were other powerful motives, besides the purely medical, behind the response of the colonial powers. King Leopold II of Belgium, probably the most ambitious imperialist in Africa, had more than one motive for protecting the human capital in his private state.[34] After all, the Congo was very much his creation. In late 1903, some eighteen years after Leopold had founded his empire, John Todd described the position thus:

> The King of the Belgians is absolute sovereign here and this is not a Belgian colony in the proper sense of the word. The King of the Belgians made the state, and it is practically his. He must be a very smart man indeed to have made use of his position as a Ruler to so successfully exploit the country. He is boss of the state both as ruler and in the same way as some of the big mine owners out West are sovereigns of certain towns. . .[35]

At the invitation of Leopold, the Liverpool School sent an expedition to study sleeping sickness in the Congo Free State. This consisted of three experienced scientists, J.E. Dutton, J.L. Todd and Cuthbert Christy, who arrived at Boma in the autumn of 1903. Officially, the expedition remained eighteen months, although Christy left much earlier and Dutton died of 'tick' fever in February 1905. In these months, the entire length of the Congo river and most of the Lualaba were examined for the disease while more general observations were made on the sanitation of the state posts. The researchers relied upon written and oral reports for vast regions of the state, but in spite of these limitations their conclusions and advice to the Congo State authorities formed the basis of a public health programme for decades to come.[36]

Leopold established a precedent for later colonial administrations by insisting upon the importance of the new field of tropical medicine, medical provision, and public health policy as essential features in the justification, sometimes rationalization, of colonization. His decision to invite British scientists to investigate sleeping sickness in his state becomes explicable in this context. So, while diseased and dead Africans were an economic loss to all involved in the Congo adventure, Leopold had a second powerful motive for his quick response to the discovery of sleeping sickness. He intended to make the most of this opportunity to combat the increasingly effective anti-Congo Free State propaganda campaign being waged in England. In March 1900, E.D. Morel, an Englishman who had worked for Jones's shipping line since 1891, wrote a series of articles exposing the scandal of 'Red Rubber' in the Congo Free State. He publicized the shocking mistreatment by the state's agents of Congolese men, women, and children, who were driven without mercy to collect rubber. In 1902, Morel made a number of public speeches and published articles in Europe where his condemnation of the 'Leopoldian system' met enthusiastic response. His book, *Affairs of West Africa*, held Leopold personally responsible for these atrocities. On 20

May 1903, a debate in the British House of Commons on the 'Congo question' resulted in a resolution indicting the Congo Free State government. As a result, on 5 June 1903, the British Consul at Boma, Roger Casement, began a tour of Upper Congo to investigate the situation.[37] The resulting 'Casement Report' was submitted to the Foreign Office in December 1903, and a heavily revised version was sent to the Congo State in early February 1904. In March 1904, the Congo Reform Association was officially established. An increasingly effective lobby, this group successfully pressured the 'Leopoldian regime' for many years. The Association was dissolved in June 1913, some five years after the Congo Free State had passed into the jurisdiction of the Belgian government as a colony.[38]

It is clear that Leopold's invitation to the Liverpool School to investigate sleeping sickness was related to his concern for his international image. It is also clear that he knew the potential propaganda value of attending benevolently to an epidemic of sleeping sickness. It was an opportunity not only to prevent dangers to his labour force, but also to take part in a prestigious, international quest. After a visit to Leopold in August 1906, John Todd made this revelation in a letter to his family:

> After we'd finished telling the old man how to make the Congo healthy and promised to administer a lovely coat of whitewash to his character in the eyes of the English, he created Boyce, Ross and myself officers of his Order of Leopold II. . . We commenced yesterday what is intended to become quite a political move — an *entente cordiale* — a renewal of the intimacy of Belgium and England, which Congo jealousy has placed under a cloud.

This scientist had no doubts about the lively connection between health, economics and politics. He added:

> The anti-Congo papers will certainly say that they [funds allocated by Leopold to the Liverpool School] represent the bribe to the School (and myself in particular) for saying nothing concerning Congo atrocities and administering a lovely coat of whitewash to the Free State.[39]

THE EPIDEMICS

Sleeping sickness remained a major preoccupation of the Belgian government throughout the six decades of their occupation in the Congo. Epidemics killed thousands of people in the Congo basin, especially in parts of Kwango and Kasai, the Semliki valley in eastern Congo, the Ubangi river region, and the Gwane district in the north.[40] In addition, there were scores of foci of the disease scattered over the colony. By 1910, when the Congo Free State passed to the jurisdiction of the Belgian government and became a colony in the true sense of the word, it is believed there may have been several hundred thousand Congolese with sleeping sickness. But it would be another ten years before the state began to develop a special sleeping sickness service. The *équipes mobiles* designed by Dr Eugene Jamot of the French colonial medical service served as a model. Mobile teams of doctors, with European and African assistants, toured designated areas with the goal of examining every single man, woman, and child in order to identify all victims of the disease. A *cordon sanitaire* was established around infected areas and a strict system of medical passports evolved in the attempt to contain the 'germ'. Special clinics were established where Africans received series of trypanocidal injections.

In 1920, the state identified and treated 15,205 victims. The number had grown to 100,000 victims in 1925, the year when one and a half million examinations took place, and, it was estimated, 15 per cent of the population had been seen. Dr Jean Burke, a Belgian scientist with long experience and who still works with sleeping sickness in Zaire, gives 1930 as the peak of the Congo epidemics. In that year, the state medical service examined 3,000,000 people and treated 104,000. In 1940, 5,000,000 people were seen and in 1955 there were 6,600,000 examinations. By 1955 the number of victims, however, had fallen to 12,117. The total population of the colony in 1951 was 11,660,798, so from the point of view of sheer organizational skills, the sleeping sickness surveys were impressive. But what were the results?[41]

THE LEGACY

When their colonial venture came to an abrupt end in June 1960, the Belgians were convinced of the success of at least one aspect of their half century of administration in the Congo. They were confident that their medical service was outstanding in all of colonial Africa. Many agreed. For instance, in 1959 an American survey reported that the Belgian programme was one of the best on the continent, with more hospital beds in the Congo than in *all* the rest of tropical Africa.[42] Their approach to the control of sleeping sickness, unlike that of the British, had been the medicalization of the entire human reservoir. The Belgians were convinced that in the area of public health their paternalistic style of administration had been a resounding success, and they often pointed to the apparent near-victory over sleeping sickness as a clear example of that success.

Some twenty years earlier, in 1940, a medical administrator, Dr A. Duren, had explained that while improving the 'dreadful state of African health' had not been Leopold's primary motive for building an empire, it was still important to 'see medical provision . . . as a justification after the fact of colonisation'. He continued:

> it is a compensation offered to the natives for certain misfortunes that colonisation brought them . . . the spread of certain scourges, like the fearsome

> sleeping sickness, venereal diseases and the introduction of certain diseases like tuberculosis, are the consequence of our presence and the interactions [among peoples] which we made possible.

Duren argued that 'medical action is thus an obligation created for the white man by colonisation'. It was Duren's opinion that the Congolese were 'indebted to colonisation' for the gift of European medicine and medical services.[43]

But was Belgian colonization a blessing for the health of the Congolese? Or was colonial health provision a powerful tool for the domination and control of African peoples which outweighed, even negated, the medical advantages, as Martin Shapiro contends was the case in Portuguese Africa? Was the cost too high, as Frantz Fanon has asserted?[44] It has been said that 'apologists for colonialism often look myopically at the medical services, proclaim their humanity and even argue that their philosophy ran counter to that of imperialism'. Another goes further, insisting that colonial doctors were, in fact, 'medical operatives', or agents of imperialism.[45] These are serious criticisms. Early this century, the Congolese suffered a series of tumultuous upheavals which profoundly altered their social and ecological relationships. One result of the colonization of the Belgian Congo was the exacerbation of endemic sleeping sickness, which became epidemic in large areas and killed thousands of people. To use the establishment of the medical service as a justification after the fact, is simply to apply another 'coat of whitewash' to the politics of medicine in the service of empire.

NOTES

This paper was first presented at the annual conference of the Society for the Social History of Medicine at Birmingham on 11 April 1985.

1. *La Belgique coloniale* (26 June 1898), 305–7; *Le Mouvement géographique* (25 August 1901), 442; Brussels, Ministère des Affaires Etrangères, Archives Africaines (hereafter MAEAA), Service de l'Inspecteur Général de l'Hygiène, 846.34, Dr Catherine Mabie, Mbanza Manteke, District des Cataractes. Response to Royal Society questionnaire on sleeping sickness, August 1903; MAEAA 846.34, Dr A. Sims, Matadi. Response to questionnaire, 11 August 1903; MAEAA 846.34, Rev. Peder Frederickson, American Baptist Missionary Union, Madimba District. Stanley Pool (Kitwa). Response, September 1903.

2. London School of Tropical Hygiene and Medicine, Library Archives, Correspondence of Dr George Carmichael Low to Patrick Manson, Director of the School, June-October 1902; Wellcome Institute for the History of Medicine, Contemporary Archives Centre, Lt. Col. A.E. Hamerton, MSS Notebook and photo-album while serving on Sleeping Sickness Commission, 1908–1910; Royal Commonwealth Society, Library Archives, Cuthbert Christy Papers, MSS Notebooks of Royal Society Commission Expedition to Uganda, 10 June 1902–12 April 1903; Wellcome Tropical Institute, Library Archives, A.J. Duggan papers, Correspondence *re* Ugandan epidemic and C. Christy, 8 October 1902–27 May 1903; Wellcome Tropical Institute, Library Archives, G. Hale Carpenter MS 'History of sleeping sickness in Uganda', 13 August 1924.

3. D.J. Bradley, 'The situation and the response', in E.E. Sabben-Clare *et al.* (eds), *Health in Tropical Africa during the Colonial Period* (Oxford: Clarendon Press, 1980), 9.

4. John Ford, 'Ideas which have influenced attempts to solve the problem of African trypanosomiasis', *Social Science and Medicine, 13B* (1979), 272.

5. MAEAA 846.1, Vice Governor-General Felix Fuchs to Secretary of State C. Liebrechts, 4 November 1902.

6. Bridget Todd Fialkowski (compiler and editor), *John L. Todd 1876–1949 Letters* (Senneville, Quebec: privately printed and circulated, 1977), letter to brother, 8 July 1903.

7. P.E.C. Manson-Bahr, *The History of the School of Tropical Medicine in London (1899–1949)* (London: H.K. Lewis, 1956), 9.

8. 'Lines by an Insomniac', *Punch* (16 September 1903), 185.

9. H. Harold Scott, *A History of Tropical Medicine*, 2 vols (London: Edward Arnold & Co., 1939); Michael Worboys, 'Tropical medicine and imperialism, 1895–1914', in 'Science and British colonial imperialism, 1895–1940' (Unpublished D.Phil thesis, University of Sussex, 1979, 127).

10. Lesley Doyal and I. Rennell, *The Political Economy of Health* (London: Pluto Press, 1979); Meredeth Turshen, *The Political Ecology of Disease in Tanzania* (New Brunswick, N.J.: Rutgers University Press, 1984); Michael Worboys; 'The "discovery" of colonial malnutrition: the colonial problem as a technical problem', in Worboys, op. cit., n. 9 above.

11. David Bruce, 'Sleeping sickness in Africa', *Journal of the African Society, 7* (1908), 249. The parasite which Bruce observed was named in his honour *T. brucei*.

12. A.J. Duggan, Director of the Wellcome Museum of Medical Science (retired), personal interview, 9 August 1983; Evan Stark, 'The epidemic as a social event', *International Journal of Health Services, 7* (1977), 681–705.

13. Fialkowski, op. cit., n. 6 above; Todd to brother, Bert, 8 July 1903.

14. ibid., Todd to mother, 13 July 1903.

15. Dr Louis Sambon, quoted in 'Tropical medicine and the Congo state', *West Africa* (22 August 1905), 195.

16. London School of Tropical Hygiene and Medicine, Library Archives, J.L. Todd, 'Tropical medicine, 1898–1924', n.d., 25th year Commemorative Talk for the United Fruit Company.

17. Gladys Philips (comp.), 'Historical Record, 1920–47' (Unpublished typescript, no date, in the Liverpool School of Tropical Medicine Library); J.L. Todd, ibid; B.G. Maegraith, 'History of the Liverpool School of Tropical Medicine', *Medical History, 16* (1972), 354–68; M.F. Lechat, 'L'Expédition Dutton-Todd au Congo 1903–05, de Boma à Coquilhatville, septembre 1903 — juillet 1904', *Annales des Sociétés Belges de Médecine Tropicale, de Parasitologie et de Mycologie, 44* (1964), 493–512.

18. W. Roger Louis and Jean Stengers (eds), *E.D. Morel's History of the Congo Reform Movement* (Oxford: Clarendon Press, 1968); MAEAA 847.356, A.L. Jones to Secretary of State, Liebriechts, 13 January 1908; E.D. Morel, *Red Rubber* (London: T. Fisher Unwin, 1906); E.D. Morel, *Great Britain and the Congo* (London: Smith, Elder, 1909); Robert Harms, 'The end of Red Rubber: a reassessment', *Journal of African History, XVI* (1975), 73–88.

19. S.J.S. Cookey, *Britain and the Congo Question 1885–1913* (New York: Humanities Press, 1968), 94–8.

20. Louis and Stengers, op. cit., n. 18 above, 50.

21. Cuthbert Christy, 'Sleeping sickness', *Journal of the African Society, 3* (1903), 4. He gave 20,000 dead. Harvey G. Soff, 'A history of sleeping sickness in Uganda' (Unpublished PhD thesis, Syracuse University, 1971), 21, 30–1. Soff explains that the statistics provided by the African chiefs showed the mortality in Busoga as 13,565 but the Commissioner, Colonel James Hayes Sadler, agreed with the Sub-Commissioner that

this figure represented only the confirmed deaths and that, in fact, 20,000 was most likely a 'low estimate' of the actual deaths.

22. Christy, op. cit., n. 21 above, 1–11; Soff, op. cit., n. 21 above, 27; John Eyers, 'A.D.P. Hodges and early scientific medicine in Uganda, 1898–1918: with a select bibliography on the early history of sleeping sickness in Uganda, 1900–1920' (Unpublished MA thesis, Loughborough University of Technology, 1982), 27.

23. Wellcome Tropical Institute (Library Archives), G.C. Low to Royal Society, 15 October 1902, Castellani had found the 'germ' causing the disease. See London School of Tropical Hygiene and Medicine (Library Archives), G.C. Low, Entebbe, to P. Manson, 15 October 1902; A. Castellani, 'Etiology of sleeping sickness', *British Medical Journal* (14 March 1903) (i) 617–18.

24. Soff, op. cit., n. 21 above, 24; On the fears for India, see Wellcome Tropical Institute (Library Archives), A.J. Duggan Papers, A.C.H. Gray, Sleeping Sickness Laboratory, Entebbe, to Col. Bruce, 15 March 1903; Lt.-Col. Bruce, Sleeping Sickness Commission, Uganda, to H.M. Commissioner-General, British East Africa, 30 June 1903.

25. The Sleeping Sickness Bureau was initiated by Lord Elgin, Secretary of State for the Colonies, and was housed temporarily at the Royal Society in 1908. From then until 1912, it issued a large number of important *Bulletins* on sleeping sickness, but in 1912, having broadened its scope to tropical diseases, it moved to the new Imperial Institute and changed its name to the Tropical Diseases Bureau. Since that time, it has published the extremely important abstracting journal, *Tropical Diseases Bulletin*. In 1926, the organization became the Bureau of Hygiene and Tropical Disease.

26. Wellcome Tropical Institute (Library Archives), Minutes of Meeting of Royal Society Malaria and Tsetse Fly Committee, 12 May 1903.

27. Wellcome Tropical Institute (Library Archives), Minutes of Meeting of the Malaria Committee, 5 December 1902.

28. G.D. Hale Carpenter, *A Naturalist on Lake Victoria with an Account of Sleeping Sickness and the Tsetse Fly* (London: T. Fisher Unwin, 1920), 7

29. D. Bruce, 'Sleeping sickness in Africa', *Journal of the African Society, 7* (1908), 251; Dr Nabarro quoted in J.L. Todd, 'The distribution, spread and prophylaxis of "sleeping sickness" in the Congo Free State', *Transactions of the Epidemiological Society of London, 25* (1905–6), 23.

30. B.W. Langlands, 'The sleeping sickness epidemic of Uganda 1900–1920', paper presented to World Health Organization course in parasitology, Makerere University College, May 1967; Wellcome Institute for the History of Medicine (Library Archives), Western Manuscripts Collection, MSS. 2268, Expedition Diary. J.L. Todd was informed on 23 April 1905 by Major E. Wangermée of the Congo Free State that within four years about 250,000 Africans had died around Entebbe. Dutton and Todd believed that most of the recent figures of deaths in both the Congo Free State and Uganda only approximated the truth because about 30 to 50 per cent of the population in many villages had trypanosomes and only a small number could be expected to recover. Therefore, one-third of the population would probably die. (J.E. Dutton and J.L. Todd, 'The distribution and spread of "sleeping sickness" in the Congo Free State with suggestions on prophylaxis. Being the Fourth Progress Report from the Expedition of the Liverpool School of Tropical Medicine to the Congo, 1903–05', Liverpool School of Tropical Medicine, *Memoir XVIII* (March 1906)). For the early demography of Uganda, see David W. Cohen, *The Historical Tradition of Busoga* (Oxford: Clarendon Press, 1972). Cohen asserts that the most important causes of the tremendous demographic upheavals in Busoga during the colonial period were famines and epidemics. The sleeping sickness epidemic continued in full force until 1910 and 'as a result, the most densely populated region of Busoga, the homeland of perhaps 200,000 persons in the late nineteenth century, was totally cleared of population in ten years' (24–5).

31. Robert du Bourg de Bozas, *Mission scientifique du Bourg de Bozas de la Mer Rouge à l'Atlantique à travers l'Afrique tropicale (Octobre 1900 — Mai 1903)* (Paris: F.R. de Rudeval, 1906), 404; A. Laveran and F. Mesnil, *Trypanosomes et trypanosomiases* (Paris: Masson, 2nd edn, 1912); G. Casati, *Ten Years in Equatoria* (London: Frederick Warne, 1891), 234.

32. J. Van Riel and P.G. Janssens, 'Lutte contre les endemo-epidemies', in *Livre Blanc, 2* (Brussels, Académie Royale des Sciences d'Outre-Mer, 1962); C. Lucasse, 'Control of human sleeping sickness at present times', *Annales de la Société Belge de Médecine Tropicale, 44* (1964), 287.

33. Brian W. Langlands, 'The sleeping sickness epidemic of Uganda 1900–1920: a study in historical geography', paper presented to the World Health Organization course in Parasitology at Makerere University College (May 1967); M.T. Ashcroft, 'A critical review of the epidemiology of human trypanosomiasis in Africa', *Tropical Diseases Bulletin, 56* (1959), 1073–93; Professor P.G. Janssens, personal interviews at Antwerp and Brussels, 10 April 1982, 20 July 1982 and 11 April 1984.

34. J.S. Galbraith, 'Gordon, MacKinnon and Leopold: the Scramble for Africa, 1876–84', *Victorian Studies, 14* (1971), 373.

35. Fialkowski, op. cit., n. 6 above; Todd to family, 2 October 1903.

36. Dutton and Todd, op. cit., n. 30 above, 25–38; MAEAA 847.143, Todd to Dr Van Campenhout, Department of Colonial Hygiene, Brussels, 23 April 1906.

37. Louis and Stengers, op. cit., n. 18 above, 158–68.

38. D. Vangroenweghe and J.L. Vellut (eds), 'Le Rapport Casement', *Enquêtes et documents, 6* (1985).

39. Fialkowski, op. cit., n. 6 above; Todd, 23 August 1906 and 27 August 1906.

40. See map, p. 246.

41. Jean Burke, 'Historique de la lutte contre la maladie du sommeil au Congo', *Annales de la Société Belge de Médecine Tropicale, 51* (1971), 468–73. The Bureau Centrale de la Trypanosomiase, established by presidential ordinance in 1968, continued the sleeping sickness surveys with thirty mobile teams specified for six endemic zones in Zaire. See Lord Hailey, *An African Survey. Revised 1956* (London: Oxford University Press, 1957), 143.

42. Foreign Area Studies Division, Washington D.C., *Area Handbook for the Republic of the Congo (Leopoldville)* (Washington, D.C.: Government Printer, 1952), 238.

43. MAEAA 4389.1090, Dr A Duren, 'Etat sanitaire des populations de Congo avant sa colonisation par la Belgique', 19 November 1943.

44. Martin Shapiro, 'Medicine in the service of colonialism' (Unpublished PhD thesis, University of California, Los Angeles, 1983); Frantz Fanon, 'Medicine and colonialism', in J. Ehrenreich (ed.), *The Cultural Crisis of Modern Medicine* (New York: Monthly Review Press, 1978), 229–51.

45. Turshen, op. cit., n. 10 above, 5. Jim Paul, 'Medicine and imperialism in Morocco', *Middle East Research Information Project (MERIP), 60* (1977), 3–12.

13

Typhus and social control: South Africa, 1917–50

Shula Marks and Neil Andersson

INTRODUCTION

In the early 1980s, epidemics of cholera and typhoid raged in the South African Bantustans.[1] Hundreds of people were known to have died from cholera alone, and probably more than 100,000 were affected. When the first cholera outbreak came to public attention, it was received with near-hysteria by the press, which predicted that it would soon affect 'white' Durban, or even Johannesburg and Pretoria. By and large the South African government was less perturbed and successfully covered up the nature and incidence of the epidemics, especially once it was realized that cholera and typhoid, like the other diseases of poverty, could be safely confined to the rural Bantustans. According to Dr G. de Klerk, head of the Medical Association of South Africa, South Africa's health services were the best in the world; the spread of epidemics in South Africa could therefore be blamed on the breakdown of health services in the neighbouring black states.[2]

Despite the fact that cholera, newly recognized as an epidemic disease in South Africa in 1980 and now endemic in at least five of the Bantustans, is more widespread than ever, it receives very little publicity.[3] The Department of Health and Welfare prefers not to describe the spread of cholera between 1980 and 1983 as a single epidemic, but as two separate ones, probably because that way the full impact of the figures is not felt immediately. Even so, official figures have been few and far between and those which have been cited have been greeted with scepticism by the medical profession: most doctors put the numbers at five times the official figures wherever these have been quoted. Through a manipulation of the statistics and by the political sleight of hand which declares that the 'Bantustans' are not part of South Africa, the extent of the epidemics could be minimized and responsibility sloughed off. In 1982, a member of the Provincial Executive Council in charge of hospital services in Natal disputed the official estimate of cholera cases in that province as 12,000: 'This figure is unrealistic. A more likely estimate is 60,000. For heaven's sake, when things go wrong why don't they say so instead of covering up?'[4]

The state's attempt to cover up news of the cholera epidemic was less than convincing. Headlines in virtually every South African newspaper chronicled the spread of the epidemic, despite the attempts to muzzle doctors communicating with the press. Nurses in rural areas told reporters of numerous and unrecorded backyard burials after people died of rapid dehydration, before they could be taken to a clinic or seen by a doctor. But while stories poured in daily of the devastation caused by cholera, health authorities first tried to blame the deaths on gastroenteritis and, when that failed, to keep quiet about the figures. According to a Department of Health and Welfare representative, the Minister of Health, Dr Lapa Munnik, 'decided several months ago that there was no point in providing the press with death rates on cholera any longer. But you can take my word for it,' she said, 'cholera is definitely on the wane and that's also why we no longer find it necessary to issue press releases of the exact figures.'[5]

The issues were clearly stated by Professor Gerry Coovadia, then Associate Professor of Paediatrics and Child Health in the Natal Medical School, when he said,

> Cholera is only a different shade on the canvas of ill-health. The cause of cholera is not to be found in biology, but in poverty. Inadequate and non-existent sanitation and the lack of piped clean water are the immediate causes of the spread of the disease. But the roots of cholera lie in an unequal distribution of resources — too much for some, very little or next to nothing for others. Many of us have been saying for years now that serious diseases which are preventible have been among black South Africans all the time.[6]

The cholera epidemic demonstrates graphically the failure of the state to provide sanitation and clean water supplies in the rural areas of South Africa. Despite a certain panic when it seemed as though cholera might cross the lines into 'white' towns, the state has been able to take its *laissez-faire* attitude because the epidemics have remained amongst South Africa's 'surplus population' within the borders of the Bantustans. The diseases of poverty have been successfully confined to the black and the poor.

Cholera in 1982 also put the spotlight on other diseases and the lack of basic facilities in the rural areas. Thus, the number of typhoid cases notified has remained more or less constant over the years: between 3,000 and 4,000 cases in the early 1980s.[7] Even one case of this disease in other developed countries is regarded as a public health failure. Yet it is commonly accepted that only about 10 per cent of all typhoid cases find their way into government records. These are alarming figures, for a disease which is supposed to be a 'thing of the past'. For blacks, typhoid is now as much a part of life as are mass removals. It is only when the disease encroaches on the 'white preserve' that it causes an uproar: thus it was declared an 'epidemic' recently and taken up by the national press when five black inmates of Weskoppies Mental Hospital in Pretoria were diagnosed as suffering from typhoid.[8]

In many ways, epidemics highlight the nature of power relations in society in the same way as heightened popular militancy serves to reveal social structures, processes, and actors normally shrouded in darkness. The better-than-average reporting which is occasioned by the outbreak of 'abnormal' and frightening levels of disease often serves to illuminate the more routine and endemic killers: the epidemic may well be the tip of the iceberg which leads to a better understanding of the major killers. While the officially recognized epidemics may not be these 'major killers' — at least since bubonic plague and smallpox no longer destroy vast numbers and major killers like tuberculosis and malnutrition are seldom recognized as epidemics — the outbreak of epidemics reveal the concerns of the state and the ruling class in society, both with their own safety and with the reproduction of the labour force. As Roderick McGrew has remarked in relation to cholera in Russia, 'Epidemics do not create abnormal situations'; they sharpen existing behaviour patterns which 'betray deeply rooted and continuing social imbalances'.[9]

In South Africa, since the late nineteenth century, the outbreak of 'epidemics' amongst whites has elicited a public health and social welfare response, in line with the development of public health policies in the United Kingdom and the 'white' dominions. As in the latter, from the second half of the nineteenth century, the usual quarantine measures against imported infections were taken at the ports. In the British colony of Natal in particular, the spread of bubonic plague from the East led to recurrent draconian measures at the ports, especially in Durban with its large Asian indentured population. From the last third of the nineteenth century, however, it was the fear of disease transmitted not across the seas but across land, from impoverished blacks moving from the countryside to the urban areas in search of work, which was to prove a far more potent spur to public health interventions.

From the time of South Africa's mineral discoveries in the last third of the nineteenth century, fears that epidemic disease 'would know no colour bar' and thus threaten whites, or that it would interfere with the reproduction of the labour force, lay behind much public health legislation and state intervention. The presence in South Africa of a conquered and colonized black working class led to the development of policies of racial segregation that also served as a public health strategy to protect white settlers. In the early twentieth century, public health officials were in the forefront of the demand for urban residential segregation. For blacks the experience of public health was, by and large, authoritarian and repressive. As in the rest of colonial Africa, the state intervened when there was danger of disease spreading to the white settlers, and was relatively unconcerned when there was not.

HISTORICAL PRECEDENTS

South Africa's contemporary health pattern is rooted in the social changes which began with the discovery of minerals in the last third of the nineteenth century:

diamonds in Kimberley in 1868, vast seams of gold at very deep levels underground on the Witwatersrand in 1886. The industrial and agrarian revolution which followed the development of the mining industry, the new concentrations of population on the mines and in the rapidly developing towns and the special hazards of the mining operations as well as growing impoverishment in the countryside were to have swift and grave implications for the physical well-being of workers, both black and white.[10]

Until the mineral discoveries, medical services were undeveloped in the colonies, republics and African kingdoms which co-existed uneasily south of the Limpopo. Africans were largely dependent on the ministrations of traditional healers and the patent medicines brought by missionaries; in the Afrikaner South African Republic (Transvaal) there were fewer than thirty medical practitioners, trained mainly in the United Kingdom. The British colony of the Cape had the most established medical profession. The vast majority were private practitioners who had trained in Britain and were registered with the British General Medical Council. The private medical practitioner has remained at the centre of personal health services for whites in the region to the present.

From 1828 certain private practitioners who had been appointed previously on an *ad hoc* basis by local magistrates as district surgeons were now appointed by the colonial state; they were expected to attend police officers, prisoners, convicts and paupers, prescribe and sell medicines, and vaccinate. According to E.H. Burrows, 'This was the begining of rural public health at the Cape.'[11] Elsewhere, the establishment of rural public health followed far later. In the British colony, Natal, district surgeoncies followed in the wake of the establishment of the sugar plantations in the late 1850s and 1860s. In the Orange Free State the State President was given power to appoint district surgeons in 1866 and the first hospital was established in 1877. In the South African Republic, there were only three district surgeons on the Cape model in 1887, the year after gold was discovered on the Witwatersrand, when a Sanitary Committee with its own inspector was appointed.[12]

With the mineral discoveries, new concentrations of population and the development of a migrant labour system drawing vast numbers of rural Africans into the urban areas led to the development of new methods of health control. The Cape was the first to set up a Public Health Department in 1897, although by then the Witwatersrand's Sanitary Committee had considerably elaborated its functions, in part as a result of the outbreak of smallpox on the Rand in 1893. It was only after the South African War (1899–1902) that the British administration in the conquered Boer Republics began to organize public health in the interior on the late-nineteenth-century British model. By the first decade of the twentieth century most towns in South Africa had municipal medical officers of health on the British model, as well as hospitals for infectious diseases, which were a municipal responsibility.

The Act of Union which brought the four colonies and ex-republics together in a political union in 1910 did not attempt to unify the varied health services and measures in the region. The statutes of the old colonies became the statutes of the respective provinces, and all the Provinces therefore inherited certain health responsibilities. Public health as such was not mentioned in the constitution. In practice, general hospitals were subject to the control of the provinces which followed the pre-1910 political divisions, while infectious diseases and sanitation remained the responsibility of municipalities. 'The isolation and treatment of cases of formidable contagious diseases mostly devolved on the Union Government', although it was only in 1919 when the first Public Health Act was passed in response to the influenza epidemic that a Department of Public Health with its own Minister was established.[13] It had general responsibility for non-personal health services in the four provinces, as well as for mental, leprosy and most tuberculosis hospitals and institutions, although the provinces and municipalities retained their earlier control over general and infectious hospitals respectively.

The 1919 Act also attempted to co-ordinate the public health legislation of the four provinces, repealed outdated statutes, and established a legislative code 'for the control of infectious diseases and environmental sanitation', placing primary responsibility for the public health on local authorities. Nevertheless, the three-tiered system remained and, according to the 1944 National Health Services Commission which tried unsuccessfully to rationalize it, 'from the very outset there was overlapping and confusion of responsibilities; each layer of public authority had some responsibility for public health, for hospitals and other health matters'.[14] It endorsed the views of the then President of the South African Medical Association when he castigated it as a ' "crazy patchwork" of public medical services, determined not by scientific principle but by the accidents of constitutional development in South Africa'.[15] In the control of 'formidable contagious disease' (a matter of statutory definition and notification), tensions were replicated between these different authorities, jealous of their powers, as we shall see, by tensions between the Department of Public Health with its ethos of social responsibility and social control and other departments of state — such as Native Affairs, Railways and Justice, which operated with very different imperatives.

THE SMALLPOX WAR IN THE CAPE COLONY

That the Cape Colony should have been the first to formulate a public health policy is not surprising. By far the largest, most prosperous and most populous of the four white-dominated colonies and republics in South Africa in the late nineteenth century, it was also most closely tied to the metropole. A major impetus to the formulation of a public health policy there was given by the outbreak of smallpox on the Kimberley diamond fields.[16] Then as now, what constituted an epidemic was to be defined by the ruling class. On that occasion, however, it was not the state but the mine magnates and the dependent medical profession, unrestrained by civil society, that played the main role in what became known as the 'smallpox war'.

In May 1882, smallpox broke out in the Cape Peninsula. Fearing the effects on the labour force if it spread to Kimberley, the British-trained private practitioners engaged by Cecil John Rhodes — already a leading mine magnate and well-known Cape politician and later to become the renowned imperial statesman — subjected anyone entering the Diggings from the Cape Peninsula to physical examination. They set up a quarantine station at the junction of the Modder and the Riet Rivers about 30 miles south of Kimberley and wholly illegally barred the highroad. Local police were stationed at the fords across the rivers to divert travellers, if necessary by force, to the quarantine station. There they had to provide evidence that they had been vaccinated, and then to undergo three minutes' disinfection in a fumigation chamber: a closed shed filled with the fumes of burning sulphur. Despite the protests of the genteel, and the charges of assault brought against the doctor and his police at the station, no smallpox got through to Kimberley from the south. Hijacking travellers for fumigation at the expense and behest of the mining companies was to provide a useful precedent for the South African state after its formation in 1910.

Although smallpox was controlled from the south, however, the mining companies made no effort to control Africans entering Kimberley from the north. In October 1883, smallpox was discovered in a party of labourers on their way from Mozambique through the Transvaal to the diamond mines. Three Transvaal doctors, qualified in Britain, who were unwilling to cause alarm, diagnosed the disease as acute chickenpox, and the party continued on its way. It finally came to rest considerably depleted by death some 9 miles from Kimberley on Felstead's farm. There, the magistrate appointed a commission of six British-trained private medical practitioners. Three of them, led by Rhodes's close colleague, Leander Starr Jameson (later to be the first Resident Commissioner of Rhodesia, leader of the disastrous filibustering campaign into the Transvaal which bears his name, and Prime Minister of the Cape Colony) denied that it was smallpox; the others were equally convinced that it was. As it rampaged through Kimberley, the medical men were bitterly divided, with those most dependent on the mines swearing that the disease from which considerable numbers were now dying was not smallpox but 'Felstead's disease' (after the farm on which the original sufferers died), the 'Transvaal disease', 'Kaffir pox', or 'a bullous disease allied to pemphigus' — anything but smallpox. The battle in the medical fraternity raged for some months, although even those doctors who refused to recognize the disease as smallpox vaccinated their patients as a 'precautionary measure'.

As Rob Turrell has remarked, the controversy

> turned on the politics of death. The issues were fairly stark and the moral question clear. On the one hand, knowledge that small-pox existed in Kimberley threatened to cut the mines off from crucial supplies of wood, wheat and labour . . . On the other hand, if the epidemic was called its rightful name, lives would be saved through preventive measures.[17]

As the Prime Minister put it in the Cape parliament, some medical men 'had declared the disease not smallpox lest the result should be injurious to the mining interest'.[18] It was in response to this situation that the Cape colonial legislature passed as a matter of emergency its Public Health Act of 1883. This made vaccination compulsory in the Cape Colony for the first time, and made wide-scale vaccination on the fields and adequate quarantine measures possible. In 1893 compulsory notification of infectious diseases was introduced in the Cape and together these Acts which were based on British precedents provided the basis for subsequent South Africa-wide public health legislation.[19]

Events in Kimberley between 1882 and 1885 provide two major themes in South Africa's subsequent handling of epidemic disease: drastic intervention in the case of diseases which it was feared 'would know no colour bar' and the turning of a blind eye on those diseases confined to blacks in rural areas. In the black rural areas, then known as reserves, the ravages of certain forms of epidemic disease could be virtually ignored by the state. In the urban areas, where black and white lived in close proximity, and the latter were dependent on the labour of the former, medical men were foremost advocates of residential segregation and vigorous measures of social control from the late nineteenth century.

As Maynard Swanson has shown, from the 1870s with the advent of industrialization and urbanization as well as the development of public health consciousness in the metropole, 'fear of epidemic cholera, smallpox and plague both roused and rationalized efforts to segregate Indians and Africans in municipal locations', especially in Natal and the Transvaal. In the early twentieth century, in the towns of the Cape Colony, as well as in Durban and Johannesburg, 'the accident of epidemic plague became a dramatic and compelling opportunity for those who were promoting segregationist solutions to social problems'. Urban public health officials played a major role in 'accounting for the ''racial ecology'' of South Africa'. The establishment of rural reserves for sole African occupation meant that certain epidemic diseases had far less impact on the white population than would otherwise have been the case.

At the same time, urban segregation was seen as a way round the contradictions posed by a welfare system geared to the needs of whites and a migrant labour system which threatened to undermine the neat divisions between urban and rural, white and black workers. The 'metaphoric equation' of blacks with infectious disease and the perception of urban social relations in terms of 'the imagery of infection and epidemic disease' provided a compelling rationale for major forms of rural separation and the removal of segregated African housing to the edges of the towns.[20] At the same time, the fear of epidemic disease led public health officials to insist on the inclusion of African locations within municipal frontiers.

Swanson deals in detail with the outbreak of bubonic plague between 1900 and 1904 in the Cape and Natal and shows how this occasioned the mass removal of Africans from the town centres. What he calls the 'sanitation syndrome' — equating 'black urban settlement, labour and living conditions with threats to public health and security — became fixed in the official mind, buttressed a desire to achieve positive social controls, and confirmed or rationalized white race prejudice with a popular imagery of medical menace'.[21]

TYPHUS AND SOCIAL CONTROL

Less well known than the outbreak of bubonic plague at the beginning of the century, or the influenza epidemic in 1918 which led to the passage of South Africa's first Union-wide Public Health Act, are the recurrent outbreaks of typhus epidemics in the rural areas of South Africa.

Perhaps because it did not afflict upper-class whites — although a certain number of poorer whites as well as medical personnel and traders in the 'native territories' did succumb annually to the disease — typhus was overshadowed by the more spectacular epidemic diseases such as smallpox and plague, or the emotionally charged issue of venereal disease. As a group of South African scientists stated somewhat bluntly:

> Typhus fever, for obvious reasons, affects the Natives chiefly, but it is so readily spread among them that it is somewhat surprising that more cases do not spread among Europeans. The probable reasons for this are: firstly there is little intimate contact between Europeans and natives, who, in every sphere of life, are separated by the colour bar; secondly, the standard of cleanliness among Europeans in South Africa is high and there is little lousiness among them. Most of the cases reported in Europeans are contracted by contact with infected lousy Natives.[22]

Nevertheless, until mid-century, typhus was 'a major public health problem in South Africa'.[23] If the disease does not seem to have caused the same degree of concern, the fear that it would spread from the rural areas, both amongst mineworkers and in the densely populated towns, nevertheless led to drastic and highly discriminatory deverminization procedures from the time of the first diagnosed epidemic in 1917. As the *Natal Witness* remarked at the time of a major outbreak in 1944,

> this is not a crisis which affects the Transkeian native alone. There are thousands of Europeans and non-Europeans who are already living on or just below the breadline in our large centres in social conditions which are anything but of the cleanest. If typhus were to jump the reserves it would find a fertile breeding ground among these people.[24]

It demanded 'energetic emergency action' and 'widespread radical measures',[25] and these indeed were generally taken when the disease threatened to move beyond the confines of the reserves. Bitterly resented by the black population, the measures taken provided a focus for political action by the African petty bourgeoisie.[26]

Louse-borne typhus is 'one of the greatest epidemic diseases of history'. As Hans Zinsser has shown in his incomparable *Rats, Lice and History*, it as been associated with nearly every great war and famine since the fifteenth century.[27] A disease of 'poverty, filth, human distress and overcrowding', it can spread through a community or ravage a continent with great rapidity.[28] The rickettsial organism responsible for the typhus infection can be transmitted to humans through ticks, rat- and mice-borne fleas, mites or lice, although the majority of cases with lethal consequence in South Africa as elsewhere was generally the louse-borne infection.[29] Of rapid onset, classically typhus is recognized by fever, severe headache and muscular pains, a characteristic rash which appears about the fifth day and nervous symptoms (nightmares, tremors and twitching, stupor and delirium). The crisis is normally reached after fourteen to sixteen days. Fatality rises with age and deficient nutrition.[30]

In South Africa the disease generally presented 'a clinical picture conforming with the well-known text book description of typhus fever' but was also believed to be 'considerably milder than classical typhus'.[31] Many medical men also emphasized 'the difficulty of detecting the rash in the dark-skinned Bantu'. According to James Gear and his fellow-workers:

> Most district surgeons, who have had a long experience of this disease, agree with this opinion, and there is no doubt that in most cases it is not possible to recognise an eruption that can be described as characteristic. However, in many cases, by examining a case closely and in good light . . . it was possible to detect the rash . . . However, only in the most obvious cases was it possible to determine the characteristic appearance and distribution.[32]

It is not at all clear when typhus entered South Africa, although according to Laidler it was introduced to the Cape from a Dutch East India Company ship in 1666.[33] It was first recorded as 'Black Fever' in 1867, a name which it retained amongst Africans in the twentieth century.[34] Its appearance amongst European armies suggests a connection with colonial military. Louse-borne typhus was prevalent in the nineteenth century in a minor form in the eastern Cape, present-day Lesotho and Botswana, the Orange Free State maize belt and northern Natal. It is significant, however, that it has only become a major scourge in the twentieth century, together with other diseases of development and underdevelopment.

The major outbreaks of typhus have thus to be seen against the progressive impoverishment of the African rural areas and their unequal incorporation into the capitalist economy. In the nineteenth century most Africans had access to land and produced sufficient and varied food for themselves and their families. The conquest of the major African chiefdoms in the late nineteenth century as the precondition for South Africa's capitalist development, and the confinement of Africans to a mere 13 per cent or less of the land together with the development of the low-wage migrant labour system, totally transformed this self-sufficient and relatively healthy population. Far from being some tropical inheritance, the diseases of twentieth-century South Africa — malnutrition, tuberculosis, typhus, cholera, typhoid, VD — are the diseases of nineteenth-century industrial Britain.

It is impossible to know the extent of typhus in nineteenth-century South Africa. Surprisingly, perhaps, in view of the number of wars on the Cape frontier, there does not appear to have been an epidemic, which would presumably have been recognized by the miliary medical men with the colonial forces. Perhaps because in the nineteenth century most Africans did not live in the huddled and overcrowded conditions which conduce to the spread of the infection, and perhaps because of the difficulty in recognizing the characteristic rash amongst Africans, typhus was not even officially recognized until 1917.[35] In that year for the first time, apparently, it reached hyperendemic proportions. This epidemic lasted until 1924; it recurred in 1933–5 and in 1944–6, also years of acute economic stress.[36]

In the epidemic of 1917–23, the disease hit the reserves of the Eastern Cape hardest, but there were also outbreaks on the coalfields in northern Natal, and it was noted as prevalent in Basutoland. In the Transkei and Ciskei, the annual number of cases reported between 1920 and 1923 was over 8,000, while in 1922 the Public Health Department maintained that 'on a conservative estimate, *the disease is killing not less than 2,500 Natives, most of them of working age, annually in the Union*' (italics in original).[37] Like cholera in the 1980s, typhus came to be regarded as endemic in the Transkei, and therefore somehow 'natural'. Its increased incidence in the war and the immediate post-war years (both the First and the Second World War saw outbreaks of the disease) and the thirties was, as Dr E.H. Cluver pointed out, the result of 'the increasing poverty of the Natives resulting from various causes'. Cluver, who was to become the Secretary for Public Health and Chief Health Officer a couple of years later, reported to the Native Economic Commission in 1930:

> I investigated this [the incidence of typhus] during the second half of 1929. The disease is endemic in most of the districts [for the Transkei] and appears to be increasing. During the year ended 30th June, 1930, the number of cases notified among Natives in the Transkei was 1530 of whom 165 died. The incidence is probably very much greater than these figures indicate, notification being very incomplete. I found the probable causes of this increased incidence to be (a) wearing off of the immunity acquired during the very extensive outbreaks which occurred some six years ago; (b) the increasing poverty of the Natives resulting from various causes such as prolonged droughts and over-population.
>
> It was noteworthy that the incidence was highest in the districts which were thickly populated and the inhabitants very poor, e.g. Glen Grey where the notifications were for year ended June 1929: 205; and for year ended June 1930: 339. In that district the children were noticeably suffering from malnutrition.

> One gained the impression in regard to both this disease and leprosy that the problem was to a very great extent an economic one. Both these diseases are associated with extreme poverty and will tend to disappear if mal-nutrition and overcrowding in huts were prevented.[38]

In 1935, when conditions had deteriorated even further as a result of the world depression and a prolonged drought, Cluver returned to this theme:

> It is possible that immunity acquired during the previous epidemic period was wearing off; but the excessive lousiness of the Bantu population [*sic*!] and their malnourishment resulting from the widespread financial depression seem sufficient to account for the rapid spread of infection.[39]

Each of the major outbreaks coincided with either depression or a sharp increase in the cost of living and drought. Drought not only undermined nutritional status; drought also affected the water supply so that 'people do not wash as often as usual . . . and their lousiness in consequence increases'. The dry cold winters saw the number of cases peaking each year, although those winters which were both cold and rainy could have a similar effect. As Gear and his colleagues pointed out,

> The year 1943, the winter of which was one of the coldest in living memory, was also noted for its frequent spells of rain. Both rain and cold tend to keep the people within their huts and cause them to don their blankets and extra clothes, and so circumstances become more favourable to the spread and propagation of lice.[40]

The specific effects of the weather and depression in fanning the disease in South Africa's rural areas into epidemic proportions should not disguise the fact, however, that the typhus epidemics were a direct consequence of impoverishment and underdevelopment of the reserves. And this in turn, as has been extensively documented, was directly related to processes of capitalist development in South Africa's metropolitan areas, and the system of migrant labour on which it was based.[41]

Nor were the ravages of the disease limited to the reserves of the Eastern Cape. By the 1930s it was felt on the white farms of the highveld. In 1933–5, the disease extended into the Orange Free State, which had 'considerable higher incidence than the whole of the Cape Province', perhaps because 'economic distress has nowhere been more severe during recent years than in the Orange Free State'.[42] By 1935, the louse was endemic in a triangular area which covered half of the Union, and a new epidemic was under way.[43] In the Free State the problems were exacerbated, according to the Assistant Medical Officer of Health, as a result of the concentrations of destitute people on the farms in search of food and work once the drought broke:

> [Their] movements took place from district to district but mainly from Basutoland which normally is the main source of supply of cheap casual labour during the harvesting season . . . Certain other factors have facilitated the spread of the infection . . . there is evidence that many employers, due probably to the busy time they were having after the drought, did not take early steps for the early discovery of cases of illness among their natives, nor did they worry themselves about the condition of temporary labourers entering their employ. The result was that deverminisation had to be carried out on a very much larger scale and with less prospect of eradicating the disease than would have been the case had primary outbreaks been reported promptly to the magistrate.[44]

It was the major outbreak of typhus in 1917 which laid the basis for the state's further reaction to the disease. Although methods of 'deverminization' were to become more sophisticated, the nature of the measures adopted and the fears for the workforce which it aroused were expressed by an Inspector appointed by the Native Affairs Department to inspect conditions of mine compounds in 1917:

> As it appears to me that this is the most menacing outbreak of disease in South Africa in the writer's experience of nearly 30 years; and as the negligence I have experienced may be general, I have deemed it my duty to report to you the danger we are in, on the Rand, owing to such laxness of supervision over 'New' natives from the Cape Colony, south of the Vaal River. I have now arranged . . . as follows:
>
> No 'new' C.C. [Cape Colony] natives to be allowed into compounds, on any pretext, either as recruits, or as visitors, until their bodies, and their *heads*, have been thoroughly cleansed, in the presence of an European. The clothing, and particularly the hat, to be boiled; or . . . put through the Thresher Vapour Disinfector. During this period the native concerned is accommodated in the convalescent wards, and furnished with two blankets, while his clothing is being disinfected and dried.
>
> 'New' Visitors who will not voluntarily accept this routine, to be refused admittance [to the compounds] . . .
>
> It has been represented to me that we ought to insist on hair being clipped . . . but in view of the known value put upon long plaited locks, by the Pondos, and others, I cannot advocate any such system . . . indeed I have forbidden it, on the Nourse, where the hospital Superintendent desired to do it . . . There is much nervousness amongst Compound Managers, as to whether all measures are adopted, on *all* mines; as they allege that laxity will render those Mines guilty of such, popular amongst the C.C. natives, after this outbreak is over.[45]

For the Department, the 'delousing' 'in mine compounds, town locations and elsewhere where the Natives are under supervision and control' was a relatively 'simple matter' compared with the situation in the African reserves.[46] There the cost of controlling the epidemic in 1922 was running at £8,000 to £10,000 in ten districts, which as the Secretary of Health remarked was either too little or too much:

> it is of little use to attempt eradicative measures in a few districts. The alternatives are either to organise a campaign on Union lines . . . or else curtail the expenditure and restrict action to measures in connection with what may be called obtrusive outbreaks causing public concerns and criticism, and concurrently to devote special attention to propaganda and educative work amongst Natives.[47]

Essentially it was the cheaper of the two options which was chosen. By 1922, as a memorandum in the Department of Health admitted, the physical measures adopted — essentially 'tent disinvestors' and 'medicaments' — 'had not succeeded in materially reducing the prevalence of the disease'. The Department went on to make further recommendations, which are more interesting in illuminating its attitudes towards South Africa's black population than for their potential utility in ending the epidemic. Thus it was suggested that certain storekeepers be allowed to sell 'pumula', naphthaline, and paraffin and oil at cost price (free to the indigent); that two inspectors, one male and one female, be appointed in each magisterial district to 'inspect for lousiness, warn, advise and report'; and that a handful of medical men be engaged to lecture 'in the Native language . . . saying plainly that Government intends forcing natives and their families to be free of vermin'. Finally, urban authorities were to be encouraged to have a free hot-water wash house, preferably attached to a municipally controlled beer-hall as in Natal. This would entail economic savings as the steam boiler could be used — and Africans could be told 'No beer for the dirty or verminous' — thus adding to the already formidable social control embodied in the establishment of the municipal monopoly over African beer. The Department saw an urgent necessity for the extension of powers to municipalities outside Natal to monopolize beer-halls on the Durban model, and its recommendation to this effect was embodied in the 1923 Urban Areas Act which was being drafted at that time.[48]

By 1935, the Department of Public Health remarked resignedly, 'Combatting lousiness among so huge a population of primitive, poverty-stricken Bantus [Africans] is a formidable proposition. All the Union Health Department can do is to deal with typhus outbreaks wherever they are reported.'[49] One way of responding to outbreaks was to curb the movement of people. Thus, according to the Secretary for Public Health and Chief Medical Officer, J.A. Mitchell, in 1922, if the disease could not be controlled at its rural source, what was necessary was 'to tighten up the control of travelling Natives, so as to prevent as far as practicable, dirty and lousy Natives leaving their kraals or locations'.[50] As Mitchell must have known by the time he was writing, precisely this 'control of travelling Natives' had already caused considerable tension between different departments of state and between the state and the African public.

It was clearly impossible to forbid African movement totally — not because of any fear of hardship this would cause the African public, but because, as the Medical Officer of Health for the Union remarked 'drastically restricting or altogether prohibiting Natives from leaving Typhus-infected districts by rail, for the Rand or elsewhere' would 'materially' affect railway revenue — and no doubt also the labour supply.[51] Nevertheless an attempt could be made to control the travelling public.

Thus, in 1917, in response to the newly declared epidemic, the Department of Public Health had issued regulations which gave 'any Station Master or any officer acting by due authority on his behalf' the authority to remove blacks — Africans, Coloureds or Asians — from trains.[52] The Department also established a 'dipping station' at Sterkstroom Junction, in the Cape Province, where all Africans on their way to the Rand from the Transkei had to be disinfected. A 'compound' (i.e. African living quarters), disinfecting station and other buildings were erected just above the railway station on land leased by the local municipality to the Chamber of Mines. The area was fenced in and the railway line extended to the compound 'so that native trains are shunted right into the compound premises where the natives alight'. There the coaches were scrubbed and disinfected, while the 'bodies, clothing and effects' of the Africans were 'expeditiously cleansed', disinfected and medically examined before being despatched onwards.[53]

As the Native Affairs Department official sent down to inspect the procedures reported at the end of 1917:

> On arrival at the compound the natives are formed into batches, recruited, voluntary[54] etc., contracts produced and travelling passes checked. The natives are then sent to room 'A' where they have to undress, tie up their clothes blankets and hand them in to room 'B', the fumigating shed, where they are thoroughly disinfected by a process of steam fumigation . . . A European official is in charge of rooms 'A' and 'B'. After this the natives proceed to room 'C', the bathroom. Here they have their hair cut and wash their bodies in a large disinfecting concrete bath . . . cold water is . . . used. After each native has been thoroughly cleansed he is sprayed with a paraffin emulsion, being a slight improvement on system [*sic*] used at the American Emigration Experimenting Station . . . After the Native has been sprayed with disinfectant, he has to rub the mixture thoroughly into his head and body, then he goes to room 'D' where a clean blanket is issued. From there he goes into compound no. 1 with his valuables and awaits medical inspection.[55]

In other words, Africans recruited for the mines were simply derailed at Sterkstroom and treated to the first of the deliberately humiliating procedures which initiated them into mining culture. The *herrschaft* of the white man was made abundantly clear, as was his disregard for African conventions and morality. Many Africans, for example, regarded it as abhorrent for the initiated male to appear naked before the uninitiated.[56] Nevertheless, the Union's Medical

Officer of Health explained, 'the removal and disinfection of Natives travelling by special native trains . . . has occasioned no difficulty'.[57] Nor was this entirely surprising, though the recruits probably bitterly resented these procedures. In general they would have been first-time recruits, illiterate and unused to white authority, travelling on special trains provided by the Native Recruiting Corporation, which by this time had a monopoly over the purchase of labour. It is unlikely that they could have communicated their fears and complaints to those in authority had they wanted to, in the absence of sympathetic interpreters. The procedures were well suited to an industry which aimed at 'total control of the worker both in and outside of his working hours'.[58]

When it came to dealing with educated Africans and Coloureds, however, the Public Health Department found it had an altogether more delicate situation on its hands. As the MOH continued:

> with passengers by ordinary trains the difficulties have all along been considerable, and are increasing. Whilst second-class Native, Coloured and Asiatic passengers are inspected (when time permits), it has not hitherto been found necessary to remove any of these for cleansing. In practice, it proved desirable to remove all third-class Native, Coloured and Asiatic passengers, and this procedure has so far been carried out, every effort being made to minimise the delay of these passengers.[59]

Despite the view of the MOH that those removed from the carriages were 'well fed, well housed, and sympathetically treated during their detention in the Disinfecting Station', the Sterkstroom Junction procedures caused endless protest, especially from the better educated and better off. The indiscriminate application of the deverminization procedures to all travellers in third-class compartments, including those whom the local magistrate called 'civilized and quite respectable and clean' was the source of the trouble.[60] Here the racist presumptions of the white Public Health officials came into headlong conflict with the class position of the African petty bourgeoisie. As a letter signed by E.M. Tunzi complained to the relatively liberal newspaper, the *Cape Times*, in 1918:

> It is not the disinfecting of our bodies that we resent, but the needless waste of our clothing and the degradation of the present system which we hate.
>
> Native women, some of whom hold their matriculation and other scholastic degrees, together with others equally civilised, are insulted most cruelly, being treated worse than animals, inasmuch as the heads of all natives are practically shaven. The Bible says, I Cor. chapter 11, verse 15: 'But if a woman have long hair it is a glory to her'. . . . It is this cruel state of affairs which is eating into our hearts, and it seems to us a very poor return for the work we are doing and have done in the war. The Government say they are fighting for the removal of injustice and oppression of the weak. All right, we believe you, but we should believe you much more if you did things in

our land as well as fought to do it in other lands.[61]

The letter was in fact written by R.M. Tunzi, a mission-educated teacher, on behalf of his wife Edith, who, five months' pregnant, had ample cause for complaint. When her train stopped at Sterkstroom on its way to Cape Town from Umtata, two officials from the Disinfecting Station entered her third-class carriage. All Africans travelling from the infected areas were obliged to obtain health certificates from their local magistrates within seven (later three) days of their departure, together with a letter from the Acting Secretary of the Interior. Despite the pass and health certificate which Mrs Tunzi carried exempting her from the typhus regulations, the officials insisted that she come off the train to be 'deverminized'. They tore up the pass and certificate and dismissed the letter as 'nonsense'. The unfortunate lady was forced to bathe in cold water and then sit around for an hour in nothing more than a blanket. Not surprisingly, she soon complained of severe stomach pains and had developed a cough. She maintained that she had been detained at the Junction in severe discomfort for four days, forced to eat food to which she was unaccustomed and to sleep on the bare floor without blankets.[62]

The Tunzi letter became a *cause célèbre*. The immediate reaction of the officials responsible was to deny any reason for complaint by Africans for any improper treatment, and the Secretary for Native Affairs 'challenged' the correspondent to substantiate his claims. Mrs Tunzi's telegrams to her husband, the intervention of Father Wallis of the Anglican mission society, a question in parliament and the personal interest of the Prime Minister and Minister for Native Affairs, General Louis Botha, led to a further enquiry by the Native Affairs Department. The Department now discovered that the local magistrate believed that the actions of the railway officials (in response to the advice of the doctor-in-charge) in removing all third-class passengers caused unnecessary hardship. Clearly indignant at the treatment meted out to educated, middle-class Africans travelling third class, the magistrate decided to meet trains personally 'and advise the Railway Officials which Natives etc., should be removed from trains . . . using the utmost discretion'.[63]

As a result of his enquiries, the Secretary for Native Affairs, Edward Dower, had 'frankly to admit that grounds for grievance had been shown to exist'.[64] Despite his initially hectoring tone towards African complainants, which led both Father Wallis and William Stuart, MLA, who accompanied them, to take exception to the way in which the enquiry into the allegations was made, Dower was forced to apologize publicly to Mr Tunzi. During the war years, when the government was facing opposition from Afrikaners and needed co-operation from blacks, the administration was forced to take account of the African intelligentsia, and to adopt a somewhat more conciliatory attitude towards them. The Prime Minister himself intervened to ensure that 'civilized natives' received more considerate treatment, and the local magistrate threatened to appeal to Botha's authority if matters did not improve.[65]

As a result of the Tunzi enquiry, the Native Affairs Department (NAD) decided to despatch one of its officers to proceed to Sterkstroom 'for the purposes of watching over the interest of Natives in connection with the disinfecting measures carried out there and seeing that the assurances given by Government as to due and proper discrimination were fulfilled'.[66] The officer delegated by the NAD was a well-known Transkeian magistrate, R. Welsh. He found a complex situation at Sterkstroom.

In a personal letter to the Director of Native Labour, H.S. Cooke, Welsh argued that the 'important question to be decided is who is to be granted authority to remove natives etc. from the trains north'.[67] He outlined the conflict of authority between the doctor, the railway officials, and the magistrate. The local Medical Officer of Health, Dr Young, had instructions from the Department of Health

> to remove all 3rd class native etc. passengers, so that these persons may be examined by him, and if dirty or verminous they have to be cleansed and disinfected, and if clean they are allowed to proceed on their journey . . . It is quite clear to me that the Station Master and the Foreman are not willing to take any responsibility in the removal of native third class passengers, and the S.M. maintains that the terms of the regulations . . . do not permit them to delegate the authority it conveys to any person not an officer of the Rlwy Admn.

In addition, according to Welsh, Dr Young alleged that

> the Magistrate has not been co-operating with him in connection with the discrimination question and allowed 133 persons from 16/20 April to proceed north without examination. Dr. Young states it is a farce, and will result in typhus spreading and he will accept no responsibility for the consequences . . . Dr. Young also wishes me to state that his position here will be untenable if the Magistrate is allowed to interfere in any direction in connection with the question of deciding who are dirty and verminious and who are clean. Dr. Young is very anxious that an official of the NA Dept be appointed. I hope I am not selected.[68]

Perhaps because of Welsh's equivocal stand, within days of his arrival there were further complaints. On 25 April 1918, Mrs Catherine Dlodlo, wife of the Reverend Velebay Dlodlo of the Free Church of Africa, travelling from Umtata and on her way to visit her sick daughter in Johannesburg, was similarly stopped and removed from the train at Stersktroom. Like Edith Tunzi she felt humiliated by her treatment and was delayed for two days before she could resume her urgent journey, and was subjected to humiliating and uncomfortable procedures — all the more irksome because as she said she was a considerable owner of property in East London and lived 'up to the Standard of Europeans' having been educated at the famous Scottish mission institute at Lovedale in the Eastern Cape.[69] This was the very situation that the local magistrate objected to, and the one that Welsh had been instructed to stop.

Despite Welsh's sympathies with the local doctor, the Medical Officer of Health at the Department of Public Health in Pretoria was forced by the Native Affairs Department to 'review and reconsider' the arrangements. He suggested as an interim measure that the only feasible course was to inspect blacks on the trains and 'exempt from removal and disinfection those found to be thoroughly clean and free from vermin'.[70] This could be done by delaying the trains a little longer than usual rather than by wholesale removals of the third-class carriages. At the same time, in response to these 'difficulties' with passengers on 'ordinary trains', a new clause was added to the regulations governing deverminization removals on railway property at the instance of the Public Health Department. As Welsh explained:

> I find it almost impossible by a casual examination, for a layman to discriminate between those persons who are clean, and those who are dirty or verminous. A Native apparently clean in body and clothing, and who may be living up to the standard of a respectable European has been found on examination by the Medical Officer to be verminous.[71]

He recommended that the regulations governing the procedures be amended, preferably empowering himself or the magistrate of the district to take action. The railway authorities, however, refused to surrender their power to decline tickets or remove anyone from trains or railway property. Nevertheless, the Public Health officials were able to extend greatly their control over the movements of blacks. New regulations published in August 1918 made it incumbent on 'every native, coloured person, or Asiatic' from areas affected by typhus fever to carry a certificate that they were free of vermin and healthy, issued not more than three days previously by a magistrate or Medical Officer of Health. The certificate could be demanded for inspection by a remarkable range of white officialdom:

> by any railway officer or employee, or by any district surgeon, health officer or sanitary inspector, or other duly authorized officer of the Government, or of a local authority, or by any members of the police, or by his employer, or the owner, occupier, or manager of the estate, farm, or premises on which he is resident.[72]

In the end, despite the objections of the local magistrate and the Native Affairs Department, the stronger line insisted upon by the Public Health Department held sway. By 1923 the Department was suggesting that 'lousy' natives be prosecuted and penalized, and 'as far as possible prevented from leaving their kraals [homesteads] and locations' — measures which still drew a strongly worded protest from the Chief Magistrate in the Transkei — but to no avail. As he pointed out, unless some assistance were provided for Africans to free themselves of vermin,

> it will be merely purposeless cruelty to penalise them wholesale for being verminous. It is not practicable to punish a large majority of the individuals of a populous territory, and when nearly all are verminous, it is difficult for the clean minority to escape collecting vermin from their natives . . . It is still more impracticable to prevent dirty or lousy Natives from leaving their kraals or locations as to do so effectively would embarass the Government and cost more in policing and lost labour than would suffice to eradicate Typhus Fever.[73]

The correspondence reflected the inevitable friction between the different authorities, as the aggressive measures taken by the Public Health officials led to African opposition which had to be coped with both by the Native Affairs Department and local railway officials. Medical officers were generally able to pose successfully their ethos of the public good — however draconian the measures — against the lingering paternalist ethos of many of the local magistrates and officials of the Native Affairs Department.

Deverminization procedures were pursued even more vigorously in Durban where the most serious outbreak of typhus was in 1924 although there were periodic outbreaks thereafter. As the MOH, Dr Gunn, described it, there the process was not dissimilar to that at Sterkstroom. In the mid-1920s, some 50,000 black men were regularly put through these municipal deverminization procedures. Africans called the process 'dipping' — by analogy with the dipping of cattle in disinfectant against East Coast Fever.[74] The humiliation of the system led to a major campaign by the African all-in union, the Industrial and Commercial Workers' Union, or ICU, led by A.W.G. Champion. As Champion put it, he objected

> to the indignity of the system. I even went so far as to suggest that this thing be done in private. The natives were marched from the Court House; there was no respect for civilised natives. There was steam, and you had to go and have a bath with other boys of different nationalities.[75]

Although Champion was temporarily able to halt the 'dipping procedures', the Durban municipality resumed the practice in the 1930s, and it remained a constant source of 'very grave dissatisfaction' amongst Coloureds and the African elite for many years.[76]

The views of less articulate and less educated Africans are hard to discern in the record, although the opposition of recruiters to the long delays at Sterkstroom after the First World War was coupled with statements that 'the boys [i.e. the workers] complain of the treatment accorded them, and they are handled, to say the least of it, very roughly. The result of the long delay encourages desertions and makes the boys very dissatisfied'.[77] By and large the dangers of the disease spreading amongst the workforce were considered to outweigh the dissatisfactions and desertions of that workforce. As late as 1944 religious leaders, the Cape

African National Congress and the Coloured political association, the African People's Organization, were protesting against the indignities of the procedures and the ban on travel arising out of public health policy towards the typhus outbreak.[78]

The drastic action against Africans travelling in 1944 was perhaps an over-reaction in response to the earlier failure by the Department of Public Health to take adequate steps to deal with the typhus epidemic which was known to be raging in the Transkei in 1943 and 1944 in semi-famine conditions. According to the Member of Parliament for the Transkei, Gordon Hemming, despite repeated requests for assistance and equipment, nothing was done. He reminded the House that 'it is common case that typhus follows in the footsteps of starvation' and that over the past couple of years the Transkei had suffered famine conditions. In 1943, 167,000 bags of maize had to be imported into the territory; in 1944 the shortfall was estimated to be 300,000 bags and the price of maize had risen 100 per cent during the war years. Yet no action had been taken. Hemming, 'an extremely able and highly respected attorney from Umtata', went so far as to accuse the department of 'almost criminal neglect'.[79] As in the case of later epidemics, there is some evidence that the state attempted to cover up the outbreak. Thus in January 1944, the *Cape Times* reported that 1,692 deaths from typhus were recorded that month, yet in April the Department of Public Health issued a press statement denying that the outbreaks signified an epidemic.[80]

According to the *Natal Witness*, 1944 departmental statements on the typhus outbreak read

> like an apologia for years of neglect to take any action to make such an outbreak impossible . . . Knowing . . . that typhus was endemic in the territories, that starvation conditions conduced to virulent outbreaks, that famine conditions which should never have existed did in fact exist, and that the maize crop is going to be seriously short this year . . . these departments with all the facts available [have] convicted themselves of sheer neglect and inertia by their failure to forestall an inevitable crisis . . . Typhus is endemic in the Transkei. Almost every winter for years there have been sporadic outbreaks. Yet so far as we can recall not a single concerted effort has ever been made to stamp out the disease. It is a scathing commentary on the attitude of officialdom that only some drastic occurrence such as this can shock it out of inertia into action. It is also an astonishing reflection on this country's sense of comparative values that while money has been poured out to eradicate East Coast fever in cattle and every attempt made, even to appointing commissions to stamp out the disease, a deadly social scourge like typhus is ignored until tragedy compels action.[81]

Despite the evidence that anti-typhus vaccine produced a high degree of immunity, the state had refused to supply it to African schoolchildren on the grounds that it was still at the experimental stage.[82] As Captain G.H.F. Strydom remarked, 'The position is deplorable. We have medicine for animals, but we have no medicine for human beings.'[83]

The state preferred to rely on the unpopular deverminization procedures. Fifteen teams were organized to undertake the deverminization campaign, but neither the equipment nor the vaccine were available initially.[84] Part of the problem undoubtedly related to wartime conditions: 25 per cent of the full-time staff of the Public Health Department had enlisted for war service. During the war years the Department of Public Health was certainly more concerned about African health than it had been previously, and was responsible for launching an anti-typhus campaign at the end of 1943.[85]

Again because it was wartime, when the greatest consensus in the African territories was desirable and the state needed the co-operation of the African intelligentsia, there was tension between the Native Affairs Department and the Public Health Department, with the former arguing that the measures of the latter were 'precipitate and unreasonable', especially as the state did not have the facilities necessary to provide the deverminization and immunization it was making compulsory.[86]

By mid-1944, however, the Minister of Native Affairs himself had been galvanized into action by a visit to the Transkei. The equipment was provided and, according to reports, 'every single hut was now being disinfected' systematically in the territory 'and no native is being allowed outside unless he has been properly disinfected'.[87]

From the late 1940s, typhus declined as a significant public health scourge. The disease appears to have been brought under control with the effective use of DDT, pioneered against body lice in Italy during the Second World War and first used in South Africa in an epidemic outbreak in the Eastern Transvaal in 1945.[88] The new tetracyclines and effective vaccines are less likely to have been in use amongst Africans but may have played a small role in the control of the disease, especially in urban areas and amongst exposed whites. Whatever the reasons, the numbers of cases had declined by the 1950s, and although there were sporadic outbreaks, especially in the Transkei in the 1950s and 1960s, there were virtually no recorded fatalities during that period.[89]

The controversies arising out of the deverminization procedures and the ban on travel for blacks but not for whites which accompanied major outbreaks of typhus, as well as the relative success of these procedures, should not obscure the fact that the state was not disposed to do much about the conditions of poverty in the reserves which contributed to both endemic and epidemic disease. Typhus has been replaced today by other diseases of poverty.

CONCLUSIONS

As typhus has given way to other diseases of poverty, so the state's response has been modified. As in the case of typhus, the approach of the state has been characterized by a lack of concern and attempted cover-up so long as the disease remained isolated in the reserves. Unlike typhus, however, which was spread from human to human by a live vector, with diseases like cholera and typhoid which are spread by poor sanitation and polluted water supplies there has been no real need for unpopular coercive action. They can be safely contained in the black rural areas, especially now that these have been handed over to so-called 'independent' Bantustan authorities, and individual cases handled when they arrive in the 'white' areas.

The recurrence of malaria — the number of notified cases trebled between 1984 and 1985 from just under 4,000 to nearly 9,500 — has caused the state's public health officials greater concern.[90] Like the louse, the mosquito 'knows no colour bar'. Ironically the state's handover of health matters to the impoverished, inexperienced and corrupt Bantustan health authorities has partly contributed to a breakdown in mosquito control mechanisms while its racially selective policy of providing expensive prophylactic drugs to whites may in part account for the enormous resurgence of resistant strains of malaria in 1985–6.

As in the past, when deverminization procedures were applied in draconian fashion to blacks but not to whites, increased knowledge on the part of public health officials is differentially applied, and follows the racial cleavage in the society. In this case, it is the whites who have the full coverage of immunization and the latest drugs, generally administered from state-subsidized supplies through private practitioners.

The sheer weight of historical evidence thrown up by outbreaks of disease defined as epidemic reveals starkly the power relations in society. From this point of view, public health policies during outbreaks of such socially defined epidemics provide a useful barometer of its political conflicts and socio-economic cleavages. The records left in the wake of the epidemic highlight ruling-class ideology, state policies, and social priorities. This should not be allowed, however, to overshadow the fact that in the subcontinent today as in the inter-war period, the real killers are not the infectious diseases which are defined by the Department of Health as 'epidemics' — but TB, measles, and malnutrition and malnutrition-related diseases.[91] This is the true violence of South Africa.

NOTES

We are grateful to Jasmine Saloojee and Lara Marks who did some of the research on which this paper has been based.

1. 'Bantustan' is the term we have preferred to use for ten rural areas or 'reserves' set aside for sole African occupation and which are in various stages of constitutional 'independence' granted by the South African government which terms them 'Bantu homelands'.

2. de Klerk, cited in C. de Beer, *The South African Disease. Apartheid, Health and Health Services* (Yeoville, Johannesburg: South African Research Service (SARS), 1984), 60. See also 'Cholera in South Africa', *South African Outlook* (November 1981), 173; and A. Zwi, 'Cholera — a tropical disease?', in *Supplement to Work in Progress*, 16 February 1981.

3. de Beer, op. cit., no. 2 above, 13.

4. *Sunday Express* (Johannesburg), 31 January 1982.

5. ibid. According to Dr G. Coovadia, 'the reported number of severely ill patients with cholera [in Natal] has been *c.* 50,000 cases . . . we believe that a more accurate incidence of cholera is greater than two million infected people' (*Sunday Times* (Johannesburg), 28 February 1982).

6. ibid.

7. World Health Organization, *Apartheid and Health* (Geneva: WHO, 1983), 126.

8. *The Star* (Johannesburg), 19 July 1982.

9. R.E. McGrew, *Russia and the Cholera, 1823–1832* (Madison: University of Wisconsin Press, 1965), ch. 1, cited in M.W. Swanson, 'The sanitation syndrome: bubonic plague and urban native policy in the Cape Colony, 1900–1909', *Journal of African History, XVII* (3) (1977), 389.

10. For an examination of the transformation of disease patterns, see S. Marks and N. Andersson, 'Industrialisation, rural change and the 1944 National Health Services Commission', in S. Feierman and J. Janzen, *Health and Society in Africa* (Berkeley: University of California Press, forthcoming).

11. E.H. Burrows, *A History of Medicine in South Africa up to the End of the Nineteenth Century* (Cape Town, Amsterdam: Balkema, 1958), 87.

12. ibid., 278.

13. For the history of South Africa's public health legislation until 1944, see UG 30–1944, Union of South Africa, *Report of the National Health Service Commission* (Pretoria: Government Printer, 1944), ch. V.

14. ibid., ch. V, para. 9, p. 18, and para. 23, p. 20.

15. ibid., ch. XIX, para. 49, p. 100.

16. This account draws heavily on Burrows, op. cit., n. 11 above, 259–62.

17. R. Turrell, 'Capital, class and monopoly: the Kimberley diamond fields, 1871–1889' (unpublished PhD thesis, University of London, 1982), 258–9. (To be published as *Capital and Labour on the Kimberley Diamond Fields, 1871–1890* (Cambridge: Cambridge University Press, forthcoming)).

18. Cited in Burrows, op. cit., n. 11 above, 262.

19. ibid., 332, 336.

20. Swanson, op. cit., n. 9 above, 387–410.

21. ibid., 410.

22. James Gear, Botha de Meillon, and D.H.S. Davis, 'Typhus fever in the Transkei', *South African Medical Journal, 18* (22 April 1944), 146. The authors were a medical researcher, an entomologist and an ecologist respectively.

23. J.H.S. Gear and N.L. Murray, 'Typhus fever in the Eastern Transvaal, with special reference to an epidemic occurring in 1945', *South African Medical Journal, 21* (12 April 1947), 214.

24. *Natal Witness* (Pietermaritzburg), 13 March 1944.

25. ibid.

26. See below.

27. Hans Zinsser, *Rats, Lice and History* (New York: Bantam edition, 1971); for the data see 163.

28. A.R.D. Adams, 'The typhus fevers', in A.R.D. Adams and B. Maegraith, *Clinical Tropical Diseases* (Oxford: Oxford University Press, 7th edn, 1980), 494.

29. South African Government Archives, Pretoria (hereafter SAGA), E.H. Cluver, 'Typhus and Typhus-like Diseases in South Africa', Report to the Pan African Health Conference, Johannesburg (November, 1935), Department of Health, Ges[ond — Health] 470–48/409/10 (hereafter Ges).

30. Adams, op. cit., n. 28 above, 495–6.

31. Gear *et al.*, op. cit., n. 22 above, 146; Cluver, op. cit., n. 29, 6.

32. Gear *et al.*, op. cit., n. 22 above, 146. Compare the far more categorical views expressed three years later in Gear and Murray, op. cit., n. 23 above, 216: 'The appearance of the rash is not of great diagnostic value in the dark-skinned African. In many cases no rash could be detected. When it was visible, it was often difficult to determine its characteristic appearance and distribution.'

33. Cited in Gear *et al.*, op. cit., n. 22 above, 144.

34. The African term was *ifiva mnyama*; ibid., 145.

35. ibid., 144. Gear *et al.* note that reports in 1909–10 of typhus in the Kentani district of the Transkei were dismissed by the official responsible in the Cape's Department of Health as 'malignant influenza'. According to J.A. M[itchell], the Secretary for Public Health and Chief Health Officer, in 1922, 'The difficulty of diagnosis arose from the fact that it is on the whole milder than European typhus, and is only rarely associated with an eruption visible on the native skin' — to Minister of Public Health, 8 December 1922 in Ges 467–292/264/181.

36. For the incidence of the disease see UG 8–1945, Union of South Africa, *Report of the Department of Public Health for the Year ended June 30th, 1944* (Pretoria: Government Printer, 1945), 14, Table 25, for the years 1917–44, and RP 28/1962, Republic of South Africa, *Department of Health Annual Report for the Year ended December 31st, 1959* (Pretoria: Government Printer, 1962), 39, Table 22 (b), which lists the annual number of cases from 1933 to 1959.

37. Ges 467–269/264/181, op. cit., n. 35 above.

38. UG 22, 1932, Union of South Africa, *Report of Native Economic Commission, 1930–32* (Pretoria: Government Printer, 1932), Memorandum to the Commission entitled 'Prevalence of typhus in Transkeian territories', cited by F.R. Lucas, Addendum, A60, 182.

39. Cluver, op. cit., n. 29 above, 7.

40. Gear *et al.*, op. cit., n. 22 above, 145.

41. We cannot elaborate on this here, but see for example, C. Bundy, *The Rise and Fall of the South African Peasantry* (London: Heinemann, 1979), and R. Palmer and N. Parsons, *The Roots of Rural Poverty in Central and Southern Africa* (London: Heinemann, 1977). For a more general elaboration in relation to health, see Marks and Andersson, op. cit., n. 10 above.

42. Cluver, op. cit., n. 29 above, 8.

43. ibid.

44. Ges 470 28/209/10, Dr L. Fourie, Assistant MOH, to Secretary for Public Health, 28 September 1934; see also UG 30, 1933, Union of South Africa, *Annual Report of the Department of Public Health for the year ending June 30th 1933* (Pretoria: Government Printer, 1933), 65. The pattern is very similar to that described by R.M. Packard, 'Maize, cattle and mosquitoes: the political economy of malaria epidemics in colonial Swaziland', Journal of African History, XXV (2) (1984), 189–212.

45. SAGA, Pretoria, Government Native Labour Bureau (hereafter GNLB), 276 309/17/103, Inspector J.E. to Acting Director, Government Native Labour Bureau, 24 August 1917.

46. Mitchell, op. cit., n. 35 above.

47. ibid.

48. Ges 467 196/268/181, 'Memo on typhus as at 24/4/22'. For the beerhalls, the Durban system and social control, see Paul la Hausse 'The struggle for the city: alcohol, the ematcheni and popular culture in Durban, 1902–1936' (Unpublished MA thesis, University of Cape Town, 1984).

49. UG 43, 1935, Union of South Africa, Department of Public Health, *Annual Report for the Year ending June 30th, 1935* (Pretoria: Government Printer, 1935).

50. Mitchell, op. cit., n. 35 above.

51. SAGA, Pretoria, Department of Railways and Harbours (Suid-Afrikaanse Spoorweë — hereafter SAS) 885 G18/13, MOH, Pretoria, to The General Manager, South African Railways and Harbours, Johannesburg, 5 April 1918.

52. *Government Gazette*, 20 November 1917, Government Notice 1581.

53. GNLB 276 309/17/103, Copy of a 'Report dated 13.2.1917 by Mr. R. Welsh on Sterkstroom Disinfecting Station'.

54. i.e. they were placed in groups based on whether they had been recruited for mine labour on a contract basis by the native Recruiting Corporation of the Chamber of Mines, or were making their way 'voluntarily' to the goldfields.

55. Welsh, op. cit., n. 53 above.

56. For the deliberately humiliating acclimatization procedures still in use in the mining industry in the 1970s, intended to initiate men into a sub-culture which is deprived of any values about human dignity', see Dunbar Moodie, *The Perceptions and Behaviour Patterns of Black Mineworkers in a Group Gold-mine* (Johannesburg: Anglo-American Corporation, 1976). Moodie discussed the debasing aspects of male nudity, 8.

57. SAGA, Pretoria, op. cit., n. 51 above.

58. Charles van Onselen, *Chibaro Mine Labour in Rhodesia, 1900–1930* (London: Pluto Press, 1976), 158. Although van Onselen was talking of Rhodesian mine labour, the policies in South Africa were similar and the mine magnates were in a more powerful position to carry them out.

59. SAGA, Pretoria, op. cit., n. 51 above.

60. GNLB 276 309/17/103 E. Tinley, Magistrate, Sterkstroom, to Native Affairs Department, Cape Town, 20 April 1918.

61. 'A Native's plea', *Cape Times*, 6 April 1918.

62. GNLB 276 309/17/103, Telegram 53 (copy), E. Tinley, Sterkstroom, to 'Natives' (i.e. Secretary for Native Affairs), Cape Town, 16 April 1918.

63. GNLB 276 309/17/103, Telegram 56 (copy), E. Tinley, Sterkstroom, to 'Natives', Cape Town, 17 April 1918.

64. GNLB 276, copy, Secretary for Native Affairs (hereafter SNA) Edward Dower, to Mr R.M. Tunzi, St Columba's House, Cape Town, 18 April 1918.

65. ibid. Cf. GNLB 276 309/17/103, E. Tinley to Director of Native Labour, 20 April 1918: 'P.S. After Mr. Welsh has had time to investigate and report to you fully on this matter, if I find that natives etc. travelling 3rd class are still being taken off without any discrimination at the Sterkstroom Railway Station I shall consider it my duty as Magistrate of this District to report the fact to General Botha.' (Botha was at that time both Prime Minister and Minister for Native Affairs.) A number of studies of the inter-war period are beginning to reveal the extent to which the administration were concerned with separating the African intelligentsia from the working class through policies of co-option and conciliation. This was particularly marked in the period of heightened militancy and radicalization immediately after the First World War. See for example, P. Bonner, in S. Marks and R. Rathbone, *Industrialisation and Social Change* (Harlow: Longman, 1982).

66. Dower, op. cit., n. 64 above.

67. 'etc.' in these documents would appear to refer to Coloureds and Asians travelling third class. The abbreviation served to cover both embarrassment and ambiguity.

68. GNLB 276, R. Welsh to H.S. Cooke, DNLB, 23 April 1918. Personal handwritten letter.

69. GNLB 276, Evidence of Catherine Dlodlo before E. Tinley, Magistrate Sterkstroom, 26 April 1918.

70. SAS 885 G18/13, MOH for the Union to The General Manager, South African Railways and Harbours, 29 April 1918.

71. GNLB 276, R. Welsh, Sterkstroom, to Director of Native Labour, Johannesburg, 22 April 1918.

72. *Government Gazette*, 2 August 1918, Government Notice 7389.

73. Ges 467 279/264/181, Chief Magistrate of the Transkeian Territories, Umtata, to SNA, Pretoria, 8 February 1923; for the measures taken, see Union of South Africa, *Annual Report of the Department of Public Health 1923* (Pretoria: Government Printer, 1924), 23.

74. *Durban Boundaries Commission*, Evidence of Dr Gunn, 184.

75. SAGA Archives, Pretoria, Commission Reports and Evidence (Kommissies), 22, vol. 4, Evidence to the de Waal Commission on Durban Riots, A.W.G. Champion, 10 July 1929, 378.

76. Ges 469 404/10, A.E. Abdurahman, Gen. Sec. African Peoples' Organisation (APO) to Sec. Health, 17 September 1944.

77. GNLB, Part I, 309/17/103, Stuart Erskine, Pietersburg, to Union Health Dept. Sterkstroom, 10 September 1919.

78. See, for example, Ges 469 404/10, A.E. Abdurahman, op. cit., n. 76 above, and P. Mbete, The Methodist Church of South Africa to Senator C.H. Malcolmess, as well as the reply of the Public Health Department on the resolutions passed by the African National Congress on the subject in the same file; see also Ges 471 128/412/10, Sam Phooko B.A. Departmental Visit. Teacher (*sic*) to Chief Magistrate, Umtata, 7 October 1944.

79. Union of South Africa, *Assembly Debates*, vol. 49, 8 May 1944, Mr Hemming, col. 6801. See also cols 6800–10. The description of Gordon Hemming from M. Ballinger, *From Union to Apartheid. A Trek to Isolation* (Cape Town, Johannesburg and Wynberg: Juta, 1969), 53.

80. *Assembly Debates*, n. 79 above. The Minister, however, strenuously contested these figures and pointed out that according to the Director of Census in the period from 1 July 1943 to 22 April 1944, 1,983 Africans had died in the Transkei and Ciskei (col. 6821). If 1,600 for January was an overestimate it is probably a considerable underestimate for the period the Minister was referring to, as vital statistics were not kept for the African population.

81. *Natal Witness*, 4 March 1944.

82. *Assembly Debates*, vol. 49, 8 May 1944, col. 6802.

83. ibid., col. 6805.

84. ibid. The Minister of Welfare and Demoblisation (H. Lawrence), cols 6816, 6822.

85. ibid., col. 6807.

86. Ges 412/10, SNA to Secretary for Public Health, 29 June 1944.

87. Ges 467 279/264/18, Chief Magistrate, Umtata, to SNA, 8 February 1924.

88. See Gear and Murray, op. cit., n. 23 above; see also UG 6, 1946, Union of South Africa, *Annual Report of the Department of Public Health, for Year ended June 30th, 1945* (Pretoria: Government Printer, 1946), 29; UG 23, 156, Union of South Africa, *South African Department of Health Annual Report for the Year ended December 31st, 1953* (Pretoria: Government Printer, 1956).

89. It should be noted, however, that fatalities in the African reserves were likely to have been missed. Into the 1950s scientists at the Rickettsial Diseases Laboratory of the South African Institute of Medical Research (SAIMR) thought that the disease 'continues to smoulder in various parts of the country'. (SAIMR, *Annual Report* (Johannesburg: SAIMR, 1951), 35; See also, SAIMR, *Annual Report* (Johannesburg: SAIMR, 1954), 45.) By the mid-1950s the annual reports of the Department of Health did not record rural fatalities.

90. *South African Medical Journal*, (1985), 67: 232. *South African Medical Journal*, (1986), 69: 272.

91. There were 150 new cases and ten to twenty deaths each day from TB in 1982 (South African Institute of Race Relations (SAIRR), *Race Relations Survey, 1983* (Johannesburg: SAIRR, 1984), 501, figures from SANTA); it is estimated that a child

dies every twenty minutes in South Africa from malnutrition or malnutrition-related diseases — some 50,000 a year (SAIRR, *Race Relations Survey, 1980* (Johannesburg: SAIRR, 1981), 560; SAIRR, *Race Relations Survey, 1983*, 504); about 11 (black) children die each day from measles, and many more are left blind for life (*The Star*, 5 August 1982).

14

Cholera and colonialism in the Philippines, 1899–1903

Rodney Sullivan

On or about 20 March 1902 two Filipinos were admitted to Manila's St John of God Hospital with violent diarrhoea, cramps, and vomiting. The news galvanized American health authorities in the Islands. A senior group of them, including Colonel Louis M. Maus, the Commissioner of Public Health, Dr Franklin A. Meacham, Chief Health Inspector, Dr Paul C. Freer, Superintendent of Government Laboratories, and Dr. R.P. Strong, Director of the Biological Laboratory, rushed to the hospital immediately they were told of the cases. They conducted their own examination of the patients, calling fruitlessly for a rectal speculum or tube, until interrupted by a telephone message advising 'that a native had just died under suspicious circumstances in one of the districts near by' and that the body was on its way to the hospital morgue. Within an hour an autopsy was under way; microscopic examination of the mucosa of the ileum revealed *Vibrio cholerae*, the deadly comma-shaped cholera bacillus identified by Robert Koch in 1883.[1] Cholera had returned to Manila. It was the beginning of 'one of the most terrible epidemics of modern times', lasting until February 1904 and taking by official estimate 109,461 lives, 4,386 in Manila. This certainly understated its real toll according to the American head of the Bureau of Non-Christian Tribes, David P. Barrows, who directly observed the epidemic in the provinces and estimated fatalities at over 200,000.[2]

The visitation was not unexpected. In the previous month Chief Health Inspector Meacham had investigated reports of cholera in Canton and Hong Kong, from whence came much of Manila's supply of green vegetables. He believed the disease was prevalent in both centres but had difficulty in documenting its occurrence. In Canton he was unable to locate mortality records and was reduced to 'visiting the undertakers' establishments and counting the coffins sold daily'. Hong Kong authorities he accused of concealing the presence of cholera in the interests of commerce. He sought out the Chinese gardeners who grew vegetables for Manila, recoiling from their 'abominable' practice of 'using the night soil of the colony for purposes of fertilization'. He painted a vivid picture of the Chinese gardener routinely diluting human faeces with water, then 'with a pail suspended from either shoulder', generously scattering the 'semi-liquid' upon 'all the growing vegetables' as he walked up and down the furrows of low-growing plants. A report in the *Manila Times*, the American community's principal newspaper, emphasized that 'these are the vegetables which we consume here in Manila', that the night soil was used in its natural state, and bore with it 'dire possibilities in the way of propagating cholera and other diseases of like nature'.[3]

On 3 March 1902 official notification was received in Manila of the presence of cholera in Canton; on March 8 it was reported at Hong Kong. Apprehension among Manila Americans heightened. On 19 March the Chief Quarantine Officer,Dr J.C. Perry, banned the import of green vegetables from Hong Kong. At the same time Manila's health inspectors 'were warned to be on the lookout for persons suffering from bowel trouble of a suspicious character'.[4]

The first cholera deaths in Manila in March 1902 punctured a buoyant mood among Americans in the city. An epidemic of bubonic plague had erupted in Manila in December 1899, an embarrassing few months after the Americans had taken control of the city. After 'energetic repressive measures' Manila was declared free of plague in January 1902; the *Manila Times* congratulated health authorities on their success 'in keeping the city clean, and thus preventing sickness'.[5] Early in January that most influential of Philippine Commissioners Dean C. Worcester, whose multifarious responsibilities included public health, was similarly optimistic, noting 'things are going very well with us'. The Philippine-American War, which began on 4 February 1899, was apparently drawing to a successful close. According to Worcester there would be 'peace throughout the archipelago' as soon as the last enclaves of Philippine resistance — in Batangas, Mindoro and Samar — could be subdued. Mindoro he noted was 'quieting down rapidly'; the 'insurrection' in Batangas he expected to end in a matter of days as the American forces had stopped their 'shilly-shallying'. The persistence of 'trouble' in Samar he attributed to the incompetence of the American field commander. At the same time Worcester described a second war on which the Americans had embarked in the Philippines. It too was not without cost, having occasioned 'a vast amount of friction', 'the destruction of much private property', and he could have added the confinement of large numbers of people. This was the 'determined campaign' to eradicate disease and establish a new American sanitary order in the Philippines.[6]

This was not cholera's first visitation to the Philippines. Reynaldo C. Ileto has shown how in the nineteenth century, the cholera epidemics of 1882 and 1888 were used by Spanish authorities, often with the support of the Filipino *principalia* class, to consolidate the colonial state, to suppress forms of disorder and irrationality, and institute modes of mass surveillance. This provoked resistance from the 'ignorant, superstitious' masses. Further conflict developed between Spanish priests and the increasingly influential Filipino physicians who, in the 1890s, were prominent in the liberal, nationalist, and separatist movements.[7] In his 'Cholera and the origins of the American sanitary regime in the Philippines' Ileto extended his analysis into the twentieth century, noting how Filipinos resisted both the incoming American troops and the new colonial state's efforts to suppress the

1902 cholera epidemic. Like their Spanish predecessors the Americans seized the opportunity afforded by cholera to mount 'search and surveillance operations' under the guise of sanitary surveys and inspections. Similarly confinement and quarantine had overlapping military and health purposes.[8] Ileto's appraisal is at odds with standard accounts of American health policy in the Philippines. Thus Cameron Forbes makes a distinction between the period of insurrection and public disorder and the beginning of the new American regime's 'effective labors in public health'. More recently Lewis Gleeck nominated health as the one area on which the American record in the Philippines was beyond reproach. It was, he wrote, 'the one accomplishment which evoked universal approval of all who knew the Philippines before and after the American occupation'. John A. Larkin makes a similar genuflection in his influential study of Pampanga, noting that 'efforts on behalf of public health paid off rapidly . . . and the American doctors could take pride in their achievements'.[9] Even Filipino historians of the nationalist school have tended to accept American celebrations of their insular health achievements at face value.[10]

To what extent is the general, self-contratulatory tone of American writing on their insular health record justified? On a number of counts it merits a degree of suspicion. Among these are the context, motives, language, images, personnel, strategies, and institutions of the public health programme launched by the Americans in the immediate aftermath of their occupation of Manila in August 1898. There is moreover the largely unexplored question of how Filipinos perceived and experienced both the cholera epidemic and American strategies to control it.

American health endeavours in the Philippines were part of a broad, perhaps ruthless, programme of Americanization of the Islands and its people. One of its earliest and most telling expressions occurred in December 1898 with the circulation of President McKinley's plan for the 'Benevolent Assimilation' of Filipinos.[11] American military and civilian leaders in the Philippines interpreted this to mean that Filipino values, traditions, and institutions were to be displaced by Americanism, that is American values, institutions, and even traditions, as attempts to have Filipinos accept 4 July as their national day showed.[12] In May 1900 General Elwell S. Otis, the retiring Military Governor of the Philippines, was explicit about the goals of Americanization and the strictly receptive role accorded to Filipinos:

> We should seek to implant and build up our institutions. Americanism is a good thing for these islands. At present there is little understanding of a real republican government, but the people are eager to learn and they readily assimilate American ideas and become Americanized. When once they generally recognize the beneficence of our institutions these people will quickly adopt them, adapting themselves to the changed conditions.[13]

In similar vein the first American Civil Governor of the Philippines, William

Howard Taft, wrote in 1902 of the necessity to teach Filipinos English so that they could be inducted into American civilization and its practice of 'self-government on Anglo-Saxon lines', a process which would take at least two generations.[14] American health programmes and disease-control measures were developed in this context of dominant military-backed Americanism. The consequent discounting of Filipino values and experience was sharpened by the American determination to use health policy as a means to safeguard their acquisition and administration of the Philippines.

One important motive for the high priority Americans gave health questions in the Philippines at the turn of the century was the fear that white people were particularly vulnerable to tropical diseases.[15] Particular anxiety was felt for the health of American troops, the indispensable engine of the American occupation of the Islands. In 1901 Colonel Charles R. Greenleaf, Chief Surgeon of the United States Army in the Philippines, had lamented that even the most robust American soldier could not survive a year's service in the tropics without marked physical deterioration.[16] The following year a volunteer army surgeon wrote that the United States' 'greatest enemies in the tropics are the unseen bullets of cholera, dysentery and malaria. They kill more white men than the fighting force of natives.'[17]

A persistent theme among early Republic Party appointees to the Philippine Commission was the necessity and desirability of boosting American commercial activity in the Islands.[18] An influential and representative manifesto was prepared by Taft: 'The investment of American capital in the islands is necessary to their proper development, and is necessary to the material, and therefore the spiritual, uplifting of the Filipino people'.[19] In turn Philippine commerce and its attraction for American investors were adversely affected by perceptions that the archipelago and its inhabitants were prone to disease and debilitation. The answer according to Major E.C. Carter, American Commissioner of Public Health in the Philippines from 1902 to 1905, lay in the cult of 'sanitary efficiency' which he reiterated was 'the key to the prosperity of these islands and thus to the success of their administration'.[20] It was important too that the health programme should encompass Filipinos as well as insular Americans. Disease eroded the capacity of the local community to supply reliable labour for colonial commercial ventures; moreover it was realized that the American community could not effectively quarantine itself from the diseases which plagued Filipinos. Dr Victor G. Heiser came to the Islands in 1903 as Chief Quarantine Officer and from 1905 served as Worcester's principal health officer. He approached health policy on the assumption 'that disease never stays at home', arguing that 'as long as the Oriental was allowed to remain disease ridden, he was a constant threat to the Occidental who clung to the idea that he could keep himself healthy in a small disease ringed circle'.[21]

The language and imagery of American health discourse in the Philippines was sharpened by the arrival of cholera. Stereotypical images of Americans and Filipinos were endlessly generated serving to show that the Filipinos were responsible for cholera; that the imposition of American rule was justified since the epidemic demonstrated an unquestionable need for not only the surveillance and control of Filipinos, but also the reconstruction of their values, behaviours, and in many cases, towns and dwellings. Americans were depicted in seemingly endless acts of selflessness and heroism, bringing scientific medicine and 'the gospel of sanitation'[22] to the Philippine Islands. Early in 1903 the *Manila Times* popularized the sanitary case for colonization when it published the poem 'Civilizing the savage'.[23] It is notable for its theme that the road to civilization was paved with soap, and the nice ambiguity that lurks about the phrase 'water cure'. After describing the 'savages' ingratitude and penchant for futile resistance the verse proceeds:

Do not despair
. . . The only remedy that's sure
Is, after all, the water cure;
Don't shoot 'em,
Loot 'em,
Cuff and boot 'em,
But lead 'em firmly to the tub
And make 'em scrub'.
Despite their howls
And growls;
Teach 'em the use of soap and towels.
For cleanliness once understood,
Creates a higher brotherhood,
It makes men willing to be good;
. . . Remember, while there's soap
There's hope.

Initially Americans believed they were much less susceptible to cholera than Filipinos. Just prior to the outbreak of the 1902 epidemic the *Manila Times* recalled the great epidemic of 1882 which claimed an estimated 30,000 victims in the city and province of Manila in under three months. It noted that while the dead 'were mostly natives' they included 'many Spaniards' but 'only one Englishman'. It concluded hopefully that 'the Anglo-Saxon constitution', even if 'out of its latitude' was especially resistant to 'this dread bacillus'.[24] Even when the first American cholera cases had been hospitalized the image of a distinctive Anglo-Saxon resistance to cholera lingered on. From his post as head of the Santiago Hospital Dr R.E. Sievers wrote that his Filipino cholera patients accepted death with a fatalistic stoicism; the contrasting American way of death epitomized heroic struggle:

> the men from the United States . . . fight this disease with a grimness that often means victory and life. There is none of that helplessness or despair so

> characteristic of the native. Despair they often feel but they never give way, and my countrymen, in this hospital as upon the battlefield, fight to the last ditch.[25]

By July 1902 the number of American cholera victims was rising sharply with reports that at least fifty soldiers were dead of the disease.[26] There were signs that the American community had jettisoned its confidence in the Anglo-Saxon constitution and was now beset by anxiety that it was especially prone to cholera, particularly after the mortality figures for July 1902 showed that the American death-rate from the disease, per 1,000 head of population, was 31.51, compared to the Chinese community's 21.74. No comfort was drawn from the rate of 108.29 recorded for Filipinos.[27] Instead allegations that Filipinos were responsible for the presence and transmission of the disease became more pointed. Earlier references to the 'pig-sty carabao barbarism' of Cebuanos, the 'stupidity and criminal carelessness' of Pampangans, or the Filipino's 'native filthy ways' sharpened with the accusation that these were responsible for American deaths.[28]

American cleanliness was being undermined by Philippine filth. The *Manila Times* lamented the cholera deaths of 'clean-lived Americans'. It identified the 'native boy' as 'the probable means of infection' since in hotels and houses he prepared and served food and drinks to unwitting Americans. The newspaper reminded its American readers that 'cholera germs exude with the sweat through the pores of the [Filipino servant's] skin' and that 'his hands may be teeming with the germs'. There were two alternatives. American employers should confine their servant 'to the house and away from his own filthy habitats' or preferably dispense with his services 'at least until the cholera is over'.[29] Two days later there was a call for greater vigilance on the part of health authorities coupled with a note of despair at apparent Filipino apathy or resistance:

> With such crass ignorance and benighted superstition as permeate the lower classes of Filipinos, ordinary preventatives and remedies are offset and rendered useless, and all efforts, even the most strenuous, seem to be almost entirely wasted. In trying to enlighten and instruct the brown masses, we have expended money, intelligence, and energy; but all to no avail. The lump is still unleavened.[30]

It is significant that the American health programme in the Philippines began as a military measure. In September 1898 Major Frank S. Bourns, Surgeon, United States Volunteers, set about organizing a public health service and a board of health for the city of Manila. The Spanish-speaking Bourns was a close friend and colleague of Dean C. Worcester, whom he had accompanied on scientific expeditions to the Islands in 1887–8 and 1890–3.[31] Bourns's responsibility for public health provided cover for his other role as head of military intelligence, a responsibility which passed to the civilian Commissioner Worcester when Bourns returned to the United States in July 1899.[32] An Insular Board of Health was established by the Taft Commission on 1 July 1901. Its chairman was the army medical corps' Colonel L.V. Maus, who was designated Commissioner of Public Health.[33] The Insular Board of Health was responsible to Philippine Commissioner and Secretary of the Interior Dean C. Worcester. Under his forceful leadership the Board in its first year of operation drafted a plethora of bills aimed at the regulation and control of health personnel, practices, and institutions in the Philippine Islands. They included legislation, quickly enacted, to regulate the practice of medicine, pharmacy, dentistry, and veterinary science throughout the archipelago. Other measures included compulsory vaccination, an anti-leprosy campaign, controls on the manufacture and sale of alcohol, and the establishment of provincial and municipal boards of health.[34] Health provided an ideal medium for the extension of the reach of the new American colonial state into some of the most private recesses of Philippine society. Worcester himself was conscious of this development and, in an unguarded moment, took pleasure in the construction of a new and penetrative state, describing it as 'great machine . . . just being put together, oiled up and set in motion'.[35]

When the presence of cholera in Manila was confirmed on 21 March 1902 Worcester seized the opportunity to exercise dictatorial powers. Governor Taft was in the United States, the acting Governor, Luke Wright, was in Leyte, and Commissioner Henry Ide, the Secretary of Finance and Justice, was in Japan. The Philippine Commission, the archipelago's legislative forum, lacked a quorum since only two of its members were in Manila, Worcester and Bernard Moses, the unassertive Secretary of Public Instruction.[36]

Worcester 'arrogated' to himself powers to which he had no legal entitlement, including the allocation of resources, the recruitment of additional health employees, and the deployment of army detachments.[37] He was responsible for the selection and implementation of a range of anti-cholera strategies and proudly reported his adoption of 'radical measures from the start'.[38] Some had already been used with apparent success in the Manila campaign against bubonic plague.[39] These included intense surveillance of people and dwellings, the detention and isolation of the ill, and the expropriation by sanitary officials of victims' bodies. Suspect dwellings and other buildings were disinfected, in some cases compulsorily reconstructed, in others burned.[40] There was little or no attempt to enlist the support or understanding of ordinary Filipinos. The language and ruthlessness of the exercise, as well as the key role played by army doctors, suggested it was another engagement of the Philippine-American War. When Major Meacham established plague stations in the crowded Manila suburbs of Binondo and Tondo it was reported in the American press that their uniformed inspectors 'would make a clean sweep of all the dirty premises in their districts . . . whether the inhabitants like it or not'.[41]

The more fearful threat posed by cholera, as well as the apparent success of the anti-plague campaign, increased the ruthlessness with which Worcester and his officials attempted to suppress it. The cholera epidemic appeared in a most virulent form with many of the early victims dying in from one to three hours after the onset of symptoms. It was a terrible death as the patient never lost consciousness, suffering agony from cramps and the convulsive loss of fluids.[42]

Worcester's first act was an attempt to secure Manila's water from contamination. He believed that the disease had arrived in Manila with vegetables imported from Canton before the quarantine had taken effect; were its *vibrio* to invade the city's water supply he estimated that there would be 100,000 cholera victims in the capital.[43] A large proportion of Manila's water supply was drawn from the Mariquina River, a pumping station being located some two miles below the riverside town of Mariquina with over 7,000 inhabitants. There were other towns on or near the upper reaches of the river, so that some 20,000 people were living on the watershed of the Manila supply. Following an archipelago-wide pattern they traditionally relied on the river or its tributaries for domestic water, bathing, washing clothes, the maintenance of the carabao, agriculturally indispensable as well as water-dependent, and the disposal of human waste. Moreover many of the inhabitants of the Mariquina Valley made daily trips to Manila, with the real possibility that cholera would accompany them on the return journey.[44]

At Worcester's request the commander of American troops in the Islands, Major-General Adna R. Chaffee, despatched a battalion of the 28th United States Infantry and a portion of the 5th Cavalry to form 'an absolute quarantine line' forbidding the 20,000 inhabitants of the Mariquina Valley access to their twin lifelines, the river and the markets of Manila. A system of army outposts was established so that the 14-mile course of the river was supposedly under observation twenty-four hours a day. Cavalry patrolled the foothills of the mountains hemming in the Mariquina Valley, which could only be entered after five days in an external quarantine camp.[45] While a water-borne cholera epidemic in Manila never materialized the consequences for the inhabitants of the Mariquina River Valley were disastrous. After consuming the available rice they were reduced to dependence on canned food supplied by the hard-pressed Philippine Commission. In October a disgruntled American soldier enforcing the quarantine wrote that with its exports of sugar and lumber halted the Valley was experiencing 'hard times' with social unrest and banditry increasing apace. Since at that time it appeared that the epidemic in Manila was subsiding, the military were withdrawn from the Mariquina Valley. The full effects of the exercise were revealed. As the soldiers departed 'ladrones' occupied the towns and 'a large number' of refugees fled to Manila where they lived without employment 'in a half-starved condition', ready prey for the upsurge in cholera which occurred in the city during November.[46]

Despite the misery inflicted on the people of Mariquina Valley Worcester's determination to safeguard Manila's water supply never wavered. It had been planned to declare Manila cholera-free on 1 November but on that very day five cases occurred, with the number of daily cases rapidly increasing to fifteen; on 14 November there were forty-three cases. More alarming for Worcester was the reappearance of cholera in the Mariquina Valley after it 'had been clear for many days and the guards along the river bank removed'. Three cases occurred among the workmen at the intake of Manila's water supply and seven in the nearby town of Mariquina. Worcester 'routed out' the American army commander Major-General George W. Davis in the middle of the night and had him rush 'a strong detachment of soldiers to the scene of the difficulty before daylight'.[47] If the suffering of the inhabitants, to which Worcester appeared oblivious, was the most regrettable feature of the Mariquina Valley exercise, from today's perspective what is more striking is its ineffectuality. This was recognized at the time by one American soldier deployed in the Valley who observed that throughout the quarantine human and other waste was being carried into the river by natural runoff. 'Every native house', he wrote, 'has a filthy breeding place for disease at its rear; about 400 houses send their quota of filth into the river every time it rains, and all the soldiers in the province cannot keep it out.'[48] Much the same point was made later in an official report by Major Carter who claimed that though 'the grosser forms of pollution' were prevented 'it is notorious that a thorough quarantine of the Mariquina River has not existed'. He noted that the Filipinos had established their own system of observation posts in the Valley which gave timely warning to inhabitants using the river of the approach of cavalry patrols. At other points bathing and washing in the River continued as before though 'under cover of darkness'. Unlike Worcester, Carter had made some attempt to empathize with the Filipinos of the Valley, recognizing the 'great discomfort and hardship' occasioned by the attempt to deny them access to their river, since 'an abundant supply of water is absolutely essential to the Filipino and his carabao'. As well he shrewdly pointed out that the Valley's 20,000 inhabitants were unwilling to sacrifice their own livelihoods for the alleged purpose of protecting an already stricken Manila from cholera.[49]

Unfortunately the Mariquina Valley episode is a typical rather than exceptional example of American anti-cholera strategies employed during the 1902 epidemic. While its impact was undoubtedly considerable it was overshadowed by events in Manila itself.

There was a striking similarity between American tactics in the Philippine-American War, especially during the bitter fighting of 1901, and Worcester's anti-cholera measures. In the second half of 1901 particularly, American troops attempted to counter Filipino guerilla tactics with brutal population reconcentrations, the burning of crops and villages, and the widespread use of the water-cure.[50] From the point of view of the Filipino masses, termed by Worcester in a suggestive phrase as the 'more ignorant of the Filipinos' the anti-cholera tactics adopted in Manila at the onset of the epidemic must have seemed straight out of the war zones.[51] There is no more enduring symbol of this than the fate of Farola and its inhabitants. The *barrio* of Farola, known as 'Shack-town', was built on the mudflats at the extreme western boundary of the San Nicolas district, extending along the Pasig River to the Manila Light. The first cholera cases were concentrated in Farola which Worcester described as 'an aggregation of overcrowded and filthy shacks'. In an effort to contain the epidemic he ordered troops to quarantine the area but found it impossible to prevent 'escapes by water under cover of darkness'. Cases of cholera multiplied among 'the imprisoned people' with Worcester directing 'that they be removed in a body to the detention camp'. Three and a half hours of one afternoon were spent transferring 1,200 fearful Farola residents to the San Lazaro detention camp.[52]

In Spanish times proceeds from the San Lazaro estate had supported the San Lazaro Hospital for lepers which was constructed of stone in 1784 and, with the exception of a brief period between 1662 and 1681, was administered by the Franciscans. As the property of the Spanish government it came into the possession of the United States military authorities in September 1898.[53] In late 1902 'a permanent detention camp, capable of accommodating 1,500 people' had been built in the grounds of the San Lazaro Hospital after the discovery of 'numerous rats' dead from infection by the plague bacilli. This was interpreted by American health authorities as a sign that a sharp increase in the incidence of bubonic plague was imminent, necessitating a commensurate increase in the number of detainees. At the outset of the cholera epidemic the detention camp's six nipa barracks each 191 by 27 feet in size, and divided into twenty-six rooms, were empty. Publicly Worcester estimated they could accommodate 1,500 persons; in private he claimed 2,000. Beyond that the camp's capacity 'was materially increased' by rows of army tents. While Worcester proudly described the detention camp as 'a model' with its 'twelve large bath houses and water closets . . . two good nipa houses for administrative officers, and a fairly good kitchen', one detail in his description helped explain the terror with which it was regarded by Filipinos: each barrack was 'separated from the others by barbed wire'. The very architecture of the San Lazaro complex must have suggested to its unhappy inmates not only imprisonment by alien soldiers but the prospect of an awful extinction by death, dissection, and cremation. On the other side of the original San Lazaro buildings from the detention camp were a 'detention hospital for persons who fall ill in the detention camp', a cholera hospital for outside victims as well as those who developed the symptoms in the detention hospital, a morgue 'where post-mortems of all cholera suspects are made', and 'conveniently at hand' a crematorium where all cholera victims were incinerated except in those few cases where relatives were able to afford 'hermetically sealed coffins'.[54]

Edith Moses, a perceptive observer, wrote that Filipinos imagined that 'all kinds of horrors' awaited them in the detention camp.[55] One can understand something of their apprehension from a journalist's description of the Santa Mesa detention camp and cholera hospital, a city of tents, to hold 'many thousand people', hastily erected in April 1902 at a site some 6 miles of rough road from Manila. His first impression was of 'a certain strange grimness':

> as if a vague cloud-shadow sliding over the landscape had settled there. It is noticed that a barbed-wire fence with diabolical ingenuity of construction encircles the camp. At the only gate armed guards are standing in grim and silent watch. A great wagon gallops up, men at the gate work the handle of a pump up and down, a spray breaks in pulverized drops against the vehicle

and an acrid odor of carbolic acid pinches the nostrils. The tent-city is the detention camp for cholera suspects and the wagon thus being disinfected has just brought a cholera-stricken contact from the camp to the hospital beyond.[56]

Cholera hospitals, particularly in the critical early days of the epidemic, did little to induce Filipino confidence or overcome the entrenched view that hospitals were places where people were sent to die. The high mortality rate among hospital patients was not reassuring. Worcester reported 90 per cent fatalities among 'early cases' of cholera. Even after the initial onslaught hospital mortality remained high. It was at least some weeks into the epidemic when Dr Sievers revealed that 80 per cent of the cholera patients received at the Santiago Hospital died. 'One day twenty-three were admitted', he wrote, 'and in twelve hours twenty-one of them were dead.'[57]

The forced confinement of the sick, whether in detention camp or hospital, affronted Filipinos who customarily cared for the sick and dying in the family home, usually crowded with sympathetic, perhaps also curious, relatives and friends. Thus an American teacher stationed in Tanjay, Negros Oriental, during the epidemic wrote that 'it is the custom of the Filipinos, as soon as anyone falls sick, to run to the house to see what the sick man looks like'. An American doctor visited a cholera patient in Bohol and found 'the entire house filled with natives' in accordance with the local practice of neighbours congregating in the house of an ill person.[58] Heiser noted 'the strong antipathy of the Filipinos to be treated elsewhere than in their homes' and how the local press harped on the 'mental agony' suffered by Filipino families when a cholera-stricken member was hospitalized.[59] But if the pain of separation was bad, the experience of a cholera hospital could be much worse, especially in the epidemic's early stages.

Worcester wrote privately of this 'great difficulty' in getting the San Lazaro Cholera Hospital 'in shape at first'. The 'army doctor' who was placed in charge of the hospital 'got badly scared, and neglected his patients disgracefully'. What lay behind this judgement and the doctor's dismissal might be now beyond reconstruction. At least one grotesquely haunting image survives. It is of dying Filipinas, enduring the last agonies of cholera with neither dignity nor the comfort of family, priests, nor even female attendants. The cholera detainees had been separated from their families, priests either boycotted the San Lazaro Hospital or were refused admission; Worcester seems to imply the former, writing 'no priest has ever been near the cholera hospital, although there are many deaths there everyday'. It took some time before nurses could be recruited and in the interregnum Worcester observed the lonely undignified deaths: 'Native women lay around there, going it at both ends, and dying with no one but rough male hospital stewards to look after them'.[60]

Even after conditions in the hastily established cholera hospitals improved the clinical isolation of the dying persisted. Dr Sievers of the Santiago Hospital described a 'scene witnessed hourly' in mid-1902. It was of an old frail Filipina allowed to pay a last visit to a dying son or husband. She sits beside and at some distance from the cot. As the final moment arrives 'love is not to be denied': she makes a rush forward but is blocked by an attendant whose duty it is to prevent the living from touching the dying. 'There is a mute appeal in the eyes of the grief-stricken woman, but she makes no struggle. Instead, she drops upon her knees, clasps her hands, and with uplifted eyes she prays.'[61]

Many Filipinos feared western medicine, preferring to counter disease with traditional remedies and practices. Dr Sievers complained that his Filipino patients believed western medicine made 'their death a certainty'. Such Filipino suspicion was widespread. Dr Charles W. Hack who made a sanitary inspection of Cebu, Bohol, Samar, and Leyte in early 1903 reported that the natives 'refuse to take medicine furnished by the board of health'; the people, 'superstitious and suspicious' put 'much more faith . . . in candles and incantations than modern medicines'. In Manila after the epidemic had passed Major Carter attempted to explain why Filipinos rejected 'the efficacy of medicines'. He attributed it in the first place to 'the native mind' with its characteristic 'fatalism, amounting to indifference'. But he also noted that Filipinos understood disease as a spiritual affliction, perhaps a retribution for sin, against which mere physical remedies were powerless. 'Scientific medication has no physiological significance to a people who believe that disease is the result of the influence of evil spirits.'[62]

There are reports, often sceptical or even contemptuous in tone, of Filipinos attempting to ward off cholera with prayers, penance, religious processions, and pilgrimages to holy shrines. William B. Freer, an American teacher who observed the latter part of the cholera epidemic in Nueva Caceres, wrote sympathetically of the great 'faith of the people in prayer' and described their 'safeguard' against cholera: nightly processions, with statues of the Virgin and saints, sacred music, singing, chanting, reciting prayers, and frequent kneeling before elaborate temporary street shrines — all a plea to God for pardon and pity. A more typical American perception of this phenomenon has been recorded by the Philippine Constabulary Officer John R. White who was stationed in Negros when the 1902 epidemic reached the island. That the people turned wholeheartedly to San Roque, the patron saint of the sick, struck him as apathy and he wrote disparagingly of how 'in each *barrio* and pueblo pathetic little processions paraded the streets, bearing banners and battered images of the saints'. In the provinces and towns of northern Luzon cholera was regarded 'as a Divine visitation of wrath', giving 'the superstitious element in the native character . . . an opportunity to display itself in the practice of various rites, some heathen, some supposedly religious'. From Pampanga came the complaint that night was rendered 'hideous by the singing of long processions of people with the evident purpose of scaring away the cholera'. In Pasig, Rizal, an American, described how every night there was 'a great parade of women and children about the various towns praying that the disease may be abated by the Almighty'. Such expression of religious faith provoked the American response that the cause of combating cholera would be far further advanced if one-tenth the cost of candles used in the processions had been invested in soap for 'cleaning the bodies, houses and clothes of the wretched paraders'.[63]

It is clear that for many ordinary Filipinos protection from cholera was best sought from God rather than from American health officers with their gospel of sanitation, 'scientific' medicine, and their horde of military, constabulary, and police enforcers.[64] The power of the Filipino understanding of disease and its remediation, as well as the determination of state authorities to suppress it, was demonstrated near the northern Luzon town of Vigan in late 1902. A Filipino priest reported he had seen San Roque descend into a well, rendering its water holy; those who bathed in it would be immune from cholera, other diseases and the deterioration of age. Within a few days some 6,000 Filipinos had gathered at the well 'anxious to try its wonderful waters'. The provincial governor, mindful of 'neglected crops and the danger of want', dispersed the crowd, leaving a constabulary guard at the well to prevent further assembly.[65]

The American attempt to use 'scientific' medicine to legitimize their attempted re-ordering of Filipino society and lives failed its first great test in the cholera epidemic of 1902. It was not only because traditional, antithetical beliefs about the nature of disease persisted. Another important reason was the inability of western medicine to demonstrate its efficacy in the cholera hospitals.

'Cholera mocks efforts of science' was an apt heading for a description of procedures at the Santiago Cholera Hospital with its 80 per cent mortality rate. What Worcester termed the 'necessary use of strychnine as a heart stimulant' provoked widespread unease among Filipinos. Even more alarming, to both Filipinos of the time and observers from today, was the ready resort to the experimental drug Benzozone (benzoyl-acetyl-peroxide). This had been developed by the Government Laboratories' Freer in collaboration with Novy, a former colleague at the University of Michigan. Diluted and administered by enema and capsule it was claimed to have antiseptic properties. Worcester deemed it 'wonderful', the 'only thing which has proved effective in cholera', arguing with dubious logic that 'practically none of our patients have recovered, except those that have been treated with it'. His enthusiasm was misplaced. Benzozone was a powerful irritant which burnt stomach and intestinal linings. When its capsule was broken by a patient's teeth the mouth was so injured 'that nourishment by mouth was seriously interfered with'. It was doubtless Benzozone which necessitated 'the use of force in administering medicine' at the Santiago Hospital. In 1905 Major Carter officially warned that 'intestinal antisepsis, by whatever means attempted' was an untrustworthy and probably harmful cholera therapy.[66]

Other provocative aspects of the American response to the cholera epidemic of 1902 have been touched upon elsewhere. These include ruthless, repetitive, and ultimately futile attempts to enforce quarantines, the burning of dwellings, the desecration of the dead, and the preferential recruitment of Americans as health officers.[67] The discrimination against the employment of Filipinos as anti-cholera operatives widened the gulf of misunderstanding between American and Filipino and inadvertently facilitated Filipino resistance. At least one mute but suggestive cameo survives: in Manila on the 26 March 1902 a 12-year-old Filipina, an iron foundry employee, was stricken with cholera at half past two in the afternoon and died at eight o'clock that night. 'Her people failed to understand the Health Authorities who tried to trace the source of the disease.'[68]

As Worcester realized, Filipino resistance was not 'confined to the more ignorant classes'. Most Spanish-speaking doctors in the Islands declined American co-option, mounting a forceful critique which highlighted the blunders, the destructive ruthlessness, and the ineffectualities of the American anti-cholera campaign. Their agitation appears to have played a part in the withdrawal of American army surgeons from anti-cholera work in Manila in July 1902.[69]

In the Philippines imperial medicine was a two-edged sword. While it offered opportunities for the legitimation of the colonial state it also afforded Filipino doctors and nationalists a platform from which they could challenge, in its own terms, the medico-sanitary justification of American government in the Philippines. To their cost the Americans in the Philippines found that the domain of health afforded more than self-legitimating images of scientific humanitarism; it also provided subversive images of bungling insensitivity and worse; Filipinos gave these wide currency in the Islands during the Taft era.[70] Imperial medicine's Philippine essay provoked a biting counter-tradition, largely ignored by subsequent historians of America in the Philippines.

NOTES

This is a revised version of a paper presented to the 57th ANZAAS Congress at James Cook University, North Queensland, Australia in August 1987. The author thanks the James Cook University's History Department for supporting the research on which this Chapter was based and acknowledges the stimulating assistance received from his Departmental colleague, Dr Reynaldo C. Ileto, with whom he is collaborating on a wider study of the impact of epidemics on Philippine society and politics between 1882 and 1913.

1. *Report of the Philippine Commission, 1904*, (Washington, D.C.: Government Printing Office, 1905), II, 111–12 (hereafter *RPC*); *Manila Times*, 22 March 1902.

2. V. Heiser, *An American Doctor's Odyssey* (New York: W.W. Norton, 1936), 105; D.C. Worcester, *A History of Asiatic Cholera in the Philippine Islands* (Manila: Bureau of Printing, 1908), 16; D.P. Barrows, *A Decade of American Government in the Philippines* (New York: World Book Company, 1914), 5.

3. *Manila Times*, 22 March 1902; 30 May 1902.

4. *Report of the Secretary of the Interior to the Philippine Commission for the Year Ending August 31, 1902* (Manila: Bureau of Public Printing, 1902), 13–14, 27.

5. *RPC, 1903*, II, 109; *Manila Times*, 17 January 1902; 23 January 1902.

6. Worcester to Kitty (C.E. Worcester), 14 January 1902, Worcester Papers, Folio: Letters to C.E. Worcester, 1902, Thetford Historical Society, Thetford, Vermont.

7. R.C. Ileto, 'The politics of cholera in the late nineteenth-century Philippines', paper presented to the 57th ANZAAS Congress at James Cook University, Townsville, Queensland, Australia, 27 August 1987.

8. R.C. Ileto, 'Cholera and the origins of the American sanitary regime in the

Philippines', in D. Arnold (ed.), *Imperial Medicine and Indigenous Societies: Disease, Medicine and Empire in the Nineteenth and Twentieth Centuries* (Manchester: Manchester University Press, forthcoming).

9. W.C. Forbes, *The Philippine Islands* (Boston: Houghton Mifflin, 1928), Vol. I, 331; L.E. Gleeck, *American Institutions in the Philippines* (Manila: Historical Conservation Society, XVIII, 1976), 146; J.A. Larkin, *The Pampangans: Colonial Society in a Philippine Province* (Berkeley: University of California Press, 1972), 163–4.

10. Ileto, op. cit., n. 8 above, 1.

11. President McKinley's Benevolent Assimilation Proclamation is recorded in *United States Senate Document 208, 56th Congress, 1st Session, 1900*, 82–3.

12. President Truman proclaimed the Philippines an independent Republic on 4 July 1946; much earlier the same date had been chosen for the inauguration of civil government under Taft in 1901. In 1962 the Philippine Government changed the National Day from 4 July to 12 June, the day in 1898 when Emilio Aguinaldo proclaimed independence for the First Philippine Republic.

13. 'General Otis reviews his work', special cable despatch, *New York Sun*, 3 May 1900. Reprinted in M. Wilcox (ed.), *Harpers History of the War in the Philippines* (New York and London, 1900), 379.

14. W.H. Taft, 'Civil government in the Philippines', in W.H. Taft and T. Roosevelt, *The Philippines* (New York: The Outlook Company, 1902), 50, 105.

15. R.J. Sullivan ' "Exemplar of Americanism": The Philippine career of Dean D. Worcester' (Unpublished PhD thesis, James Cook University, 1986), 287–8.

16. *Manila Times*, 26 January 1902.

17. ibid., 7 October 1902.

18. Sullivan, op. cit., n. 15 above, 265–7.

19. Taft, op. cit., n. 14 above, 103–4.

20. *RPC, 1902*, II, 64: *RPC, 1904*, II, 84.

21. Heiser, op. cit., n. 2 above, 37.

22. The term was used by Major Carter. *RPC, 1904*, II, 133.

23. *Manila Times*, 6 March 1903.

24. ibid., 18 March 1902.

25. ibid., 25 September 1902.

26. ibid., 2 August 1902.

27. ibid., 26 August 1902.

28. ibid., 30 April 1902; 4 May 1902; 13 May 1902.

29. ibid., 18 July 1902.

30. ibid., 20 July 1902.

31. Forbes, op. cit., n. 9 above, vol. I, 331–2; Sullivan, 'Exemplar of Americanism', 17–45.

32. Sullivan, op. cit., n. 15 above, 147.

33. *Reports of the Philippine Commission, the Civil Governor and the Heads of the Executive Departments of the Civil Government of the Philippine Islands 1900–1903* (Washington, D.C.: Government Printing Office, 1904), 176; Forbes, op. cit., n. 9 above, vol, 332.

34. *Report of Secretary of Interior, 1902*, 6–7.

35. Worcester to Kitty (C.E. Worcester), 14 January 1902, n. 6 above.

36. Sullivan, op. cit., n. 15 above, 208. Moses soon fled to the relative safety of Baguio. See Worcester to Taft, 5 April 1902, William H. Taft Papers, Series 3, Reel 35, Manuscripts Division, Library of Congress, Washington D.C.

37. ibid., Worcester, op. cit., n. 2 above, 17.

38. Worcester to Taft, 5 April 1902, n. 36 above.

39. For an indication of the continuity between the anti-plague and anti-cholera campaigns, see ibid.

40. *Report of Secretary of Interior, 1902*, n. 4 above, 11–13; Heiser, op. cit., n. 2 above, 86–7.

41. *Manila Times*, 3 January 1902. See Ileto, op. cit., n. 8 above, for the coincidence of war and cholera especially in southwestern Luzon.

42. Worcester to Taft, 5 April 1902, n. 36 above; Heiser, op cit., n. 2 above, 100.

43. Worcester to Kitty (C.E. Worcester), 20 November 1902, n. 6 above.

44. *RPC, 1903*, II, 75–8, 221; extracts from the pamphlet 'Asiatic cholera' by Major Charles Lynch, Surgeon, US volunteers, published in *Manila Times*, 7 May 1902; *Report of Secretary of Interior, 1902*, n. 4 above, 14.

45. 'Sanitation in Manila', *Manila Times*, 28 February 1903.

46. *RPC, 1903* II, 75; *Manila Times*, 7 October 1902; 22 October 1902; 28 October 1902; 14 November 1902.

47. Worcester to Kitty (C.E. Worcester), 20 November 1902, n. 6 above.

48. *Manila Times*, 22 October 1902.

49. *RPC, 1904*, II, 75–6.

50. For a full and unusually frank account of the Philippine-American War, see S.C. Miller, *'Benevolent Assimilation': The American Conquest of the Philippines, 1899–1903* (New Haven: Yale University Press, 1982).

51. *Report of Secretary of Interior, 1902*, n. 4, above, 15. On the overlapping military and cholera campaigns see especially Ileto, op. cit., n. 8 above.

52. Sullivan, op. cit., n. 15 above, 208–9; *Manila Times*, 25 March 1902; 3 September 1902; *Report of Secretary of Interior, 1902*, n. 4 above, 15–16; Worcester to Taft, 5 April 1902, n. 36 above.

53. *RPC, 1904*, II, 188.

54. *Report of Secretary of Interior, 1902*, n. 4 above, 12; *RPC, 1903*, II, 173; Worcester to Taft, 5 April 1902, n. 36 above; Worcester, op. cit., n. 2 above, 18.

55. E. Moses, *Unofficial Letters of an Official's Wife* (New York: Appleton, 1908), 223.

56. Worcester to Taft, 5 April 1902, n. 36 above; for the description of Santa Mesa see *Manila Times*, 30 April 1902.

57. *Manila Times*, 30 April 1902; D.C. Worcester, *The Philippines Past and Present* (New York: Macmillan, 1914), vol. I, 442.

58. 'Teachers and cholera in the Philippines II', *Nation, 77*, no. 1998 (15 October 1903), 298; *RPC, 1903*, II, 231.

59. V. Heiser, 'The outbreak of Cholera in the Philippines in 1905', *Journal of the American Medical Association, XLVIII*, 10 (9 March 1907), 859.

60. Worcester to Taft, 5 April 1902, n. 36 above.

61. *Manila Times*, 25 October 1902.

62. ibid., *RPC, 1903*, II, 231; *RPC, 1904*, II, 87–8, 133.

63 .W.B. Freer, *The Philippine Experiences of an American Teacher* (New York: Charles Scribner's Sons, 1906), 142–4; J.R. White, *Bullets and Bolos: Fifteen Years in the Philippine Islands* (New York: The Century Co., 1928), 121; *Manila Times*, 28 July 1902; 4 July 1902; 9 May 1902,

64. On the role of cholera and/or sanitary police, see *Manila Times*, 25 March 1902; 17 April 1902; *RPC, 1900–1903*, n. 33 above, 555; *ROPC, 1904*, II, 186.

65. *Manila Times*, 17 November 1902.

66. *Manila Times*, 25 October 1902; Worcester, op. cit., n. 2 above, 18; *RPC, 1904*, II, 117; J.A. Le Roy, 'The Philippines health problem', *Outlook, 71*, 13 (26 July 1902), 780; Worcester to Taft, 5 April 1902, n. 36 above; J.B. Van Hise, 'American contributions to Philippine science and technology' (unpublished PhD thesis, University of Wisconsin, 1957), 116; *RPC, 1905*, II, 103; Ileto, op. cit., n. 8 above.

67. Sullivan, op. cit., n. 15 above, 207–17; Ileto, op. cit., n. 8 above.

68. *Manila Times*, 27 March 1902.

69. *Secretary of Interior's Report, 1902*, n. 4 above, 19; *Manila Times*, 13 July 1902; 17 July 1902, 27 July 1902.

70. Sullivan, op. cit., n. 15 above, 218–26.

15

The 'health of the race' and infant health in New South Wales: perspectives on medicine and empire

Milton Lewis

INTRODUCTION

For a long time medicine was widely perceived as an enterprise expressive of some of the highest values of Western civilization: scientific enlightenment, benevolence, and humanitarianism. Moreover, it was seen to possess a body of objective knowledge and a superior effectiveness in the curing of disease and the restoration of health. This view of medicine has been challenged by historians and sociologists who have drawn attention to the political, economic, and social forces shaping the development of medicine, and to the ideological ends which medicine has served.[1] Scholars — in earlier essays in this volume — have extensively explored the professionalization of medicine in Europe or America, and in Australia, and have shown how control of a special body of knowledge has been used by the profession to bolster claims to privileged status and economic advantage.[2] This chapter enquires into the ways in which 'domestic' medicine in Australia was influenced by ideological and political forces generated by imperialism. It explores how interest in infant health quickened with the emergence of concern about population and state power in a world marked by growing imperial rivalry.[3] If tropical medicine was a response to the problems associated with more vigorous economic exploitation of empire at the periphery, then rising interest in infant health was in part a result of fears that an unfit metropolitan people (including the white Dominions) would be unable to defend and develop imperial possessions.

As political and economic competition among Western nations and empires intensified in the last years of the nineteenth century, a search developed for means by which to increase national and imperial power. Quantity and quality of population became matters of concern. Infant lives lost were no longer seen as inevitable hardships in a Malthusian world of scarcity. Babies were valuable assets in the emerging struggle for supremacy. In Australia, New Zealand, and Britain, as in France, Germany, and the United States — at the outer edge of white settlement and at the centre of empire — doctors joined politicians in advocating communal action to promote infant health. The 'health of the race' and infant health became linked.

RACE AND EMPIRE

The 'new imperialism' and the heightened nationalism of the late nineteenth century brought with them a significant emphasis on race. A social Darwinist struggle for survival among races became a common vision of the future. In the 1880s, in New South Wales, the nationalist *Bulletin* welcomed T.H. Huxley's suggestion that the struggle had shifted from the level of the individual to the level of the collectivity. In the 1890s, C.H. Pearson, University Professor and Minister for Education in Victoria, whose book *National Life and Character* was well known in Britain and the United States, pessimistically forecast that 'inferior' coloured races would come to dominate the white race and that mankind would fall back to a lower stage of evolution.[4] The loyalty of race was widely proclaimed: Sir Henry Parkes, veteran New South Wales politician and advocate of colonial federation, spoke for most Australians when he proclaimed in 1893, 'we are all one family, all one blood, all one faith.'[5]

In Britain, as in America and Europe, there was much discussion of what constituted an ascendant racial group. In 1899, Colonial Secretary Joseph Chamberlain publicly canvassed the idea of a triple alliance of Britain, the United States, and Germany built on racial affinity, rather than common interest. Professor Karl Pearson, biometrician and eugenicist, envisaged a large-scale conflict in which efficient races — those superior in scientific and military terms — would overwhelm races whose physical and moral fitness had dangerously declined. Although extreme racialism was not widespread in Britain, its assumptions became part of the vocabulary of imperialism. Conflict and struggle for supremacy, accepted as inevitable and even desirable, became dominant images of human affairs.[6] In such a vision, a large and robust population was a vital resource, and there was reason to fear that Britain lacked what rival powers possessed.

Could the hundreds of thousands of able-bodied, loyal soldiers the Empire required be obtained from a stunted working class? This seemed an especially serious problem to the *fin-de-siècle* statesmen who heard repeated warnings about war as a natural law of history, and who saw in Imperial Germany a 'national organism' determined to prove itself the fittest.[7]

A DECLINING BIRTH-RATE

Fitness was one aspect of the population question. The decline of the birth-rate was another. Indeed, Britain was to inform the Imperial Conference of 1907 that the mother country could not afford to allow more than 300,000 migrants a year to settle in the overseas dominions. Concern about population marked almost every official enquiry into emigration until the Second World War.[8] The average size of completed families began to decline in most Western European countries and in English-speaking communities overseas from about 1875. This process of fertility decline was a momentous event which started in France and continued in many Western countries in the 1930s. The process began in Australia in the 1880s, a decade later than in England, but the economic depression of the 1890s was associated with a reduction in marital fertility of one-fifth, a greater decline than that of England or the United States in the early phase of their fertility transition.[9]

In France, fears of the growing power of Germany led to advocacy of measures to stimulate population growth. The Alliance National pour L'accroissement de la Population Française was formed in 1896 and in 1902 the establishment of an extra-parliamentary commission on population decline was achieved. The pronatalist movement won a further victory when the Conseil Supérieur de la Natalité was created to enquire into matters of fertility and mortality. From 1902, the Ligue Contre la Mortalité Infantile concerned itself with the specific problem of infant mortality.[10] In Germany, the declining birth-rate evoked various proposals aimed at promoting population growth: allowances for families with three or more healthy children, suppression of contraceptive information, extra taxation of the childless, and severe penalties for induced abortion. Infant welfare work received imperial patronage. The Kaiserin Auguste Victoria Haus in Berlin was established as a model institution for research on infancy, for training of nurses, and for care of parturient women and sick babies.[11]

In the United States, the declining birthrate, referred to as a 'race suicide', was the subject of national debate in the early 1900s.[12] President Theodore Roosevelt took a leading role in the debate, and was quoted in other countries, including Australia, where the question was discussed. As in Britain and Australia, national efficiency was much in vogue, and Rooseveltian progressivism saw health as an important ingredient in national economic, political, and military strength: 'Progressives cared desperately for the health of the race. Accordingly, enormous attention went to the welfare of mothers, babies and children. The stress on youth reinforced vitalism and complemented progressive education.'[13] Irving Fisher, a Yale economist, prepared for Roosevelt's Commission on the Conservation of Natural Resources a report on national vitality, strongly advocating measures to improve the health of mothers and children. In 1909 the American Academy of Medicine convened a conference from which grew the American Association for the Study and Prevention of Infant Mortality. Three years later, the United States Government created the Federal Children's Bureau, which was given the task of enquiring into 'all matters pertaining to the welfare of children and infant life'.[14]

THE AUSTRALIAN RESPONSE TO THE DECLINING BIRTH-RATE

Concern about population growth in Australia had both national and imperial dimensions which, like the dual loyalties of most Australians, were closely interwoven. The New South Wales Royal Commission on the Birth-rate and on Infant Mortality of 1903–4 served to focus this concern, and gave expression to widely held national ambitions to develop the resources of the island continent while maintaining British control of its destiny. The Birth-rate Commission warned,

> The future of the Commonwealth, and especially the possibility of maintaining a 'white Australia', depends on the question whether we shall be able to people the vast areas of the continent. . . . This can only be done by restoring . . . a high rate of natural increase or by immigration. . . . With the maintenance of a high rate of natural increase is inseparably connected the preservation of infant life.[15]

Concerning the new nation's regional ambitions, the Commission said that 'patriotic ardour' must cool in the face of the fact that while Russia and Japan, Australia's rivals for supremacy in the Western Pacific, had populations to support overseas expansion, Australia would have to wait 46 years to double her population, and 168 years before her numbers reached the existing population of Japan.[16]

The emergence of Japan as a modern power, and the flood of Japanese immigration into California and British Columbia in the 1890s, revived old fears of the 'yellow peril'. T.A. (later Sir Timothy) Coghlan, New South Wales Statistician and publicist for the declining birth-rate, spoke for many Australians when he wrote in 1908, 'The most serious objection to the coloured races . . . is the ethnical; the economic objections might perhaps be waived were the other non-existent'.[17] The leaders of the infant welfare movement in New South Wales clearly believed that white population growth was vital to the defence of 'white Australia'. C.K. (later Sir Charles) Mackellar, prominent doctor and conservative member of the Legislative Council, expressed through his work on the Birth-rate Commission and elsewhere his belief in the critical importance of population growth. Others shared his belief. Neville Mayman, President of the Benevolent Society, the state's long-established major source of social services, said to Holman's Nationalist government, in his report on infant welfare in New Zealand: 'The State is deeply interested in the increase of its population, more particularly in a young country. Every baby born is a prospective tax-payer and wealth producer'.[18] He recommended state support for infant welfare work.

Major charitable bodies, carrying out infant and maternal work, appealed for funds from the public in similar terms. In 1918 the Benevolent Society asked for support for its Renwick Hospital for Infants and its Royal Hospital for Women; 'Healthy, happy children make a strong and virile race. Australia needs every baby it can save. . . . The Mothers of our race deserve the best we can provide for them, as the future of the nation is in their keeping'.[19] Appealing for funds in 1925, the management of St Margaret's Hospital, a leading maternity hospital in Sydney, declared:

> In the last four years, 122,990 infants have died . . . more than twice the number of Australian soldiers killed during the war. . . . Just as surely as the white races took Australia by force from the aboriginals, so surely will the coloured races take Australia by force from the descendants of the present race unless something is done towards self-preservation.[20]

The expansion of Japanese power and the increasing instability of the international order kept interest in population growth alive in the inter-war period.

THE EMERGENCE OF INFANT WELFARE IN BRITAIN AND NEW SOUTH WALES

Public provision for infants in Britain before the end of the century involved shelter for abandoned and unwanted babies, and protection of infants from abuse or neglect. In 1870 the Infant Life Protection Society was founded by J.B. Curgenven, Surgeon and Honorary Secretary of the Harveian Society, and W.T. Charley, Conservative MP for Salford, and soon after a Select Committee of the House of Commons investigated infant abuse.[21] The Committee found that paid fostering of babies, known as baby-farming, had led to widespread abuse of infant life and it recommended that all persons fostering two or more infants for reward be registered. The Infant Life Protection Act of 1872 implemented the recommendation but the protection offered by the legislation was less than complete. Public disquiet about the case of Mrs Dwyer, a foster mother, executed for the murder of her charges in 1896, led to the passing of new legislation. The Infant Life Protection Act of 1897 gave local authorities the power to remove a child from premises when inspection was refused. It raised the age limit to five years, and under improper care it specifically included danger to the health of the child.[22]

The development of collective concern about the welfare of infants followed a similar path in New South Wales. Emphasis was placed on the protection of illegitimate babies from baby-farming and on the provision of shelter for orphans. In 1874 the Sydney Foundling Hospital was established to save illegitimate babies from 'hideous maltreatment' by baby-farmers.[23] The Benevolent Society provided refuge for unmarried mothers and abandoned infants. The Society's Asylum housed a lying-in establishment which, until the 1880s, was the only public maternity accommodation in Sydney. Law reformers sought protective legislation similar to that enacted in Britain. In 1886, J.M. Creed, a senior member of the medical profession, persuaded the Legislative Council of New South Wales to create a Select Committee on abuse of infant life. Both Creed and C.K. Mackellar were members of the Committee. Like Mackellar, Creed publicly stated his concern about population increase and maintenance of a racially homogenous Australia. He believed that it was a matter of the 'highest moment' for the Empire that tropical Australia be settled by British stock in such a way that it did not result in 'race deterioration'. Proposing tax incentives to raise the birth-rate, Creed proclaimed that 'it is in the interest of the State that the population of white British subjects in it should increase'.[24]

Creed's Committee heard that illegitimate babies were often buried as stillborn when such was not the case, and that many private maternity homes neglected to report births and deaths occurring on their premises.[25] Creed introduced a bill based on the Committee's findings, but it was not passed. Against a background of publicity about baby-farming in Sydney, the Children's Protection Act was passed in 1892. This outlawed lump-sum payments for fostering, required notification of deaths of fostered infants, and obliged keepers of private maternity homes regularly to furnish lists of births in their establishments. In the early 1900s, C.K. Mackellar introduced further protective legislation. The Infant Protection Act of 1904 was intended to enable the single mother to keep her baby in the early critical stage of life. Mackellar hoped that the very high mortality of illegitimate babies would thus be reduced. The Private Hospitals Act of 1908 introduced official supervision of private lying-in establishments. Mackellar intended that supervision would not only promote better hygiene, but would also help to put down the practice of induced abortion. Behind his concern about the well-being of illegitimate and disadvantaged babies, a strong interest in the general health of infants was developing. Humanitarianism was a moving force but concern about population was manifestly important.

INFANT HEALTH, POPULATION AND STATE POWER

Around the turn of the century there was a marked change in attitudes towards the health of infants and children in Britain. While the last two decades of the nineteenth century saw growing domestic pressures for social reform, they produced little political benefit. In 1899, however, Britain was plunged into war in South Africa, and widespread physical disability among the working-class recruits was revealed. Behind the immediate challenge presented by the Boers, there loomed the menace of Imperial Germany, which was thought to be more 'efficient' than Britain in major areas of national life. The chimera of 'national efficiency' ranged through politics, education, commerce, and industry, but basic to all was the concept of physical efficiency. In this climate of opinion, a falling birth-rate and fitness of the population become significant issues. Social reform now possessed imperial significance: 'Imperialism and the "condition of the people" question became linked. Only an efficient nation could hold a vigorous expanding empire'.[26] Lord Milner told a conservative audience in 1906 that raising the efficiency of the people was not philanthropy, but good business.[27]

In 1901, two publications drew Britain's attention to the problem of national fitness. Arnold White's *Efficiency and Empire* revealed that three out of five volunteers at the Manchester depot in 1899 had been rejected as unfit, and Seebohm Rowntree's study of poverty in York showed that more than 26 per cent of recruits at the York, Leeds, and Sheffield depots between 1897 and 1900 had been similarly rejected, and that another 29 per cent had only been accepted provisionally. However, it was an article by General Sir John Frederick Maurice, published in 1902, which really stirred public opinion.[28] Maurice pointed out that when the rejectees were added to the recruits later lost because of poor fitness, only two out of five men became useful soldiers. The Inspector General of Recruiting laid before parliament a report on manpower which confirmed the alarming picture. In July 1904, the Balfour Government received a report from its Interdepartmental Committee on Physical Deterioration, which recommended the extension of public health measures, the instruction of girls in child care and domestic arts, the encouragement of physical education and the creation of a system of school inspection and school meals.[29] Above all, the problem of physical deterioration would be attacked by improving the health of the young. What had been philanthropy or Socialism, now became a vital 'national' interest. Thus in 1905, when proposing various reforms including provision of school canteens, free transport, and baths for school children, T.J. Macnamara, a Liberal Member of parliament, could claim,

> All this sounds terribly like rank socialism . . . but I am not in the least dismayed. Because I know it also to be first rate Imperialism . . . because . . . it is out of the mouths of babes and sucklings that the strength is ordained which shall still the Enemy and the Avenger.[30]

During 1903 and 1904, the *British Medical Journal* published material on the question of physical deterioration: 'now, more than at any time in the history of the British people do we require stalwart sons to people the colonies and to uphold the prestige of the nation'.[31] The British Medical Association urged the government to introduce medical inspection and physical training in schools. One of the principal medical advocates of improved state provision was Arthur (later Sir Arthur) Newsholme, Chief Medical Officer to the Local Government Board from 1908 to 1918. Infant health was an enduring concern of Newsholme's long career in public health. While at the Local Government Board he produced five reports on infant mortality, each of which emphasized the importance of infant welfare work to the British population.[32] His contemporary, G.F. McCleary, saw fears about depopulation motivating the pioneers of infant health work.[33] McCleary himself became chairman of the National Council for Maternity and Child Welfare, and chairman of the National Association of Maternity and Child Welfare Centres and for the Prevention of Infant Mortality.

With the appointment of Newsholme to the Local Government Board and the passing of the Notifications of Births Act, 1907, central government began to assume a direct role in the campaign to reduce infant mortality. Local government provided the actual services for mothers and babies, while voluntary effort also played a significant part. In 1917 the Local Government Board reported that in England and in Wales, local authorities operated 396 infant welfare centres, while voluntary bodies operated another 446 centres. Sanitarians like Newsholme were only too well aware that while public health measures helped reduce the general death-rate, they had little effect on the infant mortality rate. For decades, public health doctors had been concerned about the high infant mortality rate in cities and the devastations of infant diarrhoeal disease. Sir John Simon had identified the infant mortality rate as a prime indicator of sanitary conditions. However, it took the concern about physical deterioration of the race generated by the revelation of poor fitness among recruits to turn the problem of infant health into a national and imperial issue.

In New South Wales, attention on infant health was focused by the Royal Commission on the Birth-rate and on Infant Mortality in 1903. The enquiry publicized the problem of infant mortality nationally.[34] The man who persuaded the Government to institute an enquiry, who became President of the Commission, and who dominated its proceedings was C.K. Mackellar. Mackellar saw Asia's fertility as a threat to Australia's survival as a white British nation.

Many in the medical profession shared Mackellar's fears.[35] As early as 1898, the New South Wales professional journal, the *Australasian Medical Gazette*, had drawn attention to the marked decline in the birth-rate over the previous decade. In an editorial of January 1901, the *Gazette* discussed the matter again, and concluded 'what with Russia, Germany and France becoming Pacific powers, and the yellow peril looming up again . . . a population sufficiently large to discount any thought of invasion is a vital necessity'. The journal accepted that the use of contraceptives should not be outlawed, so it turned its attention to the reduction of infant mortality as the most promising way to promote population growth.[36] A substantial part of the Birth-rate Commission's report was devoted to the problem of infant mortality, and a number of its recommendations were implemented. More important than its specific proposals was its impact on public opinion. Through the population question, it articulated the connection between infant health and national power and imperial strength.

In the early years of Federation, this connection was observed time and again in both medical and lay press. In 1907 the *Australasian Medical Gazette* took up a position against contraception, in the interests of population growth and national well-being. When this proved difficult to achieve, it praised public health authorities and 'philanthropists' who turned to effective means of reducing infant mortality.[37] In 1913 the *Gazette* reported approvingly the Bishop of Riverina's address to an Anglican conference, on the 'dark blot of race suicide' which had 'infected the Christian nations like the plague'.[38] Australian Protestant and Catholic doctors shared a strong pro-natalist position, displaying a common opposition to contraception and abortion. In a period when the Catholic minority in Australia sought to identify with the nation, Catholic doctors were influenced by nationalist as well as by moral and doctrinal considerations.[39] The conservation of infant life became a new area of organized effort by medicine and the state.

MODERN INFANT HEALTH WORK

Organized infant health work was initiated in Australia in the early 1900s by W.G. Armstrong, Sydney's first Medical Officer of Health. Armstrong had been influenced by the work of Newsholme in England, and of Pierre Budin at the Charité Hospital in Paris. In 1904 Armstrong introduced a domiciliary service in the inner city. In 1914 the New South Wales Labor government established the first clinic. By 1918, there were twenty-eight clinics in operation. With some justification, the clinics could claim to have played an important part in the eradication of diarrhoeal mortality. In 1915, the New South Wales government introduced the Early Notification of Births Act, similar to that which operated in Britain. This legislation was intended to improve contact between the infant health authorities and the mothers of new-born children. Infant health and 'white Australia' went hand-in-hand. Welcoming the Bill, J.J. Morris, then Labor Member for King (but later a Nationalist) argued that the coloured races were reproducing more prolifically than the white race, and thus presented a threat to European supremacy. W.R.C. Bagnell, Labor Member for St George (later a Nationalist) congratulated the government on its efforts to save infant lives at a time when so many young men — potential fathers — were dying at the front; there was no proper substitute for native-born citizens.[40]

The loss of men in the Great War evoked demands in both Britain and Australia for greater effort to conserve infant life. The UK Maternity and Child Welfare Act of 1918 confirmed the legality of local government expenditure on infant and maternal welfare services, and a maternity and child welfare section was created within the new Ministry of Health. To co-ordinate the activities of voluntary bodies, nine organizations came together in 1917 to form the National League for Health, Maternity and Child Welfare. In New South Wales, the Holman government sent Neville Mayman, deputy chairman of the Clinics Advisory Board, as a Commissioner to investigate work in New Zealand. Mayman reported favourably in 1918 on Dr Truby King's Plunket Society, and spoke of the 'imperative obligation' on New South Wales and the other Australian States to initiate immediate measures to conserve infant lives.[41] A Royal Society for the Welfare of Mothers and Babies was formed in New South Wales with official support.[42] But when the performance of the Society in reducing infant mortality was compared unfavourably with the achievements of the Plunket Society in 1926, on the recommendation of the Director General of Public Health, control of the State's network of baby clinics passed from the Royal Society to the new Division of Maternal and Baby Welfare within the State Department of Health.

INFANT HEALTH IN NEW ZEALAND

By the end of the nineteenth century, New Zealand had enjoyed a remarkably low level of infant mortality, and in this respect was the envy of other Western nations. In 1891–5, when the New South Wales rate was 111 per thousand live births, the New Zealand rate was only 87; and in 1901–5 the rates were 97 and 74 respectively. Moreover, the New Zealand rate was falling substantially well before Truby King began his campaign in 1907.

King had been much impressed by General Maurice's warnings about physical deterioration in Britain and had become determined to teach proper care and, especially, the practice of breast-feeding for the development of a worthy imperial race. He admired Japanese military prowess which he believed rested ultimately on the fitness of peasant babies enjoying prolonged breast-feeding.[43] In 1909 he admonished New Zealanders to remember that 'Ancient Greece and Rome and modern France had become second-class powers because of increasing selfishness . . . [and] a disinclination for the ties of marriage and parenthood.'[44] Like Mackellar in New South Wales, King reflected the imperialism of New Zealand's colonial upper and middle classes. The military power of the Empire clearly depended upon a population of healthy boys who would become fit young soldiers and on healthy girls who would be capable mothers. King wanted an Antipodean Utopia where workers and employers could live in health, happiness and social order. King's influence spread to Australia and Britain.[45] He was appointed first Director of Child Welfare in New Zealand in 1921, and by 1930 about 65 per cent of all non-Maori babies were under the care of his Plunket Society. Mackellar shared King's belief that this Utopia was possible in the new Dominions, with their abundance of resources, and where Europe's heritage of poverty and class conflict was unknown.[46]

In 1920, Margaret Harper, a Sydney paediatrician, recommended to the Royal Society for the Welfare of Mothers and Babies that it establish a training school on the model of King's Karitane Hospital school. But this was the high point of King's influence in New South Wales.[47] Although the Australian Mothercraft Society, which strictly followed King's principles of child-care, was launched in Sydney in 1923, it remained small and never seriously challenged the hegemony of the Royal Society.

CONCLUSION

Mackellar in New South Wales, King in New Zealand and McCleary and Newman in Britain shared similar ideas about population and infant health. These ideas continued to be influential into the 1930s. At the first meeting of the Federal National Health and Medical Research Council in 1937, the Australian Minister for Health (and former Prime Minister) W.M. Hughes, who in the 1930s was obsessed by the problem of defence, said, 'We can only justify our claim to this great and fertile country by effectively occupying it. Australia must advance and populate or perish.'[48] In 1930, the British Ministry of Health agreed that the maternal and infant mortality rates determined 'the survival of a nation'.[49] In 1937 the Conservative Government in Britain introduced a Population (Statistics) Act, to increase the collection of information about fertility. A meeting of the Primrose League passed a resolution saying that the tendency of the population to decline constituted a grave menace to the standard of living and the security of the nation.[50]

Not all doctors who promoted infant health work were so manifestly influenced by the idea of population as a national and imperial resource. Armstrong, for example, did not employ the rhetoric of population and power. But others did lend the weight of medical science to an ideology widely shared among members of the elite, and collective support for infant health was much advanced in this ideological climate. In the Antipodean Dominions, a local nationalism, in which deep fear of Asian (especially Japanese) expansionism was a prominent element, affected thinking about population growth and infant health. The nationalism co-existed with a strong imperial patriotism.

In 1909, J.S.C. Elkington, Commissioner of Public Health in Tasmania and later an influential member of the Federal Health Department, told the patriotic Australian Natives' Association that the high level of infant illness was a threat to the racial efficiency and the survival of the nation.[51] 'The skilled and earnest infant visitor is the very best of all missionaries if we desire to glorify, dignify and purify motherhood among those who furnish the very bones and sinew of our body politic'.[52] Elkington revealed again the connection between medicine and the contemporary social context. Medicine was not simply a body of scientific knowledge and a source of increasingly effective practice, immune from the dominant ideological influences generated in its socio-economic and political environment. Indeed, the origins of modern infant health policy reveal the important links between the roles set for medicine and the political, economic, and social assumptions of nineteenth-century imperialism.

NOTES

The author wishes to thank Dr Jay Winter and Professor Roy MacLeod for their comments on an earlier draft of this chapter.

1. See, for example, M. Worboys, 'The emergence of tropical medicine: a study in the establishment of a scientific specialty', in G. Lemaine, *et al.* (eds), *Perspectives on the Emergence of Scientific Disciplines* (The Hague: Mouton, 1976, 75–98). E.R. Brown, 'Public health in imperialism: early Rockefeller programs at home and abroad', *American Journal of Public Health, 66* (1976), 897–903. N.Stepan, 'The interplay between socio-economic factors and medical science: yellow fever research, Cuba and the United States', *Social Studies of Science, 8* (1978), 397–423.

2. See, for example, E. Freidson, *Profession of Medicine: A Study of the Sociology of Applied Knowledge* (New York: Harper & Row, 1970). M.J. Peterson, *The Medical Profession in Mid-Victorian London* (Berkeley: University of California Press, 1978). T.S. Pensabene, *The Rise of the Medical Practitioner in Victoria* (Canberra: Australian National University Press, 1980). M. Lewis and R. MacLeod, 'Medical politics and professionalisation

of medicine in New South Wales, 1850–1901', *Journal of Australian Studies* (1988); E. Willis, *Medical Dominance: The Division of Labour in Australian Health Care* (Sydney: Allen & Unwin, 1983).

3. A well-known history of paediatrics links the emergence of paediatrics as a medical specialty with concern about population. I.A. Abt and F.H. Garrison, *History of Pediatrics* (Philadelphia: Saunders, 1923), 130. Recently, M.S. Teitelbaum and J.M. Winter have examined the ramifications of concern about population decline in Europe and the United States over the last century. They point to the recurrent waves of alarm over decline, relating this to demographic change and to perceptions of connections between population change and economic, social, and political power. They also point to the ideological element underlying many perceptions. *The Fear of Population Decline* (London: Academic Press, 1985), 1–2 and 129–33. R.A. Solway has discussed the often contentious debate about the declining birth-rate in England in his *Birth Control and Population in England, 1877–1930* (Chapel Hill: University of North Carolina Press, 1982). He notes that the population question intruded into most contemporary issues, including imperialism (ibid., XII). The debate in Australia has been analysed by N. Hicks in *'This Sin and Scandal': Australia's Population Debate, 1891–1911* (Canberra: Australian National University Press, 1978). A. Davin has explored the connections in Britain between the population question, interest in infant welfare work, and imperialism in 'Imperialism and motherhood', *History Workshop, 5* (Spring 1978), 9–65. She identifies a strong ideological element in public health doctors' discussions of infant health problems (ibid., 55). Attitudes to motherhood in Australia in this period are discussed in M. Lewis, '"Populate or perish": aspects of infant and maternal health in Sydney, 1870–1939' (Unpublished PhD thesis, Australian National University, 1976), ch. 9.

4. C.D.W. Goodwin, *Economic Enquiry in Australia* (Durham, N.C.: Duke University Press, 1966), 335–8, 344, 347–9.

5. Quoted in D.L. Cole, 'The problem of "nationalism" and "imperialism" in British settlement colonies', *Journal of British Studies, 10* (1971), 168. For racism in Australian and other white-settler colonies, see D.G. Baker, 'Australian and Anglo racism: preliminary explorations' in F.S. Stevens and E.P. Wolfers (eds), *Racism: The Australian Experience*, 3 vols (Sydney: Australia and New Zealand Book Company, 1977), vol. 3, 19–38.

6. G.R. Searle, *The Quest for National Efficiency: A Study in British Politics and Political Thought, 1899–1914* (Oxford: Blackwell, 1971), 95–6.

7. B. Semmel, *Imperialism and Social Reform: English Social-Imperial Thought, 1895–1914* (London: Allen & Unwin, 1960), 23.

8. W.D. Borrie, *The Growth and Control of World Population* (London: Weidenfeld & Nicolson, 1970), 221.

9. L.T. Ruzicka and J.C. Caldwell, *The End of Demographic Transition in Australia* (Canberra: Australian National University Press, 1977), 1–7. In Australia, the average completed size of family in 1891 was seven children. In 1891–1911 it was only five, and for families started in 1911, it was somewhat less than four.

10. D.V. Glass, *Population: Policies and Movements in Europe* (London: Frank Cass, 1967), 147–50.

11. ibid., 270–2. Abt and Garrison, op. cit., n. 3 above, 161. Until the rise in natality under the Nationalist Socialist regime, scores of studies appeared about the *Geburtenrückgang*. J.E. Knodel, *The Decline of Fertility in Germany*, 1871–1939 (Princeton: Princeton University Press, 1974). 6.

12. L. Gordon, 'Race suicide and the feminist response: birth control as a class phenomenon in the US', *Hecate. A Women's Interdisciplinary Journal, 1* (1975), 41.

13. M.Roe, *Nine Australian Progressives: Vitalism in Bourgeois Social Thought, 1890–1960* (St Lucia: University of Queensland Press, 1984), 14.

14. Abt and Garrison, op. cit., n. 3 above, 163–4.

15. *Report of the Royal Commission on Decline of Birth-Rate and on Mortality of*

Infants in New South Wales, vol. 1, 1904, 53, *NSW Parliamentary Papers*, vol. 4, 2nd sess., 1904.

16. ibid.

17. Quoted in A.T. Yarwood, *Asian Migration to Australia: The Background to Exclusion, 1896–1923* (Melbourne: Melbourne University Press, 1967), 26.

18. *Report of Commissioner, Mr. Neville Mayman, on Inquiry into Welfare of Mothers and Children in New Zealand*, 1918, 11, *NSW Parliamentary Papers*, vol. 5, 1918.

19. *Charities Gazette and General Intelligencer* (January 1918), 4–5.

20. *The Romance of St Margaret's Hospital: Behind the Little Green Gate* (Sydney, 1925).

21. The work of Curgenven and other reformers such as Ernest Hart, editor of *The British Medical Journal*, is discussed in G.K. Behlmer, *Child Abuse and Moral Reform in England, 1870–1908* (Stanford: Stanford University Press, 1982), ch. 2. Behlmer suggests that Curgenven and Hart as social 'outsiders' were motivated by the desire for social recognition as well as humanitarianism.

22. J.S. Heywood, *Children in Care: the Development of the Service for the Deprived Child* (London: Routledge & Kegan Paul, 1966), 94–109.

23. *Second Annual Report of the Infants' Home (late Sydney Foundling Hospital), 1876*, 8.

24. J.M. Creed, *My Recollections of Australia and Elsewhere, 1842–1914* (London; H. Jenkins, 1916), 206 and 215.

25. *Report of Select Committee on Registration of Births, Deaths and Marriages*, 1886, 3–4, 7 and 11, *Journal of NSW Legislative Council*, vol. 40, 4 (1885–6).

26. B.B. Gilbert, *The Evolution of National Insurance in Great Britain: The Origins of the Welfare State* (London: Michael Joseph, 1966), 60–1.

27. Searle, op. cit., n. 6 above, 63.

28. Gilbert, op. cit., n. 26 above, 85.

29. ibid., 90–1.

30. Quoted in Davin, op, cit., n. 3 above, 17.

31. *British Medical Journal* (July 1903) (ii), 208.

32. J. Lewis, 'The social history of social policy: infant welfare in Edwardian England', *Journal of Social Policy, 9* (1980), 463.

33. Davin, op. cit., n. 3 above, 14–15.

34. In 1907, O.C. Beale, successful businessman and member of the Royal Commission on the Birth-rate, saw published the report of his own Royal Commission on Secret Drugs, which continued investigation of the population question. Beale had persuaded Prime Minister Alfred Deakin to appoint him Royal Commissioner. In 1910, Beale's book, *Racial Decay*, was published. This appears to have contained everything that could not be included in the Royal Commission Report, and is alleged to have reawakened Theodore Roosevelt's interest in 'race decline'. Hicks, op. cit., n. 3 above, 100–1 and 125.

35. Six of the thirteen Commissioners were prominent members of the medical profession in Sydney: Sir Normand McLaurin, Joseph Foreman, J.B. Nash, Thomas Fiaschi, R.T. Paton, and Mackellar himself. After building a prosperous physician's practice in the 1870s, Mackellar became President of the New South Wales Board of Health. He resigned from the Board in 1885 to become a member of the Legislative Council. He was a director of a number of leading companies. In 1902 he was made Chairman of the State Children's Relief Board. Because of his work in the post and in the Legislative Council, he was seen as an authority on infant and child welfare. MacLaurin, like Mackellar, was an Edinburgh graduate and a Member of the Board of Health from 1882. He was a Legislative Councillor from 1889 and served with Mackellar on the boards of the Mutual Life and Citizen's Assurance Company, the Bank of New South Wales and the Colonial Sugar Refining Company. Foreman went to Europe in 1881 to study women's diseases

at Berlin, Vienna, London and Edinburgh. He became lecturer in obstetrics and gynaecology at Sydney University Medical School in 1896. Nash, another graduate of Edinburgh, became a member of the Legislative Council in 1900. Paton joined the Public Health Service in 1890 and was a member of the Board of Health. He was to succeed to the post of Senior Medical Advisor to the Government. Fiaschi was an Italian graduate who became a leading surgeon in Sydney. For the backgrounds of other members of the Commission and their connections with Mackellar, see Hicks, op. cit., n. 3 above, 1–17.

36. *Australasian Medical Gazette* (November 1898), 502–3 and (January 1901), 43–4.

37. *Australasian Medical Gazette* (November 1907), 587 and (December 1908), 675.

38., *Australasian Medical Gazette* (October 1913), 354.

39. Hicks, op. cit., n. 3 above, 48–9 and 75–6. For changes in medical attitudes to contraception in England, see J. Peel, 'Contraception and the medical profession', *Population Studies, 18* (1964), 133–45. For a general discussion of the attitudes of the Christian Churches to birth control, see F. Campbell, 'Birth control and the Christian churches', *Population Studies, 14* (1960), 131–47. For an attempt to assess the effect of Catholic doctrine on contemporary natality in a number of countries, see L.H. Day, 'Natality and ethnocentrism: some relationships suggested by an analysis of Catholic-Protestant differentials', *Population Studies, 22* (1968), 27–50.

40. *NSW Parliamentary Debates*, vol. 57, 10 February 1915, 2386–7.

41. Mayman Report, n. 18 above, 12.

42. The Holman government introduced legislation in 1919 to incorporate the Society and provide it with funds.

43. For an account of King's work, see M. King, *Truby King: The Man. A Biography* (London: Allen & Unwin, 1948).

44. Quoted in E. Olssen, 'Truby King and the Plunket Society: an analysis of a prescriptive ideology', *New Zealand Journal of History, 15* (April 1981), 4.

45. One historian has suggested that King's influence in Britain was extensive, claiming that he was the 'Spock of that generation' and that he provided the 'theoretical underpinning for much of the advice on childcare', but she casts doubts on the extent of his influence in working-class homes. Davin, op. cit., n. 3 above, 417.

46. Mackellar wrote in 1917: 'we have a healthy climate, a well paid and vigorous young people who are subject to none of the unfavourable conditions which so largely contribute to the excessive mortality of the people of older countries, with their teeming population, often crowded in insanitary tenements, and a majority of them working ten hours a day or more, in ill-ventilated workrooms amidst the grime and the dust engendered by manufacturing processes'. C.K. Mackellar, *The Mother, the Baby and the State* (Sydney: Government Printer, 1917), 15. Mackellar strongly opposed the entry of women into the workforce: 'Women come into the industrial arena to the detriment . . . of their social and natural duties — the care and nurture of children', C.K. Mackellar, *The Child, the Law and the State* (Sydney: Government Printer, 1907), 33.

47. When, in 1922, King sent a large consignment of his infant food from New Zealand to Sydney, the Society refused to take delivery.

48. Quoted in C. Thame, 'Health and the state: the development of collective responsibility for health care in the first half of the twentieth century' (Unpublished PhD Thesis, Australian National University, 1974), 154. Official concern about the declining birthrate continued into the 1940s. See J.H.L. Cumpston, *The Health of the People: A Study in Federalism* (Canberra: Roebuck Press, 1978), ch. XV.

49. Ministry of Health, *Interim Report of Departmental Committee on Maternal Mortality and Morbidity* (London: HMSO, 1930), 103.

50. D.V. Glass, *Numbering the People: the Eighteenth Century Population Controversy and the Development of Census and Vital Statistics in Britain* (Farnborough: D.C. Heath, 1973), 173.

51. Elkington sought public health facilities in northern Australia so that Europeans might safely develop the tropical area. See J.S.C. Elkington, *Tropical Australia: Is it Suitable for a Working White Race?* (Melbourne: State Government Printer for the Commonwealth Government, 1905).

52. Quoted in Roe, op. cit., n. 13 above, 96.

Bibliography

The literature on the relationship between European medicine, medical practice, and colonialism is vast and growing. At this stage, any well-intentioned attempt to do more than provide an introductory bibliography could founder in the complexities and diversities of imperial experience. Nevertheless, it is useful to indicate some of the leading primary sources which anyone new to this subject will find important; and some of the more important secondary sources (chiefly still in journals and monographs) which must inform any general treatment of this subject.

For this purpose, sources appearing before 1939 and listed below are considered 'primary'. This arbitrary distinction locates such well-known 'secondary' texts as Crawford on India and Scott on tropical medicine, and the early writings of important post-war figures, in this category. There are other points the reader will observe. Given the nature of this volume, our bibliography suffers from the inevitable limitations of an Anglo-Saxon (and particularly British) perspective, in both scholarship and subject matter; and from a perspective shaped by our historical interest in social structures, organizations, professions, and demographic trends. Medical anthropology, recently conscious of indigenous systems of medical practice — and the 'fatal impact', in Alan Moorehead's classic phrase, delivered to native regimes by European medicine, as well as by European-borne diseases — is notably absent from our coverage, and would require a large volume in itself. Equally, there is a vast literature on the historical epidemiology and demography of colonial health, much of which has direct bearing on our case studies; and its absence from this bibliography reflects the editorial limits of this volume, not the limits of our vision. Medical history in the imperial context is essentially a field with moving frontiers, and closer contact between epidemiologists, historians, and medical planners must lie high on our future agenda.

We have made no attempt to include here the principal unpublished or archival sources, but of course there are many relevant collections in Europe and North America. In the British context, the archives of the Wellcome Institute for the History of Medicine and the London School of Tropical Medicine (especially the Ross Papers) are well known; the Liverpool School of Tropical Medicine, while perhaps less studied, has considerable archival material awaiting further work. Nancy Stepan and David Fisher have drawn attention to the wealth of Spanish and American materials, particularly in relation to Central and Latin America, which will merit attention for years to come. The essays in this volume on French and German possessions suggest the vast reservoir of archival sources yet to be tapped for research in an area long viewed as unfashionable, as empires are today prone to be, among European social, economic, and medical historians. Indian, African, Asian, and Latin American historians have as yet only begun to address the subject, but there are signs that this is changing. The growth of interest on the 'periphery' in questions viewed traditionally from the 'metropolis' — no less evident in Australia and the Pacific, as in the more established centres of imperial history — indicates that the subject is at last considered too important to be left to Europeans alone.

PRIMARY SOURCES

Balfour, Andrew, *War Against Tropical Disease: being Seven Sanitary Sermons Addressed to all Interested in Tropical Hygiene and Administration*, London: Baillière, 1920.

—— 'Some British and American pioneers in tropical medicine and hygiene', *Transactions of the Royal Society of Tropical Medicine and Hygiene, 19* (1925), 189–229.

Balfour, A. and Scott, H.H., *Health Problems of the Empire: Past, Present and Future*, London: Collins, 1924.

Barrett, J.W., *The Twin Ideals: An Educated Commonwealth*, 2 vols, London: H.K. Lewis, 1918.

Bell, John. *An Inquiry into the Causes which Produce and the Means of Preventing Diseases amongst British Officers, Soldiers and Others in the West Indies, containing observations on the mode of action of spirituous liquors on the human body: on the use of malt liquor and on salted provisions, with remarks on the most proper means of preserving them*, London, 1791.

Bethune, C.R. Drinkwater, *The Observations of Sir Richard Hawkins, Knt., in his Voyage into the South Seas in the year 1593*, London: Hakluyt Society, 1847.

Blacklock, D.B., 'The prevention of disorders and disease in tropical countries', *Journal of State Medicine, 39* (1931), 204–18.

Boyce, Sir Robert W., *Mosquito or Man?*, London: H.K. Lewis, 1909.

—— *Health Progress and Administration in the West Indies*, London: John Murray, 1910.

Boyle, James, *Letters on the Prevention and Cure of Diseases Peculiar to Hot Climates*, London, 1823.

—— *A Practical Medico-Historical Account of the Western Coast of Africa, etc.*, London: S. Highley, 1831

Brau, Paul, *Trois siècles de médecine coloniale française*, Paris: Vigot Frères, 1931.

Breinl, Anton, 'The influence of climate, disease and surroundings on the white race living in the tropics', Stewart Lecture of the University of Melbourne (1913), Melbourne: McCarron, 1914.

—— 'Figures and facts regarding health and diseases in northern Australia influencing its permanent settlement by a white race', *Transactions of the Australasian Medical Congress*, 11th Session (Brisbane, 1920), 558–69.

Brocklesby, Richard, *Economical and Medical Observations, in two parts, From the year 1758 to the year 1763, inclusive. Tending to the improvement of Military Hospitals, and to the cure of camp diseases, incident to soldiers. To which is subjoined, an appendix, containing a curious account of the climate and diseases in Africa, upon the great river Senegal*, London: T. Becket and P.A. De Hondt, 1764.

Burg, C.L. van der, 'L'Alimentation des Européans et des travailleurs indigènes aux pays chauds', *Janus, 10* (1905), 88–94.

Burnett, Sir William and Bryson, Alexander, *Report on the Climate and Principal Diseases of the African Station*, London: Admiralty, Medical Department, 1847.

Buzacott, A., *Mission Life in the Islands of the Pacific*, London: John Snow, 1866.

Canniff, William, *The Medical Profession in Upper Canada, 1783–1850*, Toronto: W. Briggs, 1894.
Castellani, A. and Chaimers, A.J., *Manual of Tropical Medicine*, London: Baillière, Tindal and Cox, 1910.
Christie, James, *Cholera Epidemics in East Africa from 1821 till 1872*, London: Macmillan, 1876.
Cilento, R.W., *The White Man in the Tropics: With Especial Reference to Australia and its Dependencies*, Commonwealth of Australia, Department of Health, Service Publication (Tropical Division), no. 7, Melbourne: Government Printer, 1925.
—— 'The white settlement of tropical Australia', in P.D. Phillips and G.L. Wood (eds), *The Peopling of Australia*, Melbourne: Macmillan, 1928.
—— 'Australia's problems in the tropics', *Report of the Australian and New Zealand Association for the Advancement of Science, 21* (Sydney, 1932), 216–33.
—— 'The conquest of climate: The Anne MacKenzie oration', *Medical Journal of Australia* (8 April 1933) (1), 421–32.
Clark, John, *Observations on the Diseases in Long Voyages to Hot Countries, and particularly on those which prevail in the East Indies*, London: D. Wilson and G. Nicol, 1773.
Coville, R., *Un médecin maritime française au XVII siècle: C. Dallon*, Paris: Jouvre, 1914.
Crawford, D.G., *A History of the Indian Medical Service, 1600–1913*, London: W. Thacker, 1914.
Creighton, Charles, *A History of Epidemics in Britain from A.D. 664 to the Extinction of Plague*, 2 vols, Cambridge: Cambridge University Press, 1891.
Daniell, William F., *Sketches of the Medical Topography and Native Diseases of the Gulf of Guinea, Western Africa*, London: Samuel Highley, 1849.
Elkington, J.S.C., *Tropical Australia: Is it Suitable for a White Working Race?*, Melbourne: Government Printer, 1905.
—— 'The Australian hookworm campaign', *Health, 3* (5) (Canberra, 1925), 141–5.
Fellowes, Sir James, MD, *Reports of the Pestilential Disorder of Andalusia which Appeared at Cadiz in 1800, 1804, 1810 and 1813; with an Account of that Fatal Epidemic as it Prevailed at Gibraltar during 1804, etc.*, London, 1815.
Fiddes, Sir George V., *The Dominions and Colonial Offices*, London and New York: G.P. Putnam's Sons, 1926.
Fischer, Alfons, *Geschichte des Deutschen Gesundheitswesen*, 2 vols, Berlin: Kommissionsverlag von Oscar Rothacker, 1933.
Fraser, Lovat, *India Under Curzon and After*, London: Heinemann, 1911.
Fremantle, Sir Francis Edward, *Study of Health and Empire*, London: John Ouseley, 1911.
George, Claude, *The Rise of British West Africa*, London: Houlston, 1903.
Grainger, James, *An Essay on the More Common West India Diseases and the Remedies which that Country Itself Produces. To which are added Some Hints on the Management of the Negroes*, London, 1764.
Great Britain, Colonial Office. *Tropical Diseases and the Establishment of Schools of Tropical Medicine*, London: HMSO, 1903.
Greenwood, Major, 'The work of the London School of Hygiene and Tropical Medicine', *Journal of the Royal Society Arts, 79* (1931), 538–53.
Hall, Henry L., *The Colonial Office: a History*, London: Longman, 1937.
Hamilton, Robert, MD, *The Duties of a Regimental Surgeon Considered*, London, 1787.
Heagerty, John, *Four Centuries of Medical History in Canada*, 2 vols, Bristol: J.L.W. Wright, 1928.
Heiser, V., *An American Doctor's Odyssey*, New York: W.W. Norton, 1936.
Heyman, Bruno, *Robert Koch*, Leipzig: Akademische Verlag, 1932.
Hillary, William, *Observations on the Changes of the Air and the Concomitant Epidemical*

Diseases in the Island of Barbadoes. To which is added a Treatise on Yellow Fever, London, 2nd edn, 1766.

Horton, James A.B., *Physical and Medical Climate and Meteorology of the West Coast of Africa*, Edinburgh, 1867.

Hunter, John, [*Observations*] *on the Diseases of the Army in Jamaica and on the Best Means of Preserving the Health of Europeans in that Climate*, London, 1788.

Huntington, E., 'Natural selection and climate in northern Australia', *Economic Record*, *5* (1929), 185–201.

Jackson, R. *A Treatise on the Fevers of Jamaica, with some Observations on the Intermitting Fever of America, and an Appendix containing Some Hints on the means of Preserving the Health of Soldiers in Hot Climates*, London, 1791.

—— *A Sketch of the History and Cure of Febrile Diseases; More Particularly as they Appear in the West Indies, among the Soldiers of the British Army*, Stockton: T & H. Ecles, 1817.

Jeffries, Sir Charles, *The Colonial Empire and its Civil Service*, Cambridge: Cambridge University Press, 1938.

Johnson, James, *The Influence of Tropical Climates on European Constitutions*, London: Thomas & George Underwood, 1819.

Jones, R. Fleming, 'Tropical diseases in British New Guinea', *Transactions of the Royal Society for Tropical Medicine and Hygiene, V* (1910–11), 93–105.

Kidd, Benjamin, *The Control of the Tropics*, New York: Macmillan, 1898.

Knowles, Robert, *The Calcutta School of Tropical Medicine, 1920–1933: An Essay Review*, Alipore: Bengal Government Press, 1934.

Lawes, W.G., 'The effect of the climate of New Guinea upon the exotic races', *Australasian Medical Gazette, 6* (1887), 185–6.

League of Nations Health Organisation, Annual Report, *Epidemiological Intelligence n. 8. Statistics of Notifiable Diseases for the year 1923*, Geneva, 1924.

—— Abbatucci, S., *Public Health Services in the French Colonies*, Geneva, 1926.

—— Cumpston, J.H.L. and McCallum, F., *Public Health Services in Australia*, Geneva, 1926.

—— Graham, J.D. *et al.*, *Health Organisation in British India*, Calcutta, 1928.

Lemprière, William, MD, *Practical Observations on the Diseases of the Army in Jamaica as They Occurred between the Years 1792 and 1797 etc.*, 2 vols, London: Longman, 1799.

Lind, James, MD, *A Treatise of the Scurvy. In Three Parts*, Edinburgh, 1753.

—— *An Essay on the Most Effectual Means of Preserving the Health of Seamen in the Royal Navy, and a Dissertation on Fevers and Infection, together with Observations on the Jail Distemper and the Proper Methods of Preventing and Stopping its Infection*, London, 1757.

—— *An Essay on Diseases Incidental to Europeans in Hot Climates, with the Method of Preventing their Fatal Consequences*, London: T. Beckett, 1768.

Lugard, Lord F.D., *The Dual Mandate in British Tropical Africa*. London: Blackwood, 1922.

MacCulloch, John, *Malaria; an Essay on the Production and Propagation of this Poison, and on the Nature and Localities of the Places by which it is Produced, with an Enumeration of the Diseases caused by it, and of the Means of Preventing or Diminishing them both at Home and in the Naval and Military Service*, London, 1827.

Macdonald, John D., *Outlines of Naval Hygiene*, London: Smith, Elder, 1881.

MacGregor, Sir William, 'Some problems of tropical medicine', address at the London School of Tropical Medicine, 3 October 1900, *Lancet* (13 October 1900) (ii), 1055–61.

Mackenzie, James, *The History of Health, and the Art of Preserving it etc.*, Edinburgh: W. Gordon, 1758.

MacWilliam, James Ormiston, *Medical History of the Expedition to the Niger, 1841–42*, London, 1843.
Manson, Sir Patrick, *Tropical Diseases, A Manual of the Diseases of Warm Climates*, London: Cassell, 1898.
—— 'Tropical medicine and hygiene', *British Medical Journal* (1917) (ii), 103–9.
Manson-Bahr, P.H., 'Notes on some landmarks in tropical medicine', *Proceedings of the Royal Society of Medicine, 30* (1937), 1181–4.
Manson-Bahr, P.H. and Alcock, A., *The Life and Work of Patrick Manson*, London: Cassell, 1927.
Martin, Sir James Ranald, *The Influence of Tropical Climates on European Constitutions, etc*, London, 1856.
Megroz, R.L., *Ronald Ross: Discoverer and Creator*, London: Allen & Unwin, 1931
Monro, Donald, *An Account of the Diseases which were Most Frequent in the British Military Hospitals in Germany, from January 1761 to March 1763. To which is added, an Essay on the Means of Preserving the Health of Soldiers, and conducting Military Hospitals*, London, 1764.
Morris, Sir Malcolm, *The Story of English Public Health*, London: English Public Health Series, 1919.
Moseley, Benjamin, *A Treatise upon Tropical Diseases; on Military Operations; and on the Climate of the West Indies*, London: T. Cadell, 3rd edn, 1792.
New Settler League of Australia (Queensland Division), 'Tropical settlement in Australia', *Edinburgh Review, 240* (1924), 186–96.
Newman, Sir George, *The Building of a Nation's Health*, London: Macmillan, 1939.
Nightingale, Florence, *Notes of Matters Affecting the Health, Efficiency and Hospital Administration of the British Army, founded chiefly on the Experience of the late War*, London: Harrison, 1858.
Price, A.Grenfell, 'The white man in the tropics', *Medical Journal of Australia* (26 January 1935) (1), 106–10.
Pringle, Sir John, *Observations on the Diseases of the Army in Camp and Garrison*, London, 7th edn, 1775.
—— *Discourse upon Some Late Improvements of the Means for Preserving the Health of Mariners*, London, 1776.
Pym, Sir William, *Observations upon Bulam, Vomito-negro or Yellow Fever, with a Review of a Report upon the Diseases of the African Coast by Sir W. Burnett and Dr. Bryson, Proving its Highly Contagious Powers*, London, 1848.
'Report of the Sub-Committee appointed by the Executive Committee of the Australian Medical Congress, 1920, in connection with tropical Australia', *Transactions of the Australasian Medical Congress*, 11th Session (Brisbane, 1920), 39–69.
Rogers, Sir Leonard, 'Climate and disease incidence in India, with special reference to leprosy, phthisis, pneumonia and smallpox', *Journal of State Medicine, 33* (11) (1925), 501–10.
Rollo, John, *Observations on the Means of Preserving and Restoring Health in the West Indies*, London: C. Dilly, 1783.
Ross, A., 'The climate of Australia viewed in relation to health, especially its influence on the constitution of European immigrants', *New South Wales Medical Gazette* (1871) 131–8; 163–87; 195–202; 227–34; 259–66.
Ross, Ronald, 'Malaria in India and the colonies', *Journal of the Royal Colonial Institute, 35* (1903), 14–25.
—— *Memoirs*, London: John Murray, 1923.
Rush, Benjamin, *An Inquiry into the Various Sources of the Usual Forms of Summer and Autumnal Disease in the United States, and the Means of Preventing Them. To which are added, Facts intended to Prove the Yellow Fever not to be Contagious*, Philadelphia: J. Conrad, 1805.

Schoute, D., *Occidental Therapeutics in the Netherland East Indies during Three Centuries of Netherlands Settlement, 1600–1900*, Batavia: Netherlands Indies Public Health Service, 1937.

Scott, H. Harold, *A History of Tropical Medicine*, 2 vols, London: Edward Arnold, 1939–42.

Severn, A.G. Milliott, 'An outline of the history of plague in Hong Kong', *Journal of State Medicine, 33* (1925), 274–84.

Towne, Richard, *Treatise of the Diseases most Frequent in the West Indies and herein More Particularly of Those which Occur in Barbadoes*, London, 1726.

Trapham, Thomas, *A Discourse of the State of Health in the Island of Jamaica, etc.*, London, 1679.

Treille, M.G. 'De l'ensignement de la pathologie tropicale dans les universités de l'Europe', *Janus, 7* (1902), 238–44, 281–7.

Tulloch, Sir Alexander Murray and Marshall, H., 'Statistical report on the sickness, mortality and invaliding among the troops in the West Indies; prepared from the records of the Army Medical Department and War Office returns', *Parliamentary Papers* (Great Britain), 1837–8, XL, 417.

Turner, J.A. and Goldsmith, B.K., *Sanitation in India*, Bombay, 1917.

Wellcome Foundation, *Spanish Influence on the Progress of Medical Science with an Account of the Wellcome Research Institution and Affiliated Research Laboratories and Museums Founded by Sir Henry Wellcome, LLD, DSC, FRS*, London: Wellcome Foundation, 1935.

Wickens, G.H., 'Vitality of white races in low latitudes', *Economic Record, 3* (1927), 117–26.

Willard, M., *History of the White Australia Policy to 1920*, Melbourne: Melbourne University Press, 1923.

Williamson, John, *Medical and Miscellaneous Observations on the West India Islands*, Edinburgh, 1817.

Worcester, D.C., *A History of Asiatic Cholera in the Philippine Islands*, Manila: Bureau of Printing, 1908.

Zinsser, Hans, *Rats, Lice and History*, Boston: Little, Brown, 1935.

SECONDARY SOURCES

Aidoo, T.A., 'Rural health under colonialism and neo-colonialism: A survey of the Ghanaian experience', *International Journal of Health Services, 12* (4) (1982), 637–57.

Alden, Davril and Miller, Joseph C., 'Out of Africa: The slave trade and the transmission of smallpox to Brazil, 1560–1831', *Journal of Interdisciplinary History, XVIII* (2) (1987) 195–224.

Arnold, David, 'Medical priorities and practice in nineteenth century British India', *South Asia Research, 5* (2) (1985), 167–83.

—— 'Cholera and colonialism in British India', *Past and Present*, no. 113 (1986), 118–51.

Banerji, D., 'Historical and socio cultural foundations of health services systems', in G.R. Gupta (ed.), *The Social and Cultural Context of Medicine in India*, New Delhi: Vikas Publishing House, 1981, 1–6.

Barrett, N.R. 'Contributions of Australians to medical knowledge', *Medical History, 11* (1967), 321–33.

Bayoumi, Ahmed, 'Medical administration in the Sudan, 1899–1970', *Clio Medica, 11* (2) (1976), 105–15.

Beck, A., 'Problems of British medical administration in East Africa between 1900 and 1930', *Bulletin of the History of Medicine, 36* (1962), 275–83.

—— *A History of the British Medical Administration of East Africa, 1900–1950*, Cambridge, Mass: Harvard University Press, 1970.

—— 'The role of medicine in German East Africa', *Bulletin of the History of Medicine, 45* (1971), 170–8.

—— 'Medical administration and medical research in developing countries: remarks on their history in colonial East Africa', *Bulletin of the History of Medicine, 46* (1972), 349–58.

Berliner, H.S. and Salmon, J.W., 'The holistic alternative to scientific medicine: history and analysis', *International Journal of Health Services, 10* (1) (1980), 134–47.

Boyd, J.S.K., 'Fifty years of tropical medicine', *British Medical Journal* (1950) (i), 37.

—— 'Sleeping sickness: the Castellani-Bruce controversy', *Notes and Records of the Royal Society of London, 28* (1973), 93–110.

Bradley, D.J., 'The situation and the response', in E.E. Sabben-Clare, D.J. Bradley and K. Kirkwood (eds), *Health in Tropical Africa during the Colonial Period*, Oxford: Clarendon Press, 1980.

Brown, E.R., 'Public health and imperialism in early Rockefeller programs at home and abroad', *American Journal of Public Health, 66* (1976), 897–903.

Browne, S.G., 'The contribution of medical missionaries to tropical medicine. Service-training-research', *Transactions of the Royal Society of Tropical Medicine and Hygiene, 73* (1979), 357–60.

Bruce-Chwatt, Leonard Jan, 'Ronald Ross, William Gorgas and malaria eradication', *American Journal of Tropical Medicine and Hygiene, 26* (1977), 1071–9.

—— 'The rise of tropical medicine: milestones of discovery and application', in C.G. Bernhard, E. Crawford, and P. Sörbom (eds), *Science, Technology and Society in the Time of Alfred Nobel*, Stockholm: Pergamon, 1982, 167–85.

—— 'Franco-British co-operation in tropical medicine', *Bulletin de la Societé de Pathologie Exotique, 76* (1983), 713–5.

Bruce-Chwatt, Leonard Jan and Glanville, W.J. (eds), *Dynamics of Tropical Disease*, London: Oxford University Press, 1973.

Bruce-Chwatt, Leonard Jan and de Zulueta, Julian, *The Rise and Fall of Malaria in Europe: A Historico-Epidemiological Study*, London: Oxford University Press, 1980.

Bryder, Linda, 'Lessons of the 1918 flu epidemic in Auckland', *New Zealand Journal of History, XVI* (1982), 97–121.

Bucco, Guiseppe and Natoli, Angelo, *L'Italia in Africa: L'organizzazione sanitaria nell' Africa Italiana*, Rome: Instituto Poligrafico dello Stato, 1965.

Burrows, E.H., *A History of Medicine in South Africa up to the End of the Nineteenth Century*, Amsterdam, Cape Town: Balkema, 1958.

Busvine, J.R., *Insects, Hygiene and History*, London, Athlone Press, 1976.

Butlin, N.G., *Our Original Aggression: Aboriginal Populations of Southeastern Australia, 1788–1850*, Sydney: Allen & Unwin, 1983.

Bylebyl, Jerome J. (ed.), *Teaching the History of Medicine at a Medical Center*, Baltimore: Johns Hopkins University Press, 1982.

Cahill, K.M., 'Symposium on American contributions in the history of tropical medicine. Introduction', *Bulletin of the New York Academy of Medicine, 44* (1968), 621–2.

Campbell, J., 'Smallpox in Aboriginal Australia, 1829–31', *Historical Studies, 20* (81) (1983), 536–56.

—— 'Smallpox in Aboriginal Australia in the early 1830s', *Historical Studies, 21* (84) (1985), 336–58.

Cantlie, Sir Neil, *A History of the Army Medical Department*, 2 vols, Edinburgh: Churchill Livingstone, 1974.

Carland, John M., *The Colonial Office and Nigeria, 1898–1914*, Basingstoke: Macmillan, 1985.

Carlson, Dennis E., *African Fever: A Study of British Science, Technology and Politics in West Africa, 1787–1864*, Canton, Mass.: Science History Publications, 1984.
Castellani, Aldo, *Microbes, Men and Monarchs: A Doctor's Life in Many Lands*, London: Gollancz, 1960.
Chalmers, A., 'Epidemiology and the scientific method', *International Journal of Health Services, 12* (4) (1982), 659–66.
Chaudhuri, R.N., 'Tropical medicine — past, present and future', *British Medical Journal* (1954) (ii), 423–30.
Chernin, Eli (ed.), 'A bicentennial sampler: milestones in the history of tropical medicine and hygiene', *American Journal of Tropical Medicine and Hygiene, 26*, Supplement (1977), 1053–104.
Childs, St Julien Ravenel, *Malaria and Colonization in the Carolina Low Country, 1526–1696*, Baltimore: Johns Hopkins University Press, 1940.
Cilento, R.W., *Tropical Diseases in Australasia*, Brisbane: Smith & Patterson, 1940, 1944.
—— 'Medicine in Queensland', *Journal of the Royal Historical Society of Queensland, 6* (4) (1961–2), 866–941.
Cilento, R.W. and Lack, C., *Triumph in the Tropics: An Historical Sketch of Queensland*, Brisbane: Smith & Paterson, 1959.
Clarke, Edwin (ed.), *Modern Methods in the History of Medicine*, London: Athlone Press, 1971.
Cleaver, H., 'Malaria and the political economy of public health', *International Journal of Health Services, 7* (4) (1977), 557–79.
Cloudsley-Thompson, J.L., *Insects and History*, London: Weidenfeld & Nicholson, 1976.
Clyde, David, *History of the Medical Services of Tanganyika*, Dar es Salaam: Government Printer, 1962.
—— *Three Centuries of Health Care in Dominica*, New Delhi: Gopal, 1980.
Corrigan, F.P., 'Political implications of global tropical medicine', *American Journal of Tropical Medicine and Hygiene, 3* (1954), 431–3.
Courtois, D., 'Naissance de l'Institut de médecine Tropicale du Service de Santé des Armées', *Médecine tropicale, 40* (6) (1980), 631–4.
Crosby, A.W., *The Columbian Exchange: Biological and Cultural Consequences of 1492*, Westport, Conn.: Greenwood, 1972.
Crowder, Michael, 'The white chiefs of tropical Africa', in Peter Duignan and Lewis Henry Gann (eds), *Colonialism in Africa, 1870–1960*, vol 2, Cambridge: Cambridge University Press, 1970, 320–50.
Crowther, James Gerald, *Six Great Doctors. Harvey, Pasteur, Lister, Pavlov, Ross, Fleming*, London: Hamish Hamilton, 1957.
Cummins, C.J., *A History of Medical Administration in New South Wales, 1788–1973*, Sydney: Health Commission of New South Wales, 1979.
Cumpston, J.H.L., *The Health of the People*, Canberra: Roebuck, 1978.
—— *Health and Disease in Australia: A History* ed. M.J. Lewis, Canberra: Australian Government Printing Service, forthcoming.
Curtin, P.D., ' "The White Man's Grave": image and reality', *Journal of British Studies, 1* (1961), 94–110.
—— *The Image of Africa: British Ideas and Action, 1780–1850*, Madison: University of Wisconsin Press, 1964, London: Macmillan, 1965.
—— 'Epidemiology and the slave trade', *Political Science Quarterly, 83* (2) (1968), 190–218.
—— 'Medical knowledge and urban planning in tropical Africa', *American Historical Review, 90* (3) (1985), 594–613.
Davies, J.N.P., 'The cause of sleeping sickness', *East African Medical Journal, 39* (1962), 81–99, 145–60.

Denoon, Donald, 'Medical services in Papua New Guinea, 1884–1984', in S. Latukefu (ed.), *Papua New Guinea: A Century of Colonial Impact, 1884–1984*, Port Moresby: University of Papua New Guinea, 1988.
Diefenbacher, Albert, *Psychiatrie und Kolonialismus. Zur 'Irrenfürsorge' in der Kolonie Deutsch-Ostafrika*, Frankfurt: Campus Verlag, 1985.
Docherty, R.L., 'The Bancroft tradition in infectious disease research in Queensland', *Medical Journal of Australia* (1978) (2), 560–3; 591–4.
Domergue, D., 'French sanitary services on the Ivory Coast', *Revue française histoire outre-mer, 65* (1979), 40–63.
Dominguez Roldan, F., 'La obra dal Doctor Carlos J. Finlay en patalogia tropical', *Revista de la Sociedad Cubana de Historia Medicina, 4* (4) (1961), 2–12.
Douglas, R.A., 'Dr Anton Breinl and the Australian Institute of Tropical Medicine', *Medical Journal of Australia* (7, 14, 21 May 1977) (1), 713–16; 748–51; 784–90.
Doyal, Lesley and Rennell, I., *The Political Economy of Health*, London: Pluto Press, 1979.
Drew, W.R.M., 'The challenge of tropical medicine', *Journal of the Royal Army Medical Corps, 110* (1964), 77–83.
—— 'Our rich tropical heritage', *Transactions of the Royal Society of Tropical Medicine and Hygiene, 65* (1971), 699–708.
Duffy, John, *Epidemics in Colonial America*, Baton Rouge: Louisiana State University Press, 1953.
Duggan, A.J., 'Bruce and the African trypanosomes', *American Journal of Tropical Medicine and Hygiene, 26* (1977), 1080–1.
Duignan, Peter and Gann, Lewis Henry (eds), *Colonialism in Africa, 1870–1960. Vol. 4: The Economics of Capitalism*, Cambridge: Cambridge University Press, 1975.
Dumett, R.E., 'The campaign against malaria and the expansion of scientific, medical and sanitary services in British West Africa, 1898–1910', *African Historical Studies, 1* (1968), 153–97.
Eckart, W., 'Der ärztliche Dienst in den Ehemaligen Deutschen Kolonien', *Arzt und Krankenhaus*, no. 10 (1981), 422–6.
—— 'Malariaprävention und Rassentrennung — Die ärztliche Vorbereitung und Rechtfertigung der Duala-Enteignung 1912/14'. *History and Philosophy of the Life Sciences, 10* (1988, forthcoming).
—— 'Medizin und Kolonialismus Der Kampf gegen die Schlarfkrankheit im deutschen Schutzgebiet Togo, 1904–1914', *Sudhoffs Archiv* (1988, forthcoming).
Eddy, T.P., 'The evolution of British colonial hospitals in West Africa', *Transactions of the Royal Society of Tropical Medicine and Hygiene, 77* (1983), 563–4.
Etherington, N., 'Missionary doctors and African healers in mid-Victorian South Africa', *South African Historical Journal, 19* (1987), 77–91.
Ewers, W.H., 'Malaria in the early years of German New Guinea', *Journal of the Papua New Guinea Society, VI* (1973), 3–30.
Eyers, John, 'A.D.P. Hodges and early scientific medicine in Uganda, 1898–1918: with a select bibliography on the early history of sleeping sickness in Uganda, 1900–1920', unpublished MA thesis, Loughborough University of Technology, 1982.
Fanon, Frantz, *A Dying Colonialism*, New York: Grove Press, 1965.
—— 'Medicine and colonialism', in J. Ehrenreich (ed.), *The Cultural Crisis of Modern Medicine*, New York: Monthly Review Press, 1978.
Faust, Ernest Carroll, 'The American Academy of Tropical Medicine. A brief sketch of its founding, its purpose and its accomplishments', *American Journal of Tropical Medicine, 29* (1949), 299–301.
Feierman, Steven, *Health and Society in Africa: A Working Bibliography*, Waltham, Mass.: Crossroad Publishing Company, 1979.
—— 'Struggles for control: the social roots of health and healing in modern Africa', *African*

Studies Review, 28 (2/3) (1985), 73–147.
Fisher, D., 'Rockefeller philanthropy and the British Empire: the creation of the London School of Hygiene and Tropical Medicine', *History of Education, 7* (2) (1978), 129–43.
Foll, C.V., 'Seventy five years old — The "Journal of Tropical Medicine and Hygiene" ', *Journal of Tropical Medicine and Hygiene, 76* (1973), 217–22.
Ford, E., 'The malaria problem in Australia and the Australian Pacific Territories', *Medical Journal of Australia* (10 June 1950) (1), 749–60.
Ford, John, 'Ideas which have influenced attempts to solve the problem of African Trypanosomiasis', *Social Science and Medicine, 13 B* (1979), 269–75.
Foskett, R. (ed.), *The Zambesi Doctors: David Livingstone's Letters to John Kirk, 1858–1872*, Edinburgh: Edinburgh University Press, 1964.
Franco-Agudelo, S., 'The Rockefeller Foundation's antimalarial program in Latin America: donating or dominating?', *International Journal of Health Services, 13* (1) (1983), 51–67.
Franz, K.H., 'Contributions of American industry in tropical medicine', *Bulletin of the New York Academy of Medicine, 44* (6) (1968), 747–58.
Fraser, K.B., 'Glimpses of yesterday north of Capricorn', *Medical Journal of Australia* (16 September 1967) (2), 531–5.
Frey, Raymond, 'Colonisation et Médecine', *Presse médecine, 63* (1955), 1245.
Gallagher, Nancy E., *Medicine and Power in Tunisia, 1780–1900*, Cambridge: Cambridge University Press, 1983.
Gandevia, B., 'Medical history in its Australian environment', *Medical Journal of Australia* (18 November 1967), (2), 941–6.
Gandevia, B., *Tears Often Shed. Child Health and Welfare in Australia from 1788*, Gordon: Charter Books, 1978.
Garnham, P.C.C., 'Britain's contribution to tropical medicine, 1868–1968', *Practitioner, 201* (1968), 153–61.
Gear, J.H.S., 'The South African contribution to medicine in a tropical environment', *South African Medical Journal, 55* (1979), 455–9.
Gelfand, Michael, *Tropical Victory. An Account of the Influence of Medicine on the History of Southern Rhodesia*, Cape Town: Juta Press, 1953.
—— *Lakeside Pioneers: A Socio-Medical Study of Nyasaland, 1875–1920*, Oxford: Blackwell, 1964.
—— *Rivers of Death in Africa*, London: Oxford University Press, 1964.
—— *A Service to the Sick. A History of the Health Services for Africans in Southern Rhodesia, 1890–1953*, Gwelo: Mambo Press, 1976.
Gibson, M., 'Sir Ronald Ross and his contemporaries', *Journal of the Royal Society of Medicine, 71* (1978), 611.
—— 'The identification of Kala Zar and the discovery of Leishmania Donovani, *Medical History, 27* (1983), 203–13.
Goff, H.G., 'Sleeping sickness in the Lake Victoria region of British East Africa, 1900–1915', *African Historical Studies, 2* (1969), 255–68.
Gordon, Douglas, *Health, Sickness and Society: Theoretical Concepts in Social and Preventive Medicine*, St Lucia: University of Queensland Press, 1976.
Gordon, S. Harvey, 'A history of sleeping sickness in Uganda: administrative response, 1900–1970', unpublished PhD thesis, Syracuse University, 1971.
Guerra, F., 'Medical colonisation of the New World', *Medical History, 7* (1963), 147–55.
—— 'The influence of disease on race, logistics and colonisation in the Antilles', *Journal of Tropical Medicine and Hygiene, 68* (1966), 23–35.
Gupta, G.R., 'Indigenous medicine in 19th and 20th century Bengal', in C.M. Leslie (ed.), *Asian Medical Systems: A Comparative Study*, Berkeley: University of California Press, 1976.
Gupta, G.R. (ed.), *The Social and Cultural Context of Medicine in India*, New Delhi:

Vikas Publishing House, 1981.
Gurner, J., *The Origins of the Royal Australian Army Medical Corps*, London: Hawthorne Press, 1970.
Harris, J.R., 'Sir James Cantlie (1851–1926). Founder of the *Journal of Tropical Medicine*', *Journal of Tropical Medicine and Hygiene, 76* (1973), 185–7.
Harrison, G., *Mosquitoes, Malaria and Man: A History of Hostilities since 1880*, London: John Murray, 1978.
Hartwig, G.W. and Patterson, K.D. (eds.), *Disease in African History*, Durham, N.C.: Duke University Press, 1978.
Headrick, D.R. 'The tools of imperialism: technology and the expansion of European colonial empires in the nineteenth century', *Journal of Modern History, 57* (1979), 231–63.
—— *The Tools of Empire: Technology and European Imperialism in the Nineteenth Century*, New York: Oxford University Press, 1981.
Heiser, V.G., 'Reminiscences on early tropical medicine', *Bulletin of the New York Academy of Medicine, 44* (1968), 654–60.
Hicks, N., '*This Sin and Scandal*': *Australia's Population Debate, 1891–1911*, Canberra: Australian National University Press, 1978.
—— 'Medical history and the history of medicine', in G. Osborne and W.F. Mandle (eds), *New History: Studying Australia Today*, Sydney: Allen & Unwin, 1982.
Hughes, C.C. and Hunter, J.M., 'Disease and development in Africa', *Social Science and Medicine, 3* (1970), 443–93.
Hume, John Chandler, 'Colonialism and sanitary medicine: the development of preventive health policy in the Punjab, 1860 to 1900', *Modern Asian Studies, 20* (4) (1986), 703–24.
Hunter, G., Frye, William W., and Swartzwelde, J. Clyde, *A Manual of Tropical Medicine*, Philadelphia: Saunders, 1960.
Hutchins, F.G., *The Illusion of Permanence: British Imperialism in India*, Princeton: Princeton University Press, 1967.
Hutchinson, Thomas J., *Impressions of Western Africa*, London: Longman, 1958.
Hyam, R., *Britain's Imperial Century, 1818–1914*, London: Batsford, 1976.
Jaggi, O.P., 'Indigenous systems of medicine during British supremacy in India', *Studies in History of Medicine, 1* (4) (1977), 320–47.
—— *Western Medicine in India: Epidemics and other Tropical Diseases*, (Delhi: Atma Ram, 1979.
Janitschke, Klaus, 'Kleine-Koch-Orenstein: the German connection with medical research in South Africa', *Adler Mus. Bulletin, 11* (2) (1985), 16–18.
Janssens, P.G., 'The colonial legacy: health and medicine in the Belgian Congo', *Tropical Doctor, 11* (3) (1981), 132–40.
Janzen, J.M., *The Quest for Therapy in Lower Zaire*, Berkeley: University of California Press, 1978.
Jeffrey, Roger, 'Recognizing India's doctors: the institutionalization of medical dependency, 1918–39', *Modern Asian Studies, 13* (2) (1979), 301–26.
Jeffries, Sir Charles, *The Colonial Office*, London: Allen & Unwin, 1956.
Jeffries, Sir Charles (ed.), *A Review of Colonial Research, 1940–1960*, London: HMSO, 1964.
Johnson, Gwendolyn, Z., 'Health conditions in rural and urban areas of developing countries', *Population Studies, 17* (1964), 293–309.
Joyce, Roger, *Sir William MacGregor*, Melbourne: Oxford University Press, 1971.
Kean, B.H., Mott, Kenneth E., Russell, Adair J., *Tropical Medicine and Parasitology: Classic Investigations*, 2 vols, Ithaca: Cornell University Press, 1978.
Kett, Joseph F., 'American and Canadian medical institutions', *Journal of the History*

of Medicine and Allied Sciences, 22 (1967), 343–56.

Kiat, Lee Yong, *The Medical History of Early Singapore*, Tokyo: South East Asian Medical Information Centre, 1978.

Kiernan, V.G., *The Lords of Human Kind: European Attitudes towards the Outside World in the Imperial Age*, London: Weidenfeld & Nicolson, 1969.

Kiple, K.F. and King, V.H., 'Deficiency diseases in the Caribbean', *Journal of Interdisciplinary History, 11* (2) (1980), 197–215.

—— *Another Dimension to the Black Diaspora: Diet, Disease and Racism*, Cambridge: Cambridge University Press, 1981.

Klein, Ira, 'Death in India, 1871–1921', *Journal of Asian Studies, 32* (4) (1973), 639–59.

—— 'When the rains failed: famine, relief, and mortality in British India', *Indian Economic and Social History Review, XXI* (2) (1984), 185–214.

Kluxen, G. and Bernsmeier, H., 'Endemic ocular infections of the South Seas in the German colonial era', *Papua New Guinea Medical Journal, 23* (4) (1980), 197–9.

Kubicek, R.V., *The Administration of Imperialism: Joseph Chamberlain at the Colonial Office*, Durham, N.C.: Duke University Press, 1969.

Kyle, J., 'The Hong Kong College of Medicine (1887–1915)', *British Medical Journal* (1979) (i), 1474–6.

Laidler, P.W. and Gelfand, M., *South Africa. Its Medical History, 1652–1898: A Medical and Social Study*, Cape Town: Struik, 1971.

Lambert, S.M., *A Doctor in Paradise*, London: J.M. Dent, 1942.

Lancaster, H.O., 'The causes of the decline in the death rates in Australia', *Medical Journal of Australia* (18 November 1967) (2), 937–41.

Lange, R.T., 'The revival of a dying race: a study of Maori health reform, 1900–1918, and its nineteenth century background', unpublished MA thesis, University of Auckland, 1972.

—— 'A history of health and ill-health in the Cook Islands', unpublished PhD thesis, University of Otago, 1982.

—— 'Plagues and pestilence in Polynesia: the nineteenth century Cook Islands experience', *Bulletin of the History of Medicine, 58* (1984), 325–46.

—— 'Changes in Rarotongan attitudes to health and disease: historical factors in the development of a mid-twentieth century understanding', *Pacific Studies, 10* (1) (1986), 29–53.

Lasker, Judith, 'The role of health services in colonial rule: the case of the Ivory Coast, *Culture, Medicine and Psychiatry, 1* (1) (1977), 277–97.

Latukefu, S. (ed.), *Papua New Guinea: A Century of Colonial Impact, 1884–1984*, Port Moresby: University of Papua New Guinea, 1988.

Lee, D.J. *The School of Public Health and Tropical Medicine, 1930–1980*, Sydney: School of Public Health and Tropical Medicine, 1980.

Leng Chee, H., 'Health status and the development of health services in a colonial state: the case of British Malaya', *International Journal of Health Services, 12* (3) (1982), 397–417.

Leuchsenring, Emilio Roig de, *Medicos y medicina en Cuba: Lisbona, Biografía, Costumbrismo*, Havana: Mus. Hist. Cien. Med. 'Carlos J. Finlay', 1965.

Lewis, M.J., 'Populate or perish: aspects of infant and maternal health in Sydney, 1870–1939', unpublished PhD thesis, Australian National University, 1976.

—— *Managing Madness: Psychiatry and Society in Australia, 1788–1980*, Canberra: AGPS for Australian Institute of Health, 1988.

Lewis, M. and MacLeod, R., 'A workingman's paradise? Reflections on urban mortality in colonial Australia 1860–1900', *Medical History*, 31 (1987), 387–402.

—— 'Medical politics and the professionalisation of medicine in New South Wales, 1850–1901', *Journal of Australian Studies* (1988).

Louw, J.H., *In the Shadow of Table Mountain: A History of the University of Cape Town*

Medical School and Its Associated Teaching Hospitals up to 1950, Cape Town: Struik, 1969.

Lyons, Maryinez, 'From "death camps" to *cordon sanitaire*: the development of sleeping sickness policy in the Uele district of the Belgian Congo, 1903–1914', *Journal of African History, 26* (1985), 69–91.

—— 'The colonial disease: sleeping sickness in the social history of northern Zaire, 1903–1930', unpublished PhD thesis, University of California, 1987.

McGrath, A.G., 'The history of medical organisations in Australia', unpublished PhD thesis, University of Sydney, 1978.

McKelvey, J.J., *Man against Tsetse: Struggle for Africa*, Ithaca, N.Y.: Cornell University Press, 1973.

McKeown, T., *Medicine in Modern Society. Medical Planning Based on Evaluation of Medical Treatment*, London: Allen and Unwin, 1965.

—— *The Role of Medicine. Dream, Mirage or Nemesis?* Oxford: Blackwell, 1979.

McKeown, T. and Record, R.G., 'Reasons for the decline of mortality in England and Wales during the nineteenth century', *Population Studies, 16* (2) (1962), 94–122.

MacLean, F.S., *Challenge for Health: A History of Health in New Zealand*, Wellington: Owen, 1964.

MacLeod, R.M., 'The frustration of state medicine, 1880–1899', *Medical History*, 11 (1967), 15–40.

—— 'The anatomy of state medicine', in F.N.L. Poynter (ed.), *Medicine and Science in the 1860s*, London: Wellcome Institute for the History of Medicine, 1968.

MacLeod, R. and Denoon, D. (eds), *Disease Never Stays at Home: Health and Healing in Tropical Australasia and Papua New Guinea* (forthcoming).

McNeill, W.H., *Plagues and Peoples*, Oxford: Blackwell, 1977.

Maddocks, I., 'Medicine and colonialism', *Australian and New Zealand Journal of Sociology, XI* (1975), 27–33.

Maegraith, B.H., 'History of the Liverpool School of Tropical Medicine', *Medical History, 16* (1972), 354–68.

—— 'Tropical medicine: what it is not, what it is', *Bulletin of the New York Academy of Medicine, 48* (10) (1972), 1210–30.

—— 'The Liverpool School of Tropical Medicine: the first seventy five years', *Journal of Tropical Medicine and Hygiene, 76* (1973), 187–93.

Manson-Bahr, P.E.C., *The History of the School of Tropical Medicine in London, 1899–1949*, London: LTSM, 1956.

—— 'The march of tropical medicine during the last fifty years', *Transactions of the Royal Society of Tropical Medicine and Hygiene, 52* (1958), 483–99.

—— 'Then and now: memoirs of colonial medicine, Part 4', *British Journal of Clinical Practice, 14* (1960), 300–1; 324.

—— *Patrick Manson: The Founder of Tropical Medicine*, London: Nelson, 1962.

—— 'The story of malaria: the drama and the actors', *International Review of Tropical Medicine, 2* (1963), 329–90.

Mattei, C., 'L'Action des médecins du Corps de Santé des Troupes de Marine et des Corps Expeditionnaires dans l'Apport Civilisateur Français Outre-Mer', *Médecine tropicale, 24* (5) (1964), 507–10.

May, S., 'Economic interest in tropical medicine', *American Journal of Tropical Medicine and Hygiene, 3* (1954), 412–21.

Mayne, A.J.C., *Fever, Squalor and Vice: Sanitation and Social Policy in Victorian Sydney*, St Lucia: University of Queensland Press, 1982.

Miles, J.A.R., 'On the observations on health in the Pacific by Cook and members of his expeditions', *Proceedings of the Royal Society of New Zealand, 97* (1969), 69–75.

Moodie, P. and Pedersen, E.B., *The Health of Australian Aborigines: An Annotated*

Bibliography with Classifications by Subject Matter and Locality, Sydney: School of Public Health and Tropical Medicine, 1966.
Morrison, R.J.G., 'Department of Tropical Medicine', *Journal of the Royal Army Medical Corps, 107* (1961), 11–17.
Mostofi, F.K., 'Contributions of the military to tropical medicine', *Bulletin of the New York Academy of Medicine, 44* (1968), 702–20.
Mulligan, H.W., 'Tropical medicine research in British overseas territories', *Transactions of the Royal Society of Tropical Medicine and Hygiene, 75* (Supplement) (1981), 9–11.
Navarro, Vicente, 'Work, ideology and science: the case of medicine', *International Journal of Health Services, 10* (4) (1980), 523–50.
—— 'Radicalism, Marxism and medicine', *International Journal of Health Services, 13* (2) (1983), 179–202.
Navarro, Vicente, (ed.), *Imperialism, Health and Medicine*, London: Pluto Press, 1982.
Nosny, P., 'Propos sur l'Histoire de la Médecine coloniale Française', *Médecine tropicale, 24* (1964), 375–82.
Parahoo, Kader A., 'Early colonial health developments in Mauritius', *International Journal of Health Services, 16* (3) (1986), 409–23.
Parmer, J. Norman, 'Health and health services in British Malaya in the 1920s', unpublished conference paper, Asian Studies Association of Australia, 6th Biennial Conference, University of Sydney, May 1986.
Patterson, K. David, 'Disease and medicine in African history: a bibliographical essay', *History in Africa, 1* (1974), 141–8.
—— *Health in Colonial Ghana: Disease, Medicine and Socio-Economic Change, 1900–1955*, Waltham, Mass.: Crossroad Publishing Company, 1981.
Paul, James, 'Medicine and imperialism in Morocco', *Middle East Research and Information Project Report*, no. 60 (1977), 3–12.
Pederson, Duncan and Baruffati, Veronica, 'Health and traditional medical cultures in Latin America and the Caribbean', *Social Science and Medicine 21*, (1) (1985), 5–12.
Pelling, M., *Cholera, Fever and English Medicine*, Oxford: Oxford University Press, 1978.
Pensabene, T.S., *The Rise of the Medical Practitioner in Victoria*, Canberra: Australian National University Press, 1980.
Peterson, M.J., *The Medical Profession in Mid-Victorian London*, Berkeley: University of California Press, 1978.
Porter, B., *Critics of Empire: British Radical Attitudes to Colonialism in Africa, 1895–1914*, London: Macmillan, 1968.
—— *The Lion's Share: A Short History of British Imperialism, 1850–1983*, London: Longman, 1975.
Radford, Anthony, J. and Speer, Albert, 'Medical tultuls and aid post orderlies: some historical notes on the use of village health workers in Papua New Guinea up to independence', *Papua New Guinea Medical Journal, 29* (2) (1986), 165–82.
Ramasubban, R., *Public Health and Medical Research in India: Their Origins under the Impact of British Colonial Policy*, Stockholm: SAREC, 1982.
Ransford, Oliver, *Bid the Sickness Cease: Disease in the History of Black Africa*, London: John Murray, 1983.
Rao, M.S., 'The history of medicine in India and Burma', *Medical History, 12* (1968), 52–61.
Reddy, D.V.S., *The Beginnings of Modern Medicine in Madras*, Calcutta: Racker, Spink, 1947.
Reid, J. (ed.), *Body, Land and Spirit: Health and Healing in Aboriginal Society*, St Lucia: University of Queensland Press, 1982.
Rice, Geoffrey, 'Christchurch in the 1918 influenza epidemic. A preliminary study', *New*

Zealand Journal of History, XIII (1979), 109–37.

Richet, P., 'L'Histoire et l'Œuvre de l'OCCGE en Afrique Occidentale Francophone', *Transactions of the Royal Society of Tropical Medicine and Hygiene, 59* (1965), 234–51.

Roddis, Louis H., *A Short History of Nautical Medicine*, New York: Paul Hoeber, 1943.

—— *James Lind: Founder of Nautical Medicine*, New York: H. Schuman, 1950.

Roe, M., 'The establishment of the Australian Department of Health', *Historical Studies, 17* (67) (1976), 176–92.

—— *Nine Australian Progressives: Vitalism in Bourgeois Social Thought, 1890–1960*, St Lucia: University of Queensland Press, 1984.

Roelants, G., 'The Belgian Society of Tropical Medicine', *Journal of Tropical Medicine and Hygiene, 77* (1974), 103–5.

Rogers, Sir Leonard, *Happy Toil: Fifty-five Years of Tropical Medicine*, London: Frederick Muller, 1950.

Roland, Charles G. (ed.), *Health, Disease and Medicine: Essays in Canadian History*, Toronto: The Hannah Institute for the History of Medicine, 1984.

Rosen, George, *A History of Public Health*, New York: MD Publications, 1958.

Ross, Robert J. and Telkamp, Gerard J. (eds), *Colonial Cities*, Dordrecht: Martinus Nijhoff, 1985.

Rowland, J., *The Mosquito Man: The Story of Sir Ronald Ross*, London: Lutterworth Press, 1958.

Russell, K.F., *The Melbourne Medical School, 1862–1962*, Melbourne: Melbourne University Press, 1977.

Sabben-Clare, E.E., Bradley, D.J., and Kirkwood, K. (eds), *Health in Tropical Africa during the Colonial Period*, Oxford: Clarendon Press, 1980.

Salomon-Bayet, Claire et al., *Pasteur et la Revolution Pastorienne*, Paris: Payot, 1986.

Saunders, K., 'The Pacific Islander Hospitals in colonial Queensland: the failure of liberal principles', *Journal of Pacific History, 11* (1976), 25–50.

Schram, Ralph, *A History of the Nigerian Health Services*, Ibadan: Ibadan University Press, 1971.

—— 'Britain's contribution to health and medicine in tropical countries through medical missions', *Transactions of the Royal Society of Tropical Medicine and Hygiene, 75*, Supplement (1981), 56–8.

Searle, G.R., *The Quest for National Efficiency: A Study in British Politics and Political Thought, 1899–1914*, Oxford: Blackwell, 1971.

Semmel, B., *Imperialism and Social Reform: English Social-Imperial Thought, 1895–1914*, London: Allen & Unwin, 1960.

Sergent, Edmond, 'La Médecine française en Algérie', *Archives de l'Institut Pasteur d'Algérie, XXXIII* (1955), 281–5.

Sergent, Edmond and Parrot, L., *Contribution de l'Institut Pasteur d'Algérie à la connaissance humaine du Sahara, 1900–1960*, Algiers: Institut Pasteur, 1961.

Sheppard, R.L., 'Brief outline of the history of the Bureau of Hygiene, and Tropical Diseases', *Tropical Diseases Bulletin, 50* (1953), 1–2.

Sheridan, R.B., 'The Guinea surgeons on the Middle Passage — the provision of medical services in the British slave trade, *International Journal of African Historical Studies, 14* (4) (1973), 601–25.

—— *Doctors and Slaves: A Medical and Demographic History of Slavery in the British West Indies, 1680–1834*, Cambridge: Cambridge University Press, 1985.

Shineberg, D., ''He can but die': missionary medicine in pre-Christian Tonga', in Neil Gunson (ed.), *The Changing Pacific: Essays in Honour of H.E.Maude*, Melbourne: Oxford University Press, 1978, 285–96.

Shortt, S.E.D. (ed.), *Medicine in Canadian Society: Historical Perspectives*, Montreal: McGill-Queens University Press, 1981.

Shryock, Richard Harrison, *The Development of Modern Medicine: An Interpretation of the Social and Scientific Factors Involved*, London: Gollancz, 1948.

Soff, Harvey G., 'A History of sleeping sickness in Uganda: administrative response, 1900–1970', unpublished PhD thesis, Syracuse University, 1971.

Spink, Wesley W., *Infectious Diseases: Prevention and Treatment in the Nineteenth and Twentieth Centuries*, Minneapolis: University of Minnesota, 1978.

Spitzer, L., 'The mosquito and segregation in Sierra Leone', *Canadian Journal of African Studies, 11* (1986), 49–61.

Squires, H.C., *The Sudan Medical Service: An Experiment in Social Medicine*, London: Heinemann, 1958.

Stark, Evan, 'The epidemic as a social event', *International Journal of Health Services, 7* (1977), 681–705.

Stepan, N., 'The interplay between socio-economic factors and medical science: yellow fever research, Cuba and the United States', *Social Studies of Science, 8* (1978), 397–423.

Stokes, Eric, *The English Utilitarians in India*, Oxford: Oxford University Press, 1959.

Subba Reddy, D.V., 'Seventeenth century Dutch writers on tropical medicine and tropical herbs', *Journal of the History of Medicine, 6* (1951), 258–60.

Sullivan, R.J., ''Exemplar of Americanism'; the Philippine career of Dean C. Worcester', unpublished PhD thesis, James Cook University of North Queensland, 1986.

Sutton, H., 'The School of Public Health and Tropical Medicine, University of Sydney', *Australian Journal of Science, 2* (1939/40), 69–71.

Swanson, M.W., 'The sanitation syndrome: bubonic plague and urban native policy in the Cape Colony, 1900–1909', *Journal of African History, XVIII* (3) (1977), 387–410.

Swellengrebel, N.H., 'A fiftieth anniversary of the Royal Tropical Institute of Amsterdam', *Tropical Geography and Medicine, 12* (1960), 193–5.

Tachon, J., 'La Revue Médecine Tropicale – retrospective', *Médecine tropicale, 40* (1980), 639–41.

Tesh, S., 'Political ideology and public health in the nineteenth century', *International Journal of Health Services, 12* (2) (1982), 321–42.

Thame, C., 'Health and the state: the development of collective responsibility for health care in Australia in the first half of the twentieth century', unpublished PhD thesis, Australian National University, 1974.

Tiglao, Teodora V. and Cruz, Wilfredo L., *Seven Decades of Public Health in the Philippines, 1898–1972*, Tokyo: South East Asian Medical Information Centre, 1975.

Toubert, J., 'Œuvre civisatrice du Corps Médical Française en pays d'outre-mer', *Progrès médical, 84* (1956), 397–8.

Turshen, Meredith, 'The impact of colonialism on health and health services in Tanzania', *International Journal of Health Services, 7* (1) (1977), 7–35.

—— *The Political Ecology of Disease in Tanzania*, New Brunswick, N.J.: Rutgers University Press, 1984.

Twumasi, Patrick A., 'Colonialism and international health; a study in social change in Ghana', *Social Science and Medicine, 15 B* (1981), 147–51.

United Kingdom, Office of Information, *Health in the United Kingdom Dependencies*, London: HMSO, 1956.

United Kingdom, War Office, *Memoranda on Medical Diseases in Tropical and Sub-Tropical Areas*, London: HMSO, 1946.

Unterhalter, Beryl, 'Inequalities in health and disease: the case of mortality rates for the city of Johannesburg, South Africa, 1910–1979', *International Journal of Health Services, 12* (4) (1982), 617–36.

Vaucel, M.A., 'Les acquisitions de la médecine tropicale dans ces cinquante dernières années', *Annales Société Belge de Médecine Tropicale, 36* (1956), 655–64.

—— 'Le Service de santé des troupes de marine et la médecine tropicale française', *Transactions of the Royal Society of Tropical Medicine and Hygiene, 59* (1965), 226–33.

Verkataratnam, R. 'A history of western medicine in India, 1664–1945', *Indian Journal of History of Medicine, 19* (1974), 5–14.

Verso, M.L., 'Airs, waters and places', *Victorian Historical Journal, 48* (1) (1977), 6–21.

Warren, K.S., 'The bench in the bush in tropical medicine', *American Journal of Tropical Medicine and Hygiene, 30* (1981), 1149–58.

Waterford, J., 'A fundamental imbalance: Aboriginal ill-health', in J. Reid (ed.), *Body, Land and Spirit. Health and Healing in Aboriginal Society*, St Lucia: University of Queensland Press, 1982, 8–30.

Wilcocks, Charles, 'A historical trend in tropical medicine', *Transactions of the Royal Society of Tropical Medicine and Hygiene, 57* (1963), 395–408.

—— 'The Tropical Diseases Bulletin, 1912–1972', *Practitioner, 209* (1972), 706–8.

—— *A Tropical Doctor in Africa and London: An Autobiography*, London: Leatherhead, 1977.

Willis, Evan, *Medical Dominance: the Division of Labour in Australian Health Care*, Sydney: Allen & Unwin, 1983.

Wilson, Charles M., *Ambassadors in White: The Story of American Tropical Medicine*, New York: Kennikat Press, 1942.

Winslow, C.E.A., *The Conquest of Epidemic Disease: A Chapter in the History of Ideas*, Princeton: Princeton University Press, 1967.

Wood, C. (ed.), *Tropical Medicine: From Romance to Reality*, London: Academic Press, 1978.

Worboys, M., 'The emergence of tropical medicine: a study in the establishment of a scientific specialty', in G. Lemaine, R. MacLeod, M. Mulkay, and P. Weingart (eds), *Perspectives on the Emergence of Scientific Disciplines*, The Hague: Mouton, 1976, 75–98.

—— 'Science and British colonial imperialism, 1895–1940', unpublished D.Phil. thesis, University of Sussex, 1979.

—— 'The emergence and early development of parasitology', in K.S. Warren and J.Z. Bowers (eds), *Parasitology: a Global Perspective*, New York: Springer Verlag, 1983.

World Health Organization, *Apartheid and Health*, Geneva: WHO, 1983.

Wright, Gwendolyn, 'Tradition in the service of modernity: Architecture and urbanism in French colonial policy, 1900–1930', *Journal of Modern History, 59* (2) (1987) 291–316.

Wright, W.H., *Forty Years of Tropical Medicine Research: A History of the Gorgas Memorial Institute of Tropical and Preventative Medicine, Inc., and the Gorgas Memorial Laboratory*, Washington, Gorgas Memorial Institute, 1970.

Wright-St. Clair, R.E., 'The Edinburgh influence on New Zealand medicine', *Proceedings of the XXIII International Congress of History of Medicine, 1* (1974), 748–53.

Yoeli, M., 'The evolution of tropical medicine: An historical perspective', *Bulletin of the New York Academy of Medicine, 48* (1972), 1231–46.

Young, J.A., Sefton, A.J., and Webb, N. (eds), *Centenary Book of the University of Sydney Faculty of Medicine*, Sydney: Sydney University Press, 1984.

Youngson, A.J., *The Scientific Revolution in Victorian Medicine*, London: Croom Helm, 1979.

Index

9781032235394